HEALTH SERVICES MANAGEMENT

Readings, Cases, and Commentary
Eighth Edition

HEALTH SERVICES MANAGEMENT

Readings, Cases, and Commentary
Eighth Edition

Anthony R. Kovner and Duncan Neuhauser
Editors

Health Administration Press, Chicago, IL
AUPHA Press, Washington, DC

AUPHA

HAP

Your board, staff, or clients may also benefit from this book's insight. For more information on quantity discounts, contact the Health Administration Press Marketing Manager at (312) 424-9470.

Library of Congress Cataloging-in-Publication Data

Health services managment : readings, cases, and commentary / Anthony R. Kovner and
    Duncan Neuhauser, editors.—8th ed.
        p.   cm.
    Eighth ed. comprises the two books of readings and commentary and case studies into
one text, with updates and new cases.
    Includes bibliographical references and index.
    ISBN 1-56793-220-7
    1. Health facilities—Administration—Case studies.   2. Health services
administration—Case studies.   3. Hospitals—Administration—Case studies.
    I. Kovner, Anthony R.   II. Neuhauser, Duncan, 1939–   .
    RA971.H434   2004
    362.1'068—dc22   200404599

The paper used in this publication meets the minimum requirements of American National Standard for Information Sciences—Permanence of Paper for Printed Library Materials, ANSI Z39.48-1984. (TM)

Acquisitions Editor: Janet Davis; Project manager: Cami Cacciatore; Cover design: Betsy Perez.

Health Administration Press   Association of University Programs
A division of the Foundation   in Health Administration
    of the American College of   2000 N. 14th Street
    Healthcare Executives   Suite 780
One North Franklin Street   Arlington, VA 22201
Suite 1700   (703) 894-0940
Chicago, IL 60606
(312) 424-2800

To Duncan Neuhauser

We have been working together on these management books for 25 years now, and we have never had an argument. I've consistently learned from what you've had to say. Together we have enjoyed beholding the healthcare enterprise, which always amazes me in its latest twists and turns. Duncan, I admire you for your integrity, sense of humor, wisdom and experience, and intellectual courage. You have always been willing to point out but softly (and not unless someone asks you) that the emperor isn't really wearing any clothes.

—Tony Kovner

To Tony Kovner

You have had the wisdom, energy, and willingness to describe your careers in health management in your autobiographical book *Health Care Management in Mind—Eight Careers* (Springer Publishing Co., 2000). You kindly let me write an "afterword" to this book where I tried to describe our successful working relationship lasting over a quarter of a century. Here is another way to describe our working relationship. It is like sailing two boats and planning to meet at the same port at the same time. This requires years of learning and a lot of skills, but not much communication once our objective is precisely defined. Done well there is no need for committee meetings, organizational overhead, or raging arguments. This trip is as enjoyable as the successful arrival. It is clear you have enjoyed the trip of your career as much as your successful arrival to the applause of our peers, as reflected in your receiving the 1999 Gary Filerman Prize for Educational Leadership of the Association of University Programs in Health Administration.

—Duncan Neuhauser

CONTENTS

PART II CONTROL

PART III ORGANIZATIONAL DESIGN

PART IV PROFESSIONAL INTEGRATION

PART V ADAPTATION

Preface to the Eighth Edition

ealth Services Management: Readings, Cases, and Commentary is distinctive in its overview of management and organizational behavior theory. The book is organized in a framework that begins with those parts of work over which managers have the greatest control—the manager himself or herself and control systems—then extends to cover parts of the work over which managers have a good deal of control (at least over the short run)—organizational design and professional integration—and concludes with those parts of the work over which managers have less control—adaptation, including implementation of strategy, and accountability to interests that supply the organization with resources. Throughout there is an emphasis on the case method approach to teaching healthcare management.

The cases take place in a variety of organizations, including a faculty practice, a neighborhood health center, a small rural hospital, an HMO, a department of pediatrics, a medical group, an academic medical center, the Veteran's Administration, a visiting nurse association, and a number of community hospitals.

An instructor's manual is available on-line that includes suggested syllabi, approaches for discussing several topics in each part—for example, on the role of the manager, suggested topics include history of the manager's role in healthcare, organizational settings here and abroad, and career planning for managers in health care—and teaching notes for the case studies, the great majority of which have been classroom-tested.

We wrote and edited "Health Services Management: Readings, Cases, and Commentary" with the idea that it will be used as a stand-alone textbook, but it can also be used as a complement to other textbooks. For this edition, we decided to unite our previous books of readings and of case studies into one textbook of readings, cases, and commentary, for the following reasons: (1) less expense for the student; (2) facilitation of course use of other textbooks; and (3) availability of the readings on the Internet, which means they don't have to be included in the textbook (although we include at least one reading for each of the text's six parts). A note for students on how to retrieve journal articles through the Internet is included in the text. Although now combined, the book can still be viewed as a casebook, but with the inclusion of the readings.

Some things have not changed through the eight editions of this text (this is now our 25th year of writing these books). The first has been the desire to have readings that build on good evidence rather than just opinion. At first, this goal was hard to achieve because of the thinness of the literature. Now it is hard to choose among many good papers. Second, is the goal of linking theory with practice; to build a bridge between the social science literature and the actual work of improvement. Third, the text has always been divided into six sections—the role of the manager, control, organizational design, professional integration, adaptability, and accountability—each with a commentary.

We welcome dialogue with our readers, and can be reached via e-mail at:

Anthony R Kovner   anthony.kovner@nyu.edu
Duncan Neuhauser   duncan.neuhauser@case.edu

HOW TO RETRIEVE JOURNAL ARTICLES FROM THE INTERNET—A GUIDE FOR STUDENTS

Many of the journal articles referenced in this text may be easily accessed and printed from the Internet free of charge, presupposing the publisher has granted your school library access to its electronic archives. The following steps are intended to guide one through the process of locating, viewing, and printing journal articles from the Internet.

1. Access your school library homepage. If you do not know the web address of your school library homepage, you can probably find a link to it on your school's homepage.
2. Locate the directory of electronic journals to which your school library subscribes. Many library homepages display a link to "Electronic Journals and Texts" or "E-Journals and Texts" or the like. If so, click on this link. If the link is not on the homepage, try searching for the directory in areas such as "research," "databases and catalogs," or "journals."
3. Locate the directory that is likely to contain the journal you are looking for. The journal directories are often stratified according to broad subject areas. For instance, if you are looking for an article in the *Harvard Business Review,* click on the "Business" directory heading. Likewise, an article in *Health Care Management Review* would be found by clicking on the "Medicine and Health" directory heading.
4. Locate and click on the journal title in the directory. Some directories offer an option to search for the journal using a key word in the title. Otherwise, find the journal title according to the first letter in the title. If you do not see the journal title you are looking for, either the publisher has not made an electronic version of the journal available or your school's library does not subscribe to the journal. (However, this does not mean that the paper version is not available in the library.)
5. Choose and click on the volume and issue number of the journal that contains the article. A table of contents of that issue will appear.

Occasionally, issues may not be included in the archive because they are either too old or too new (e.g., *New England Journal of Medicine* articles, which become available electronically six months after the original publication date).

6. Choose and click on the article you wish to print. The article will appear.

7. Print the article by clicking on your web browser's Print button or by choosing "Print" from the File menu.

LEARNING THROUGH THE CASE METHOD

Anthony R. Kovner

A challenge for many graduate programs in health services management is bridging the gap between theory and skills and their application by students to health services organizations. Part of the problem lies in the difficulty of attracting and retaining skilled teachers who can integrate perspectives and apply concepts across disciplines in responding to managerial problems and opportunities.

A second challenge is to prepare graduate students to communicate effectively, both in writing and orally, and to assist them in working effectively in groups. This includes helping students to assess the effects of their personalities or behavioral styles on others—are they perceived as abrasive, wishy-washy, manipulative? Are they aware of how others interpret not only their words but their tone and body language?

Students in health services management graduate programs must understand their own values and those of others who differ in educational background, political and religious orientation, clinical experience, or familial exposure to careers and lifestyles.

A "case" is a description of a situation or problem facing a manager that requires analysis, decision, and planning a course of action. A decision may be to delay a decision, and a planned course of action may be to take no action. A case takes place in time. A case must have an issue. As McNair says, "There must be a question of what should somebody do, what should somebody have done, who is to blame for the situation, what is the best decision to be made under the circumstances."[1] A case represents selected details about a situation; it represents selection by the case writer.

The case method involves class discussion that is guided by a teacher so that students can diagnose and define important problems in a situation, acquire competence in developing useful alternatives to respond to such problems, and improve judgment in selecting action alternatives. Students learn ways both to diagnose constraints and opportunities faced by the manager in implementation and to overcome constraints given limited time and dollars.

Teachers can transmit great quantities of data to students more effectively and certainly more efficiently by lecture. The teacher is assumed to be correct in presenting facts, and the student transcribes key points of the lecture and transmits them back to the teacher at examination time. In contrast, in a case course, the teacher's job is to engage the students in a management simulation so that they can think independently, communicate effectively, and defend their opinions logically with reference to underlying assumptions and values. Often a case does not have one right answer because at least two sides are present in the issue at hand.

Students often have difficulty adjusting to a classroom without an authority figure, without lectures from which to take notes, and in which little information is offered by the teacher, at least until the class discussion has ended. Some students find it irritating to have to listen to their peers when they are paying to learn what the teacher has to say.

In a case course, students learn how to use information at the point of decision. Many students dislike "putting themselves on the line" when they are "only" students saying what they think. If no "right" answers can be reached, students quickly learn in a case course that many "wrong" answers can be eliminated because of faulty logic or assumptions that are challenged or contradicted by their peers. Students fear looking foolish and being downgraded accordingly by the teacher, and they must pass the course;[2] but students should consider such self-exposure to be little enough cost to pay in relation to the benefit of appearing mature and skillful after graduation and in the professional environment. It is hoped that they will have gained the ability to make logical judgments and learned how to behave and to communicate their opinions to others.

As Cantor[3] says, "You don't learn from anybody else's experience or from your own experience unless you go through the experience to learn." This is what the case method has to offer students—an experience in learning that involves testing opinions and conclusions against the reality of the case and the judgment of peers and teacher.

How do cases bridge the gap between theory and skills and their application by managers? Problems that health services managers face do not come neatly packaged as separate questions of statistics, economics, organization theory, or policy analysis. Rather they are organizational, multidisciplinary problems, sometimes difficult to define as well as to resolve. Problems may include negotiating a new contract with the chief of radiology, responding appropriately to patient complaints, or taking responsibility for quality assurance in relation to a surgeon's poor performance.

Student performance in a case course is typically assessed on class participation and on written analysis of case materials. A lack of sufficient time by the teacher in analyzing a student's evaluation may be partially corrected by allowing peer evaluation as well. Often teachers ask students to collaborate on complex cases or to evaluate each other's performance. The presenting student should be told if personal style or mannerisms interfere with a case analysis presentation or with its perception by others, as these issues could create conflicts in their professional careers.

In a case course, students are often asked to adopt the perspectives of certain characters in the case, to play certain roles. To deny someone of something or to persuade someone to do something requires an understanding of that person's needs and perceptions of the decision maker. Role-playing can promote a better understanding of viewpoints that otherwise may seem irrational given a student's prior understanding of what should be done in a particular situation. Students can better understand their own values and underlying assumptions when their opinions are challenged by peers and teachers.

To conclude, it is important to understand what a case is not and what case method cannot teach. Cases are not real life—they present only part of a situation. Writing or communicating a case may be as difficult as or more difficult than evaluating someone else's written case. Like many a consultant, the student can never see the results—what would have happened if the case participants had followed his advice.

Some aspects of management can be learned only by managing. How else can one understand when someone says one thing but means another? How else can one judge whether to confront or oppose a member of the ruling coalition when that member's behavior appears to threaten the long-range interests of the organization? Students and managers have to form and adopt their own value systems and make their own decisions. A case course can give students a better understanding of the nature of the role they will be playing as managers—an understanding that can help them to manage better, if not well.

Notes

1. R. Towl, *To Study Administration by Cases* (Boston: Graduate School of Business Administration, Harvard University, 1969), p. 67.
2. Ibid., p. 68.
3. Ibid., p. 155.

A SHORT HISTORY OF THE CASE METHOD OF TEACHING

Karen Schachter Weingrod and Duncan Neuhauser

Teaching by example is no doubt as old as the first parent and child. In medicine it surely started with a healer, the first apprentice, and a patient. The ancient Greeks codified medical principles, rules, and laws. University education in medicine started about 800 years ago, focused on abstract principles and scholastic reasoning, and was removed from practicality. By 1750 in England, the professions aspired to gentlemen status.[1] The gold-headed cane of the English physician, for instance, was the clear symbol that his hands were not expected to touch patients, unlike the hands of apothecaries and barber surgeons. Later, the American sociologist Thorstein Veblen, in *The Theory of the Leisure Class*, used the example of the cane as symbolic that a gentleman need not work with his hands.[2] In the late 1700s in France, medical education moved into hospitals or "the clinic," where patients in large numbers could be observed, autopsies performed, and the physiological state linked back to the patients' signs and symptoms.[3] This was one step in the departure from the abstract medical theorizing in universities (often about the "four humours"), which may have had no bearing on actual disease processes.

Education in law also became increasingly abstract, conveyed through the erudite lecture. It built theoretical constructs and was logically well reasoned. The professor spoke and the student memorized and recited without much opportunity for practical experience or discussion. This had become the standard by the late 1850s.

It is only by comparison with what went on before in universities that the case method of teaching represented such a striking change. The historical development of the case method can be traced to Harvard University. Perhaps it is not surprising that this change occurred in the United States rather than in Europe, with the American inclinations toward democratic equality, practicality, and positivism, and the lack of interest in classic abstract theorizing.

The change started in 1870 when the president of Harvard University, Charles William Eliot, appointed the obscure lawyer Christopher Columbus Langdell as dean of the Harvard Law School.

Langdell believed law to be a science. In his own words: "Law considered as a science, consists of certain principles or doctrines. To have such a mastery of these as to be able to apply them with constant faculty and certainty to the ever-tangled skein of human affairs, is what constitutes a good lawyer; and hence to acquire that mastery should be the business of every earnest student of the law."[4]

The specimens needed for the study of Langdell's science of law were judicial opinions as recorded in books and stored in libraries. He accepted the science of law, but he turned the learning process back to front. Instead of giving a lecture that would define a principle of law and give supporting examples of judicial opinions, he gave the students the judicial opinions without the principle and by use of a Socratic dialogue extracted from the students in the classroom the principles that would make sense out of the cases. The student role was now active rather than passive. Students were subjected to rigorous questioning of the case material. They were asked to defend their judgments and to confess to error when their judgments were illogical. Although this dialectic was carried on by the professor and one or two students at a time, all of the students learned and were on the edge of their seats, fearing or hoping they would be called on next. The law school style that evolved has put the student under public pressure to reason quickly, clearly, and coherently in a way that is valuable in the courtroom or during negotiation. After a discouraging start, Langdell attracted such able instructors as Oliver Wendell Holmes, Jr. They carried the day, and now the case method of teaching is nearly universal in American law schools.

The introduction of the case method of teaching to medicine is also known. A Harvard medical student of the class of 1901, Walter B. Cannon, shared a room with Harry Bigelow, a third-year law student. The excitement with which Bigelow and his classmates debated the issues within the cases they were reading for class contrasted sharply with the passivity of medical school lectures.

In 1900, discussing the value of the case method in medicine, Harvard President Charles Eliot described the earlier medical education as follows:

> I think it was thirty-five years ago that I was a lecturer at the Harvard Medical School for one winter; at that time lectures began in the school at eight o'clock in the morning and went on steadily till two o'clock—six mortal hours, one after the other of lectures, without a question from the professor, without the possibility of an observation by the student, none whatever, just the lecture to be listened to, and possibly taken notes of. Some of the students could hardly write.[5]

In December 1899, Cannon persuaded one of his instructors, G. L. Walton, to present one of the cases in written form from his private practice as an experiment. Walton printed a sheet with the patient's history and allowed the students a week to study it. The lively discussion that ensued in class made Walton an immediate convert.[6] Other faculty soon followed, including Richard C. Cabot.

Through the case method, medical students would learn to judge and interpret clinical data, to estimate the value of evidence, and to recognize the gaps in their knowledge—something that straight lecturing could never reveal. The case method of teaching allowed students to throw off passivity in the lecture hall and integrate their knowledge of anatomy, physiology, pathology, and therapeutics into a unified mode of thought.

As a student, Cannon wrote two articles about the case method in 1900 for the *Boston Medical and Surgical Journal* (later to become *The New England Journal of Medicine*).[7] He sent a copy of one of these papers to the famous clinician professor Dr. William Osler of Johns Hopkins University. Osler replied, "I have long held that the only possible way of teaching students the subject of medicine is by personal daily contact with cases, which they study not only once or twice, but follow systematically."[8] If a written medical case was interesting, a real live patient in the classroom could be memorable. Osler regularly introduced patients to his class, asked students to interview and examine the patient and discuss the medical problems involved. He would regularly send students to the library and laboratory to seek answers and report back to the rest of the class.[9] This is ideal teaching. Osler's students worshipped him, but with today's division of labor in medicine between basic science and clinical medicine, such a synthesis is close to impossible.

The May 24, 1900 issue of the *Boston Medical and Surgical Journal* was devoted to articles and comments by Eliot, Cannon, Cabot, and others about the case method of teaching. In some ways this journal issue remains the best general discussion of the case method. This approach was adopted rapidly at other medical schools, and books of written cases quickly followed in neurology (1902), surgery (1904), and orthopedic surgery (1905).[10]

Cannon went on to a distinguished career in medical research. Cabot joined the medical staff of the Massachusetts General Hospital, and in 1906 published his first book of cases. (He also introduced the first social worker into a hospital.[11]) He was concerned about the undesirable separation of clinical physicians and pathologists; too many diagnoses were turning out to be false at autopsy. To remedy this, Cabot began to hold his case exercises with students, house officers, and visitors.

Cabot's clinical/pathological conferences took on a stereotypical style and eventually were adopted in teaching hospitals throughout the world. First, the patient's history, symptoms, and test results would be described. Then an invited specialist would discuss the case, suggest an explanation, and give a diagnosis. Finally, the pathologist would present the autopsy or pathological diagnosis and questions would follow to elaborate points.

In 1915, Cabot sent written copies of his cases to interested physicians as "at home case method exercises." These became so popular that in 1923 the *Boston Medical and Surgical Journal* began to publish one per issue.[12] This journal has since changed its name to *The New England Journal of Medicine*, but the "Cabot Case Records" still appear with each issue.

A look at a current *New England Journal of Medicine* case will show how much the case method has changed since Langdell's original concept. The student or house officer is no longer asked to discuss the case; rather, it is the expert who puts her reputation on the line. She has the opportunity to demonstrate wisdom, but can also be refuted in front of a large audience. Although every physician in the audience probably makes mental diagnoses, the case presentation has become a passive affair, like a lecture.

Cabot left the Massachusetts General Hospital to head the Social Relations (sociology, psychology, cultural anthropology) department at Harvard. He brought the case method with him, but it disappeared from use there by the time of his death in 1939.[13] The social science disciplines were concerned with theory building, hypothesis testing, and research methodology, and to such "unapplied" pure scientists perhaps the case method was considered primitive. Further, the use of the case method of teaching also diminished in the first two preclinical years of medical school as clinical scientists came more and more to the fore with their laboratory work and research on physiology, pharmacology, biochemistry, and molecular biology. Today problem-solving learning in medical schools is widespread and replacing the passive learning of traditional lectures..

In 1908, the Harvard Business School was created as a department of the Graduate School of Arts and Sciences. It was initially criticized as merely a school for "successful money-making." Early on an effort was made to teach through the use of written problems involving situations faced by actual business executives, presented in sufficient factual detail to enable students to develop their own decisions. The school's first book of cases, on marketing, was published in 1922 by Melvin T. Copeland.[14] Today, nearly every class in the Harvard Business School is taught by the case method.

Unlike the law school, where cases come directly from judicial decisions (sometimes abbreviated by the instructor) and the medical school, where the patient is the basis for the case, the business faculty and their aides must enter organizations to collect and compile their material. This latter mode of selection offers substantial editorial latitude. Here more than elsewhere the case writer's vision, or lack of it, defines the content of the case.

Unlike a pathologist's autopsy diagnosis, a business case is not designed to have a right answer. In fact, one usually never knows whether the business in question lives or dies. Rather, the cases are written in a way that splits a large class (up to 80 students) into factions. The best cases are those that create divergent opinions; the professor becomes more an orchestra leader than a source of truth. The professor's opinion or answer may never be made explicit. Following a discussion, a student's question related to what really happened or what should have been done may be answered, "I don't know" or "I think the key issues were picked up in the case discussion." Such hesitancy on the part of the instructor is often desirable. To praise or condemn a particular faction in the classroom can discourage future discussions.

The class atmosphere in a business school is likely to be less pressured than in a law school. Like a good surgeon, a good lawyer must often think very quickly, but unlike the surgeon his thinking is demonstrated verbally and publicly. He must persuade by the power of his logic rather than by force of authority. Business and management are different. Key managerial decisions—What business are we in? Who are our customers? Where should we be ten years from now?—may take months or even years to answer.

The fact that the business manager's time frame reduces the pressure for immediate answers makes management education different from physician education in other ways. Physicians are required to absorb countless facts on anatomy, disease symptoms, and drug side effects. Confronted with 20 patients a day, the physician often has no time, even over the Internet, to consult references. The manager has a longer time horizon for decision making in business. Therefore, managerial education focuses more on problem-solving techniques than does standard medical education.

Not all business schools have endorsed the case method of teaching. The University of Chicago Business School, for example, rarely uses cases and focuses on teaching the "science" of economics, human behavior, and operations research. The faculty are concerned with theory building, hypothesis testing, statistical methodology, and the social sciences. Stanford Business School uses about half social sciences and half case method. Each school is convinced that its teaching philosophy is best and believes others to be misguided. Conceptually, the debate can be broken into two aspects: science versus professionalism, and active versus passive learning.

There is little question that active student involvement in learning is better than passive listening to lectures. The case method is one of many approaches to increasing student participation. However, only a skilled instructor, for example, can stimulate a lively discussion by social sciences students on the theoretical assumptions, methodological problems, and use or abuse of statistical analysis in an *American Journal of Sociology* assignment.

Academic science is not overly concerned with the practical problems of the world, but professionals are and professional education should be. The lawyer, physician, and manager cannot wait for perfect knowledge; they have to make decisions in the face of uncertainty. Science can help with these decisions to varying degrees. To the extent that scientific theories have the power to predict and explain, they can be used by professionals. In the jargon of statistics: the higher the percentage of variance explained, the more useful the scientific theory, the smaller the role for clinical or professional judgment, and the lesser the role for case method teaching as opposed to, for example, mathematical problem solving.

It can be argued that the professional will always be working at the frontier of the limits of scientific prediction. When science is the perfect predictor, then often the problem is solved, or the application is delegated to computers or technicians, or, as in some branches of engineering, professional skills focus on the manipulation of accurate but complex mathematical equations.

Scientific medicine now understands smallpox so well that it no longer exists. Physicians spend most of their time on problems that are not solved: cancer, heart disease, or the common complaints of living that bring most people to doctors. In management, the budget cycle, personnel position control, sterile operating room environment, and maintenance of the business office ledgers are handled routinely by organizational members and usually do not consume the attention of the chief executive officer. In law, the known formulations become the "boiler plate" of contracts.

The debate between business schools over the use of cases illustrates the difference in belief in the power of the social sciences in the business environment. Teaching modes related to science and judgment will always be in uneasy balance with each other, shifting with time and place. Innovative medical schools have moved away from the scientific lectures of the preclinical years and toward a case problem-solving mode. On the other side of the coin, a quiet revolution is being waged in clinical reasoning. The principles of statistics, epidemiology, and economics, filtered through the techniques of decision analysis, cost-effectiveness analysis, computer modeling, and artificial intelligence, are making the Cabot Case Record approach obsolete for clinical reasoning. Scientific methods of clinical reasoning are beginning to replace aspects of professional or clinical judgment in medicine.[15]

This does not mean that the professional aspect of medicine will be eliminated by computer-based science. Rather, the frontiers, the unknown areas calling for professional judgment, will shift to new areas, such as the development of socio-emotional rapport with patients—what used to be called "the bedside manner."[16]

The cases that make up this book are derived from the business school style of case teaching. As such they do not have answers. The cases can be used to apply management concepts to practical problems; however, these concepts (scientific theory seems too strong a term to apply to them) may help solve these case problems but will not yield the one "right" answer. They all leave much room for debate.

Notes

1. Harold J. Cook, *The Decline of the Old Medical Regime in Stuart London* (Ithaca, NY: Cornell University Press, 1986).

2. Thorstein Veblen, *The Theory of the Leisure Class* (1899; reprinted New York: Mentor, 1953).

3. Michel Foucault, *The Birth of the Clinic* (New York: Vintage, 1973).

4. C. C. Langdell, *Cases and Contracts* (1871), cited in *The Law at Harvard*, by Arthur E. Sutherland (Cambridge, MA: Harvard University Press, 1967), p. 174.

5. Charles Eliot, "The Inductive Method Applied to Medicine," *Boston Medical and Surgical Journal* 142, no. 22 (24 May 1900): 557.

6. Saul Benison, A. Clifford Barger, and Elin L. Wolfe, *Walter B. Cannon, The Life and Times of a Young Scientist* (Cambridge, MA: Harvard University Press, 1987), pp. 65–75, 417–418.

7. W. B. Cannon, "The Case Method of Teaching Systematic Medicare," *Boston Medical and Surgical Journal* 142, no. 2 (11 January 1900): 31–36; and "The Case System in Medicine" 142, no. 22 (24 May 1900): 563–64.

8. Benison et al., *Walter B. Cannon,* p. 66.

9. Alan M. Chesney, *The Johns Hopkins Hospital and the Johns Hopkins University School of Medicine*, vol. 11, 1893–1905 (Baltimore, MD: The Johns Hopkins Press, 1958), pp. 125–28.

10. Benison et al., *Walter B. Cannon,* p. 418.

11. Ibid., p. 145. Although not the first hospital-based social worker to work with Cabot, his best-known social worker colleague was Walter Cannon's sister, Ida Cannon.

12. These cases start October 25, 1923.

13. Paul Buck (ed.), *The Social Sciences at Harvard* (Boston, MA: Harvard University Press, 1965).

14. For more on the history of the case method of teaching managers see Roy Penchansky, *Health Services Administration: Policy Cases and the Case Method* (Boston, MA: Harvard University Press, 1968), pp. 395–453.

15. Louis B. Barnes, C. Roland Christensen, Abby J. Hansen, *Teaching and the Case Method*, 3rd Edition (Boston, MA, Harvard Business School Press, 1994).

16. A proposal to increase the problem-solving content of medical education is found in Association of American Medical Colleges, *Graduate Medical Education: Proposals for the Eighties* (Washington, DC: AAMC, 1980). Also reprinted as a supplement in *Journal of Medical Education* 56, no. 9 (September 1981, part 2).

Overview

Why do we do what we do
How do we know it works?
How can we do it better?
—John Bingham, Twin Falls, Idaho

Creating and maintaining a health services organization in which these three questions are constantly asked and answered is the role of the health services manager. This book, in its eight editions, has attempted to select from the best current literature on health services management to help learners understand the role of the manager, organizational design and control, the blending of organization and health professionals, change (adaptation), and responsiveness (accountability). The central focus is on the role of health services managers and how they modify and maintain an organization within its context. The organizations described include hospitals, nursing homes, ambulatory care, HMOs, and integrated delivery systems, which may combine many of these components.

Levels and Issues

The role of managers can be conceptualized in many different ways according to what they need to know and what they do.

The manager's role can be categorized by listing knowledge areas for the general managers, as seen in Figure 1, which lists 12 areas.[1] This general knowledge needs to be applied in a specific management context, in this case health services.

An organization such as a hospital, a group practice, or a nursing home can also be conceptualized in many different ways. One can use an organization chart; draw sociometric diagrams; indicate the flow of production based on inputs, process, and outputs; write its history; describe its key policies; and so forth. Each of these is appropriate, depending on the questions being asked. We use the following conceptualization.

The organization can be viewed as a set of concentric rings (see Figure 2). At the center is the senior manager and his or her role, in the immediate managerial context (the manager). In the second ring going outward,

FIGURE 1
Knowledge
Areas for
General
Management

Knowledge Area	Relevant Part of This Book
1. Organizational behavior	
2. Labor and human resource policy	I. Role of the Manager
3. Accounting	
4. Management statistics	
5. Information and decision systems	II. Control
6. Operation research	
7. Operations management	
8. Organization design theory	III. Organizational Design
9. Marketing	IV. Professional Integration
10. Finance	V. Adaptation
11. Economics	
12. Policy, law, ethics	VI. Accountability

All the above needs to be used within the specific features of health services

SOURCE: Modified from R. E. Boyatzis, S. S. Cowen, D. A. Kolb, and Associates. 1995. *Innovation in Professional Education*, 57. San Francisco: Jossey-Bass.

the manager undertakes to design the structure of the organization, to specify procedures, to use resources, and to provide a feedback mechanism to evaluate performance (control and organizational design). The third ring (professional integration) represents the interaction between management and professional members of the organization, including physicians. The fourth ring (adaptation) is concerned with how the organization can and must respond to fit its present and future environment. The fifth ring (accountability) signifies how the environment imposes requirements for responsiveness on the organization.[2]

Figure 2 makes the manager the "sun" in a heliocentric view of the organization. Although another diagrammatic perspective would be used if this were a book for patients, physicians, or trustees, we use this particular conceptualization because our book is written for those who are, or wish to be, health services managers. However, we do not deny the usefulness of other ways of viewing the organization.

The outline of this book follows the form of Figure 2, starting from the center and moving outward. The parts, described below, focus on key problems and issues at each level in the organization.

Part I, "The Role of the Manager," is concerned with the immediate context within which managers work, how they spend their time, the importance of judgment, the kinds of problems they are challenged by, and the opportunities and constraints they face in implementing change and sustaining the organization.

FIGURE 2
Manager,
Organization,
and
Environment

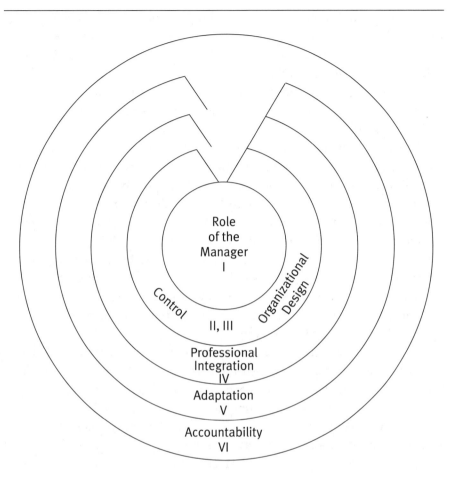

Part of Book	Key Issues	Organizational Space	Activity and Mind-Set[3]
I	Role of the Manager	The manager	Managing self (reflection)
			Managing relationships (collaborative)
II, III	Control, Organizational Design	Management, internal organization	Managing the organization (analytic)
IV	Professional Integration	Internal organization	
V	Adaptation	Organization, environment	Managing change (action)
VI	Accountability	Environment, organization	Managing external (worldly) context

Parts II and III cover "Control" and "Organizational Design." In large organizations, managers cannot work face-to-face with all employees. Rather, they must specify their activities indirectly, relying on other managers, formal rules, hierarchy, budgets, information systems, and impersonal techniques for control and evaluation. Managers will be successful to different degrees in structuring and monitoring the organization to achieve their view of organizational purpose.

Similarly, organization members will respond to these efforts in various ways with independent actions, resistance, or cooperation. A critical problem is the degree to which professionals, especially physicians, are integrated into the organization. This is addressed in Part IV, "Professional Integration."

Managers must adapt both to changes in the organization's internal structure and function and to the organization's specific environment, as discussed in Part V, "Adaptation." Managers must be accountable to the community or publics served, as indicated in the readings in Part VI, "Accountability." These last two parts are concerned with the health services organization's interface with suppliers of needed resources such as manpower, funding, legitimacy, and information.

At the center of the circle, managers are able to influence what happens. Moving toward the periphery, their influence steadily declines and is replaced by other forces. This is shown schematically in Figure 3, where managers' influence flows in diminishing strength from left to right. The influence of others (government, patients, professionals, employees, co-managers, and so on) flows with diminishing strength from right to left. The slope and height of the diagonal line, reflecting the balance of these forces, should be viewed as variable through time and dependent on the manager, the organization, and the environment.

Figure 4 presents, in an oversimplified way, examples of issues and problems at various levels of the organization that are within or outside the manager's sphere of influence. A more accurate representation would indicate that each of these issues and problems is more or less influenced by the manager at

FIGURE 3

The Flow of Influence Within a Health Services Organization

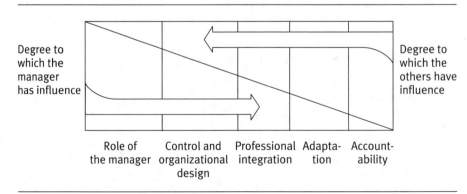

Degree to which the manager has influence

Degree to which the others have influence

Role of the manager | Control and organizational design | Professional integration | Adaptation | Accountability

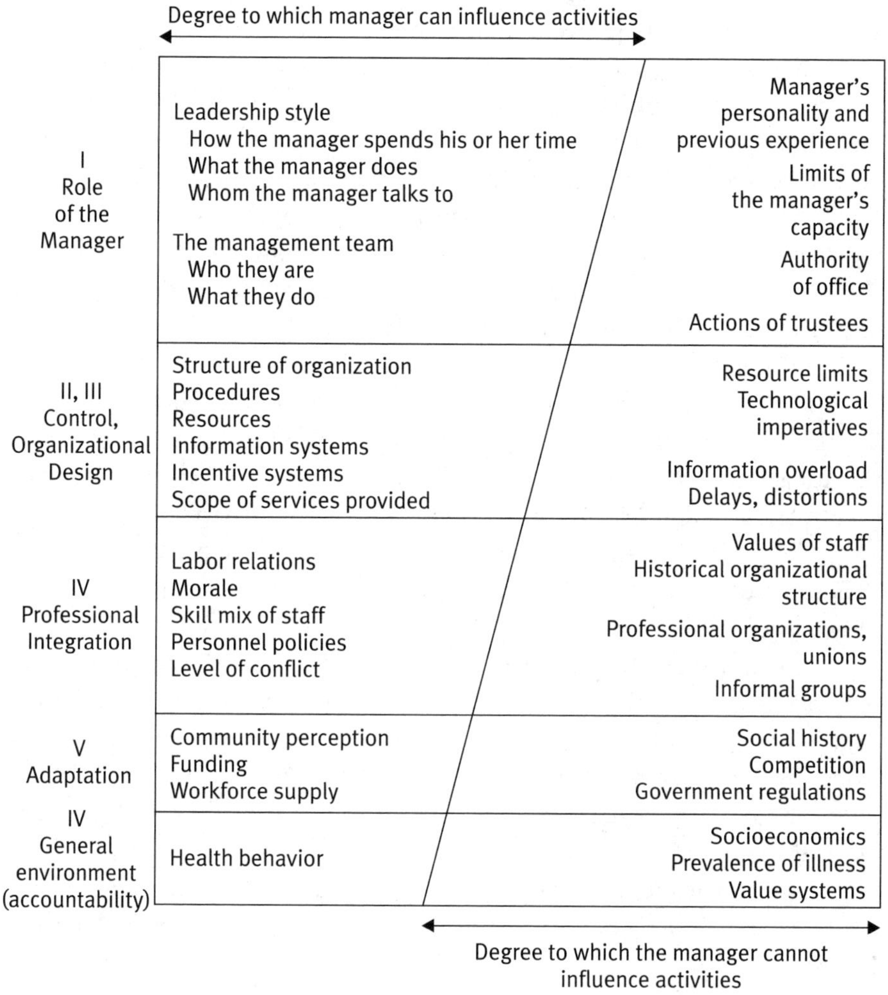

FIGURE 4

Examples of Issues and Problems Associated with Different Levels of the Organization

Degree to which manager can influence activities

Level	Can influence	Cannot influence

I
Role
of the
Manager
	Leadership style
	  How the manager spends his or her time
	  What the manager does
	  Whom the manager talks to
	
	The management team
	  Who they are
	  What they do
		Manager's personality and previous experience
		Limits of the manager's capacity
		Authority of office
		Actions of trustees

II, III Control, Organizational Design	Structure of organization Procedures Resources Information systems Incentive systems Scope of services provided	Resource limits Technological imperatives Information overload Delays, distortions
IV Professional Integration	Labor relations Morale Skill mix of staff Personnel policies Level of conflict	Values of staff Historical organizational structure Professional organizations, unions Informal groups
V Adaptation	Community perception Funding Workforce supply	Social history Competition Government regulations
IV General environment (accountability)	Health behavior	Socioeconomics Prevalence of illness Value systems

Degree to which the manager cannot influence activities

different times and to varying degrees in certain types of organizations facing certain types of environments.

Managers have most control over the structure and function of their own office (the role of the manager). They also exert some control over the authority of their office and the actions of their co-managers and trustees. They can, to a considerable extent, decide how to spend their time, what problems to address and in what order, who should be on the management team and what they should do, and so forth. However, managers' experience, work background, physical capacity, and personality are to some degree fixed and beyond their ability to change.

At the next level, managers can impose structure and specify control and information systems, but only within the limits of resource availability and technological imperatives. Information and control systems cannot be complete, exhaustive, or immediate in their effects; they are not error-free and are often costly in terms of money and managerial time.

Managers' design and control efforts will be met with different levels of acceptance by workers, professionals, and patients, all of whom sometimes act independently of, and are at odds with, managers. Often managers can do little to change the attitudes of physicians, union officials, and patients.

At the environmental level, managers have some modest influence on legislation, regulation, third-party financing, community values, and other organizations' actions. However, much of the specific behavior of groups and organizations in their environment, and most of the general environment as well, is beyond the control or influence of a manager.

Skills representative of a good manager are summarized in Figure 5. Boyatzis et al. list these as "subthemes" under the overall leadership goal of "creating economic, intellectual, and human value."[4] These subthemes have been reorganized in Figure 5 to align them with the six parts of this book.

The role all managers have is to directly supervise a team of people. This requires supervisory skills at a face-to-face level. A list of these skills is shown in Figure 6.[5]

Griffith and White, in their book *The Well-Managed Healthcare Organization*,[6] create another classification of health services management knowledge and skills. They organize this book under three large managerial objectives of governing, caring, and learning. For Griffith and White, governing consists of making the health services organization responsive to its environment. Caring means building a quality clinical service, and learning integrates meeting, planning, marketing, finance, and information needs. Griffith's and White's typology is matched to the structure of this book in Figure 7.

FIGURE 5
Skills of the
Good Manager

Part	Issue	Skills of the Good Manager
I	Role of the Manager	Understanding one's self Be a leader and team member
II	Control	Innovate in the use of information
III	Organizational Design	Innovate in the use of technology
IV	Professional Integration	Stimulate professional integrity
V	Adaptation	Manage change in a complex, diverse, and interdependent world
VI	Accountability	Show integrity and social responsibility

FIGURE 6
The Role of
the Manager

Supervisory Skills

Supervisory Skills and Domains	Relevant Content
Leadership style	Self-awareness, delegation, participatory management, constancy of purpose
Communication	Verbal, non-verbal, written
Time management	
Continuing education	For self and team members
Motivation	
Measurement and appraisal of team member performance	Performance reviews
Human resource policies	Hiring, pay raises, dismissed union agreements, coping with the problem or troubled employee Personnel rules
Creating a positive work environment	Morale, praise, criticism, motivation, justice, fairness
Running effective meetings	
Budgeting	
Knowledge of relevant laws	
Ability to use relevant technology appropriately	Knowledge of the work of the department
Management of change	Understanding customer needs, planning, quality improvement
Decision making, analytic reasoning	System thinking, quantitative analysis, social objectivity

Quality Improvement

The terms continuous quality improvement (CQI), total quality management (TQM), and quality improvement (QI) are often used interchangeably in North America, although they mean different things to some people. These ideas are defined in at least three ways. One is by the writings of Walter Shewhart, W. Edwards Deming, Joseph Juran, and like-minded thinkers, which concern reducing variation in standard operations processes. A second way defines CQI as a way to answer these three questions: Why do we do what we do? How do we know it works? How can we do it better? The third definition is very similar to the second, promoting customer-mindedness, statistical-mindedness, and organizational transformation.

FIGURE 7

Organizational
Conceptual
Frameworks

		Griffith/White	Kovner/Neuhauser
	Governing	Relating to the Environment	Adaptation, Accountability
		Governing Board	Role of the Manager
		Executive Office	Role of the Manager
		Organization Design	Organizational Design
		Performance Management	Control
	Caring	Quality and Economy of Care	Organizational Design
		Physician Services	
		Clinical Support Services	
		Nursing Services	Professional Integration
		Prevention and Non-acute Service	
	Learning	Planning	
		Marketing	
		Financial System	Control, Adaptation
		Information Services	
		Human Resources System	
		Plant System	Professional Integration

Customer-mindedness (accountability) focuses on meeting customer needs and desires. In the health field this has led to asking such questions as, "What is good care for people with high blood pressure or asthma in the population we serve?" It has led to increased use of patient-satisfaction surveys and their comparison across hospitals. Statistical-mindedness is concerned with measurement throughout the organization to understand processes, outcomes, and variation in those outcomes. What percent of inpatient meals are cold when eaten and why? Reducing variation (fewer cold meals) is an example of process improvement by reduction in variation, which can be seen as improving organizational control through improved design.

Organizational transformation occurs through managerial leadership (adaptation). Leading this change is central to the role of the manager and requires defining a clear mission, encouraging everyone to work on improvement, and creating a climate free of fear. How can everyone in a health services organization join in this common effort (professional integration)? The answer is related to what Peter Senge[7] describes as a learning organization in which people change behavior after reflecting on their experience.

CQI is also described by reference to Deming's 14 points (see Figure 8).[8] Behind these points are a number of assumptions. Production is a process with inherent variation. Understanding the causes of variation and changing the process to reduce variation will result in improved quality. Changing the way meals get from kitchen to patient rooms could reduce the number of

FIGURE 8
Deming's 14
Points

Book Part	Issue	Deming's Points
I	Role of the Manager	(1) Create constancy of purpose for improvement of product and service (2) Adopt the new philosophy of quality improvement (7) Institute leadership
II	Control	(3) Cease reliance on inspection (10) Eliminate slogans and (11) quotas (4) Do not award business on price alone
III	Organizational Design	(5) Improve constantly and forever the process for planning, production, and service
IV	Professional Integration	(6) Institute on-the-job training (continuing education) (8) Drive out fear (9) Break down barriers between staff areas (teamwork) (12) Encourage pride of workmanship
V	Adaptation	(5) Improve constantly (13) Promote education and self-improvement for everyone (14) Put everyone in the organization to work to accomplish this transformation
VI	Accountability	All 14 points drive to better meeting the needs and wishes of those we serve.

cold meals. Inspection, fear, quotas, and slogans will not help—education, pride of workmanship, teamwork, participation, and leadership will. All this transformation is intended to better meet the needs and wishes of those we serve.

Despite the fact that the active use of CQI methods in health services is less than 20 years old, it is now a worldwide movement.

Performance Requirements

All organizations can be described as having four performance requirements: goal attainment, system maintenance, adaptive capability, and values integration.[9]

Goal attainment is the requirement that organizations achieve at least enough of their goals to justify their support. The care has to be good enough for patients to come. The earnings have to be large enough to replace capital over time and to ensure money to meet the payroll.

System maintenance concerns organizational performance in self-renewal. Are the organization's members and suppliers stable over time, or are these relationships in the process of disintegrating? System maintenance includes the degree to which revenues match expenses, new staff match departing staff, deteriorating equipment is replaced, and incentive systems are appropriate to the level of effort required. It includes the maintenance of rules, procedures, and information systems. Alternative terms for system maintenance are *integration*, *structure*, *stability*, and *homeostasis*.

Adaptive capability involves organizational performance in changing to meet and cope with new conditions. Organizations must be innovative (proactive) and responsive (reactive). One indicator of adaptive capability is the presence or absence of specialized units that are primarily concerned with this function, such as long-range planning groups. Change is necessary for the organization to continue to survive and achieve its goals. Other terms specifying adaptive capability include *change orientation* and *organizational responsiveness*.

Values integration deals with organizational performance relative to congruence of the values of organizational members with the organization's goals and of organizational values with larger societal values—for example, the extent to which management and health services professionals are committed to the ideals of high-quality care, team effort, compassion, and continuing education. To the extent that the values of personnel are consistent with organizational goals, there may be less misuse of organizational resources. To the extent that organizational goals are consistent with societal goals, the organization may find it has higher prestige and access to more resources.[10] The concept of "corporate culture" has received a lot of attention. The specific cultures of different organizations have been described, in particular how they relate to goal attainment and innovation. Hospitals and medical centers often have strong cultures built on long histories, religious traditions, and notable individuals.

Conclusion

Organizations and their management can be described in many ways. Good management practices and organization survival skills are such perennially popular topics that new books fill whole shelves in local book stores. This book uses several classifications. The first defines the six parts of this book: the role of the manager, control, organizational design, professional integration, adaptation, and accountability. Of these, professional integration is a distinctive emphasis for the health field because of the prominent semi-independent nature of the many highly skilled professionals who play important roles in care.

A second classification used here is goal attainment, system maintenance, adaptive capability, and values integration.

A third way of looking at organizations is through quality improvement, which focuses on systems thinking. Customer-mindedness, statistical-mindedness and organizational transformation are concepts that can focus our understanding.

This overview has introduced these classifications and linked them to others, particularly in the figures. With these ways to organize one's thoughts about health services organizations, the reader is ready to proceed to the readings, cases, and commentary that follow in this 8th edition—and 25th anniversary issue—of this book.

Notes

1. R. E. Boyatzis, S. S. Cowen, D. A. Kolb, and Associates, *Innovation in Professional Education* (San Francisco: Jossey-Bass, 1995) p. 57.
2. The idea for Figure 2 comes from Robert Sutermeister, who put the production workers at the center of his circle. *See* Robert A. Sutermeister, *People and Productivity*, 2nd edition (New York: McGraw-Hill, 1969).
3. H. Mertzberg and J. Gosling, "Educating Managers Beyond Borders." *Academy of Management Learning and Education* 2002, 1 (1): 64–76 (see p 68).
4. Boyatzis et al., op cit 57.
5. The idea for Figure 6 comes from C. McConnell, *The Effective Healthcare Supervisor* (Rockville, MD: Aspen) 1982.
6. J. R. Griffith and K. R. White, *The Well-Managed Healthcare Organization*, 5th edition (Chicago: Health Administration Press, 2002).
7. P. Senge, *The Fifth Discipline* (New York: Doubleday, 1990).
8. W. E. Deming, *Out of the Crisis* (Cambridge, MA: Massachusetts Institute of Technology, Center for Advanced Engineering Study, 1982).
9. N. Mouzelis, *Organization and Bureaucracy* (Chicago: Aldine, 1971), chapter 7.
10. A. Etzioni, *A Comparative Analysis of Complex Organizations* (New York: Free Press, 1961).

Selected Bibliography

Argyris, C. *Knowledge for Action: A Guide to Overcoming Barriers to Organizational Change*. San Francisco: Jossey-Bass, 1993.

Barnard, C. *Functions of the Executive*. Cambridge, MA: Harvard University Press, 1964.

Bass, B. M. *Leadership and Performance Beyond Expectations*. New York: The Free Press, 1985.

Becker, S., and D. Neuhauser. *Organizational Efficiency*. New York: Elsevier, North Holland, 1975.

Berwick, D. M., A. B. Godfrey, and J. Roessner. *Curing Health Care*. San Francisco: Jossey-Bass, 1990.

Bolman, L., and T. Deal. *Modern Approaches to Understanding and Managing Organizations*. San Francisco: Jossey-Bass, 1990.

Boyatzis, R. E., S. S. Cowen, D. A. Kolb, and Associates. *Innovation in Professional Education*. San Francisco: Jossey-Bass, 1995.

Caplow, T. *Principles of Organization*. New York: Harcourt, Brace & World, 1964.

Deal, T. E., and A. A. Kennedy. *Corporate Cultures*. Reading, MA: Addison-Wesley, 1982.

Deming, W. E. *Out of the Crisis*. Cambridge, MA: Massachusetts Institute of Technology, Center for Advanced Engineering Study, 1982.

Drucker, P. F. *Managing the Non-Profit Organization*. New York: Harper Collins, 1990.

Feldstein, P. *Health Policy Issues: An Economic Perspective*, 4th edition. Chicago: Health Administration Press, 2003

Glouberman, S., and H. Mintzberg. "Managing the Care of the Health and the Cure of Disease—Part I: Differentiating." *Health Care Management Review* Winter 2001, pp 56–59.

Glouberman, S., and H. Mintzberg. "Managing the Care of the Health and the Cure of Disease— Part II: Interjection." *Health Care Management Review* Winter 2001, pp 70–84.

Greenberg, J., and R. A. Baron. *Behavior in Organizations,* 7th Edition. Upper Saddle River, NJ: Prentice Hall, 2000.

Griffith, J. R., and K. R. White. *The Well-Managed Healthcare Organization*, 5th edition. Chicago: Health Administration Press, 1999.

Guillen, M. F. *Models of Management*. Chicago: University of Chicago Press, 1994.

Handy, C. *Understanding Organizations*. New York: Oxford University Press, 1993.

Institute of Medicine. *To Err Is Human: Building a Safer Health System*. Washington, DC: National Academy Press, 2000.

Institute of Medicine. *Crossing the Quality Chasm*. Washington, DC: National Academy Press, 2001.

Joint Commission on Accreditation of Healthcare Organizations (JCAHO). *Striving Toward Improvement: Six Hospitals in Search of Quality*. Oakbrook Terrace, IL: JCAHO, 1992.

Juran, J. M. (ed.). *A History of Managing for Quality: The Evolution, Trends and*

Future Directions of Managing for Quality. Milwaukee, WI: ASQC Quality Press, 1995.

Kelly, D. *Applying Quality Management in Healthcare*. Chicago: Health Administration Press, 2003.

Langley, G. J., K. M. Nola, T. W. Nolan, C. L. Norman, and L. P. Provost. *The Improvement Guide: A Practical Approach to Enhancing Organizational Performances*. San Francisco: Jossey-Bass, 1996.

Lawrence, P., and J. Lorsch. *Organization and Environment*. Cambridge, MA: Graduate School of Business Administration, Harvard University, 1972.

Meyer, M. *Environments and Organizations*. San Francisco: Jossey-Bass, 1978.

Mick, S. S., and M. E. Wyttenbach (eds). *Advances in Health Care Organization Theory*. San Francisco: Jossey-Bass, 2003.

Morgan, G. *Images of Organization*. Beverly Hills, CA: Sage Library of Social Research, 1986.

Nystrom, P. C., and W. H. Starbuck. *Handbook of Organization Design*. New York: Oxford University Press, 1981.

Parsons, T. *Structure and Process in Modern Societies*. Glencoe, IL: Free Press, 1960.

Parsons, T. "Suggestions for a Sociological Approach to the Theory of Organizations." *Administrative Science Quarterly* June 1956, 1: 63–85, 224–39.

Peters, T. J. *Thriving on Chaos*. New York: Knopf, 1987.

Quinn, R. E. *Beyond Rational Management*. San Francisco: Jossey-Bass, 1985.

Schein, E. H. *Organizational Culture and Leadership*. San Francisco: Jossey-Bass, 1985.

Scott, W. R. "The Organization of Medical Care Services: Toward an Integrated Theoretical Model." *Medical Care Review* Fall 1993, 50 (3): 271–303.

Scott, W. R. *Organizations, Rational, Natural and Open Systems*, 2nd edition. Englewood Cliffs, NJ: Prentice-Hall, 1987.

Selznick, P. *Leadership in Administration*. Evanston, IL: Row Peterson, 1957.

Senge, P. M. *The Fifth Discipline*. New York: Doubleday, 1990.

Shortell, S. M., and A. D. Kaluzny. "Organizational Theory and Health Services Management." In *Health Care Management*, 4th edition. Albany, NY: Delmar, 2000, pp. 4–33.

Shortell, S. M., R. R. Gillies, and D. A. Anderson. *Remaking Health Care in America*. San Francisco: Jossey-Bass, 1996.

Slee, V. N., D. A. Slee, and H. J. Schmidt. *Slee's Health Care Terms*, 3rd Comprehensive Edition. St. Paul, MN: Tringa Press, 1996.

Sloane, R., B. Sloane, and R. Harder. *Introduction to Healthcare Delivery Organizations*, 4th edition. Chicago: Health Administration Press, 2003.

I

THE ROLE OF THE MANAGER

A leader is best
When people barely know that he exists
Not so good when people obey
And acclaim him,
Worst when they despise him.
Fail to honor people,
They fail to honor you;
But of a good leader, who talks little,
When his work is done, his aim fulfilled,
They will say, "We did this ourselves."

—Lao Tzu

COMMENTARY

How does one compare the management of healthcare organizations (HCOs) with that of other organizations? Relative to other sectors, more HCOs are not-for-profit and small, and more health services managers have been generalists rather than specialists. The goals of HCOs are often more complex than those of car manufacturers, banks, or police forces. These goals may include patient care, research, teaching and community service. Translating such goals into measurable objectives is difficult in healthcare, as the objectives of most healthcare organizations cannot be reduced to greater profits or market share. Healthcare is labor intensive and the work is often complex and involves many professionals working together. The healthcare manager must gain consensus from stakeholders, who often do not agree on the organization's goals and often unstated objectives.

What Do Healthcare Managers Do?

Like other managers, healthcare managers do what they are supposed to do, what they want to do, and what they can do. They confront reality, develop agendas and networks, think strategically about their work, and learn how to manage themselves effectively to accomplish their goals. Because they usually lack ownership in the firm, healthcare managers are often risk averse. They worry about their own survival as well as goal attainment. They reflect upon trade-offs between trying to improve patient care versus trying to break even financially and keep the clinicians from being discontented.

A dilemma that healthcare managers face is this: key internal stakeholders may neither particularly desire nor see the need for strategic interventions, yet managers know that external stakeholders who supply the organization with necessary resources are demanding change. Thus, health services managers must adapt their organizations to meet the demands of those who provide resources, while mobilizing the support of, or placating, internal groups.

The healthcare enterprise is increasingly concerned with measured results. Purchasers of care are demanding lower prices, documented quality and responsive services. At the same time, competition from existing or new organizations is increasing, and health services managers must be concerned with organizational adaptation to these pressures.

The service provided by most healthcare organizations is medical care. Medical care is only one of the factors affecting improved patient or population health or patient functioning; and, sometimes, more medical care may not be good for the patient, either because the treatment is unnecessary or because it is provided in such a way that the patient is injured or otherwise negatively affected. Medical care is provided by doctors and nurses and other clinicians who may view managers primarily as support staff for their work. This image may be at variance with the manager's view of herself as "relating the organization to its environment" or "coordinating processes of care to achieve measurable objectives." Managerial work is accomplished in large part through "memos and meetings," which many clinicians may regard as a waste of time (at least for them to read or attend), as they could be more usefully involved in providing patient care.

Financing is complex for most healthcare organizations, in part because one in five Americans lacks adequate health coverage. Managers must understand and generate sources of funds from varied payers. The product of healthcare is difficult to measure; therefore, managers must have patience and show creativity in applying quantitative techniques, which may be more relevant to the structure and process—rather than to the outcomes—of medical care. Change is often resisted because there is no standardized output against which it can be measured. For example, if managers wish to lower the skill level of the nursing staff or to eliminate health screening tests with low cost-benefit ratios, then recommendations must be legitimated in the face of physician objections that this would lower the quality of care. Sometimes there is no expert consensus concerning the outcomes of many clinical procedures.

Other than financing, there is no organizational factor that is unique to health services. Although the features of HCOs can be found elsewhere, the combination of such features make HCOs unique. Healthcare is a large part of the U.S. economy: 1 in 10 Americans is employed in the health services industry and $1 out of every $6 is spent on healthcare.

The role of the health services manager has changed substantially over time. Medicare and Medicaid, introduced in 1965, both reflected and fostered the growing complexity and costs of healthcare. New organizations appeared, such as health maintenance and preferred provider organizations (HMOs and PPOs), skilled nursing homes, and ambulatory surgery and neighborhood health centers. Healthcare management was no longer primarily hospital acute care management, and the hospital manager had to adapt to a more complex environment.

In the twenty-first century, the healthcare manager's work is being transformed not only by the information revolution, but by a revolution in performance expectations as well. Performance goals are being increasingly specified in terms of measurable objectives that may be shared with key stakeholders. Healthcare organizations are larger and more complex, and in many large systems there are fewer managers per dollar of sales, each with a broader scope of responsibility and a bigger paycheck.

Organizational Settings

The work of healthcare managers varies by the setting in which they practice. These settings include components of an academic medical center such as a faculty practice, the department of medicine and the breast service; a neighborhood health center; a small rural hospital; an urban Medicaid HMO; a large public hospital; a visiting nurse service; a Veterans Administration hospital network; a community hospital; and a health department. We can compare the challenges that managers face relative to the organization's stage in the growth cycle (growing, maturing, declining). Of course many managerial challenges—such as improving quality, lowering unit costs, and generating revenues—are the same across organizational settings. A simple comparison is shown in Table I.1.

Setting	Growth Cycle	Managerial Challenges
Academic Medical Center		
Faculty Practice	Mature	Choosing a new manager
Dept of Medicine	Mature	Decreasing length of stay
Breast Service	Growing	Recruiting surgeons
Neighborhood Health Center	Mature	Developing critical indicators of performance
Small Rural Hospital	Declining	Developing an affiliation with a larger hospital
Urban Medicaid HMO	Growing	Expanding marketing staff
Large Public Hospital	Mature	Decreasing patient cycle time in the emergency department
Visiting Nurse Service	Mature	Integrating services regionally
Community Hospital	Mature	Supporting physician businesses
Health Department	Mature	Focusing departmental operations

TABLE I.1
Managerial Challenges by Organizational Setting and Stage in the Growth Cycle

Expectations of Healthcare Managers

Healthcare managers are expected to support quality improvement, lead revenue generation and cost containment, and manage relationships with important stakeholder groups. Managers are challenged by situations such as having inadequate resources to provide high-quality care. Greater performance expectations are being placed on managers in the face of limitations on what HCOs can charge for their services, while costs increase at a faster rate.

Top management gets top performance from hiring great people, creating a performance culture that links rewards with results, demanding shared values, and believing that everyone counts. This is how General Electric does it. And GE wants managers with high energy, who can energize the people around them, who have an "edge" in that they can make tough decisions, and who can execute decisions.[1]

Ullian says that being a successful manager means picking the right boss. Effective managers can communicate the "bad" news, are accountable for performance, respect others, have the courage to take action, and can learn from their mistakes and weaknesses. Successful managers are self-confident and cheerful.[2]

In confronting reality, healthcare managers should ask themselves: Who are the dominant stakeholders affecting goal implementation? What do these stakeholders really want? How satisfied are they with current performance? How do I effectively communicate what I am trying to achieve, and by what means? Based on the responses to these questions, a healthcare manager's recommendations should always be financially and politically feasible. This means that the manager knows where the money is going to come from to finance program initiatives and where the buy-in is going to come from to support making and implementing the decisions.

Managers should reflect upon what it is that they want to accomplish over the next period of time, say 12 months, and determine the network through which such goals can be accomplished. Managers should consider what, if anything, will happen if these goals are not achieved. Whose cooperation does the manager need to get the critical tasks accomplished? How will the manager attain such cooperation? What information does the manager need to set goals and accomplish targets? How will the manager get the information that she needs? How does the manager spend her time and presence? Is she merely reacting to the overload of claims made on her attention, or does she spend time appropriately initiating and accomplishing her agenda?

Every manager should consider her resume as her lifeline and keep it current. She should ask herself: What results did I achieve last year? Will I achieve results this year that I can take credit for and add to my resume? In general, managers average six years on the job, according to Handy,[3] and should consider themselves as independent contractors in charge of their own careers. Managers should take ownership of their own careers, and never accept a position without an exit strategy. This means determining in advance the conditions under which they would no longer be willing to work in their current positions, and what steps they would take once they have reached that decision.

Thinking Strategically About the Job

Managers should understand the flexibility of their positions. Each managerial job has three characteristics: (1) the demands of the job that the manager must actively carry out; (2) the constraints on the position, or those activities that the manager is not allowed to carry out; and (3) the options or choices that the manager makes concerning how she is going to spend her time and presence.[4] The manager should reflect upon how she can strengthen relationships with the people upon whom she depends; managing one's self is essential for high performance.

Goleman emphasizes the importance of emotional intelligence for management success,[5] suggesting that it is more important than a high IQ and great technical skills in performing well, and that it can be learned. The five components of emotional intelligence are

1. self-awareness (how managers see themselves being seen by others),
2. self-regulation (thinking before speaking),
3. motivation (the drive to achieve results),
4. empathy (seeing others as they see themselves), and
5. social skills (in listening and responding).[6]

How can managers acquire the evidence they need to make effective decisions? The relevant skills include, as Kovner, Elton, and Billings point out:

> Identifying emerging opportunities, precisely defining management challenges or opportunities, data collection, proficiently searching and critically appraising relevant information from published and non-published sources and then deciding whether and how to use this information in practice. Also necessary is an understanding of the process of change including an understanding of reliable information regarding stakeholder expectations and capacity, and the ability to conduct and evaluate natural experiments in which new methods are piloted or considered as pilot demonstrations.[7]

McCall and others have suggested the following framework for management development: (1) find out about shortcomings; (2) accept responsibility for any shortcomings that result because of a lack of knowledge, skills or experience, or because of personality, limited ability, or being a situational misfit; then, (3) decide what to do about it accordingly. Either: (1) build new strengths, such as finding ways to get help and support while learning; (2) anticipate situations, such as seeking advice or counsel; (3) compensate, for example, by avoiding certain situations; or (4) change yourself (which is very difficult to do) either through intensive counseling and coaching or through personal change effort.[8]

Notes

1. J. Hogan, "Thriving in Health Care . . . Learning Every Day," *Journal of Health Care Administration*, 2001, 63–68.
2. E. Ullian, Presentation at the National Summit on the Future of Education and Practice in Health Management and Policy. Orlando, FL, Feb 8–9, 2001.
3. Handy, *The Hungry Spirit* (New York: Broadway Books, 1998) p 64.
4. R. Stewart and N. Fondas, "How Managers Can Think Strategically About Their Jobs," *Journal of Management Development* 1992, 11 (7): 10–17.
5. D. Goleman, "What Makes a Leader?" *Harvard Business Review*, 1998 (Nov-Dec) 76 (6): 93–102.
6. Goleman, *op. cit.*
7. A. R. Kovner, J. Elton, and J. Billings. "Transforming Health Management: An Evidence-Based Approach," *Frontiers of Health Services Management*, 2000 (Summer) 16 (4): 3–24.
8. M. W. McCall, M. M. Lombardo, and A. M. Morrison, *The Lessons of Experience: How Successful Executives Develop on the Job* (Lexington, MA: Lexington Books, 1988).

THE READINGS

The required reading for Part I is "Evidence-Based Management," by Kovner, Elton, and Billings. The authors suggest that healthcare organizations are having to make quicker, riskier decisions in a competitive and regulated environment. Chief executives often make these decisions with the advice of management consultants; however, top management, generally, lacks adequate internal support to rigorously evaluate strategic interventions or consultant recommendations and to learn from industry-wide best practices. Healthcare organizations generally underinvest in management support, both in evaluating best practices within the organization, and in learning from past strategic interventions. The authors suggest forming evidence-based management collaboratives as a possible means to facilitate evidence-based management.

Transforming Health Management: An Evidence-Based Approach

Anthony R. Kovner, Ph.D.; Jeffrey J. Elton, Ph.D.; and John Billings, J.D.
From *Frontiers of Health Services Management* 16 (4), Summer 2000.

The Challenge: Making Better-Informed Strategic Decisions

What information should management regularly provide to hospital and health system boards? How should health systems determine capital allocation priorities? How should primary care be organized for vulnerable populations? How should health plans pay specialists and primary care physicians? When should health systems merge, compete, or cooperate? How do the answers to these questions differ depending on the mission and financial and market circumstances of a particular health system? Once an intervention has been adopted, how best can the constraints to implementation be overcome, or, if these cannot be overcome, how best can managers implement a strategic withdrawal?

This article suggests that managers in large healthcare organizations are deciding on more and riskier strategic interventions based on evidence that is not systematically gathered or assessed. Often managers rely on consultants for assistance in making and implementing important strategic decisions but managers do not rigorously challenge the information upon which such recommendations are based.

Although the problem in many cases involves a lack of managerial resources to marshal and evaluate available evidence, more often the problem relates to the mind-set of managers.[1] Many are simply not trained nor experienced in the use of empirical evidence in making management decisions. Paradoxically, the increasing size of many health systems permits the gathering of empirically based information on many operational decisions made within the system. For smaller organizations, or for major strategic decisions where intra-organizational experience is not relevant (e.g., mergers, paying physicians, building or buying satellite centers), evidence-based management cooperatives are proposed as an approach to generating and assessing the required management information for deciding on interventions.

This article reviews the barriers to gathering and assessing management evidence, discusses management research in healthcare, and reviews approaches to generating better evidence in medicine and industry. Case vignettes are presented as examples of availability of evidence and of managerial use of such evidence. An evidence-based management cooperative approach is described, and other approaches are suggested as complementary ways to improve strategic management.

The ability of healthcare managers to develop and execute strategy depends on the generation and analysis of relevant data both from best practice and from research. Strategy is most likely to succeed when it is based on events that actually happened and that are reliably reported, is implemented in a timely way, and has clear and measurable objectives (Griffith 1999). Enhanced capacity to generate and assess relevant management data is expected to result in an increased internal analysis of evidence with less reliance on consultants, more focused and accountable contracting with consultants, and improved management skills and communication in gathering and arraying data.

Five main barriers have hindered efforts to base important management decisions in healthcare organizations on research and on best practices:

1. *Little evidence has been generated about best management practices and such evidence is not widely shared.* The research conducted on healthcare management is limited compared to the research in other industries and relative to research on disease prevention and treatment and on performance improvement. Neither has research on existing best practices been sufficiently conducted. Evaluation of strategic interventions is not widely shared, even within the same system, and consultants

consider such evaluation data as proprietary. Health systems traditionally underfund support services for decision making and internal management research, yet some spend millions of dollars on consultants for strategic recommendations based on data that has not received careful enough review.

2. *Historically, healthcare organizations have lacked sufficient size and critical mass to conduct and assess applied research.* In the past, most health systems have not been large enough to carry out management research. Applied research often involves quasi-experimental models where comparisons are made between different approaches. Such comparisons may require multiple settings or experience involving enough numbers to draw generalizable conclusions with any confidence. A single institution or system may lack the critical mass to benefit from conducting such applied research. In larger systems, management practice has not yet taken advantage of increased system size to regularly gather and array evidence on best management practices.

3. *Health systems have traditionally focused on operating margins and past budgets.* Support for decision making and research is typically viewed as a budgeting expense with little or no return on investment, as the period for review of return on operating investments is typically one year. Budgeting is often considered a forum for discussing ways to increase departmental revenues or decrease costs, rather than as a way to reallocate resources among operating units based on best practices and applied research to optimize value over the longer term.

4. *Healthcare managers lack training and experience in collaborating with health services researchers and lack commitment to the values of applied research.* Healthcare managers have not been trained to make strategic decisions based on evidence as have those with specialized training in research methods. Distracted by local and continuing operating crises, managers do not commit time to search for best practices, develop evidence, or analyze the evidence used by consultants to generate recommendations.

5. *Nonprofit healthcare organizations lack accountability.* Nonprofit organizations often lack market discipline in growing or discontinuing lines of business and rely in part on boards of trustees to provide such discipline. Yet board members do not always require of executive management the same rigor of "case evidence" in their own corporations, where board and management are more accountable to shareholders. Many board members do not come from corporate management and are not selected based on their skills and experience in requiring best evidence for strategic decisions.

TABLE I.1
Journals
Reviewed

1. Frontiers of Health Services Management
2. Health Affairs
3. Health Care Management Review
4. Health Services Research
5. Journal of Healthcare Management
6. Journal of Health Care Finance
7. Journal of Health Policy Politics and Law
8. Medical Care
9. Journal of the American Medical Association
10. Harvard Business Review[*]

*The *Harvard Business Review*, although not a health journal, was included in the analysis to determine the incidence of health management articles in a prominent general management journal. The author found that there was no evidence of healthcare management articles published in HBR over the 33-month period.

Management Research in Healthcare

Management research is published in a variety of journals, including ones not specifically devoted to healthcare. Ten journals (see Table I.1) were identified in which management research appears or might appear, and issues from January 1997 through September 1999 (over 33 months) were reviewed. Of the 300 articles (only 90 to 110 per year in a trillion-dollar health industry) identified as healthcare management articles, 209 were determined to be methodology-based studies.[2] The most common setting for studies was hospitals (109 studies, or 52 percent).

Funding sources were identified for 114 of the 300 articles and it was found that 60 (53 percent) were funded by one of the five following sources: Agency for Health Policy Research (30), The Robert Wood Johnson Foundation (12), the Commonwealth Fund (6), the Veteran's Administration (6), and the Health Care Finance Administration (6). No other identified source funded more than four of the articles published in these journals. Of the 300 management articles, two-thirds were on the following topics: financing or financial management (103), quality and performance management (53), and organizational design (44). Fifty-six articles were published on professional integration, internal systems, patient perspectives, and organizational staffing/training. Less than 15 percent of the 300 management articles were published on organizational adaptation (27); managerial functions such as leadership, ethics, and performance (12); and governance (5).

Based on these data, and assuming that the published articles reviewed for this study reflect the actual research being done, we draw the following conclusions:

1. Relatively few studies on the topics listed above have been published.
2. A particular dearth of studies exists on the role and contribution of managers and governance to the effectiveness and efficiency of healthcare organizations.

3. The main funders of research in healthcare, government agencies, and foundations do not see management research as one of their main priorities.[3]
4. Large health systems fund little, if any, published management research.
5. Most of the healthcare management research published is based on questions that are expenditure-related rather than value-driven.
6. Most of the healthcare management research that was done two to four years ago focused on the hospital setting, rather than ambulatory or chronic care.

Approaches Related to Evidence-Based Management

Approaches to generating and using better evidence have been pioneered and are widely used in medicine and in business.

Evidence-Based Medicine

Evidence-based medicine has been defined by Sackett et al. (1996) as "the conscientious, explicit and judicious use of current best evidence in making decisions about the care of individual patients." Best evidence includes data-based research, best practice, and expert consensus. For example, the relevant skills involved in practicing evidence-based medicine have been specified as "precisely defining a patient problem, proficiently searching and critically ap-praising relevant information from the literature, and then deciding whether, and how, to use the information in practice." Ellrodt et al. (1997) cite six reasons why evidence-based medicine should be used in disease management:

1. It allows the acquisition of valid and current information by the practicing physician.
2. Greater consensus can be reached when evidence becomes the neutral arbiter of practice.
3. Changing clinician behavior can be incorporated into disease management programs.
4. Variation around optimal practice can be reduced.
5. No specific recommendations are made if inadequate research is available.
6. Gaps in knowledge can be identified, which can help formulate a prioritized research agenda.

Axelsson (1998) reports that a great deal of medical research is con-ducted as randomized trials on patients in clinical settings. This allows the research results to be more easily communicated to clinicians and new meth-ods to be more quickly integrated into clinical practice. Most medical schools today are training physicians in the skills of evidence-based medicine. Man-agement can follow this direction, using more systematic searches for evidence related to strategic interventions, conducted by an organized unit or person given responsibility and held accountable for results.

Continuous Improvement and Knowledge Management

Continuous quality improvement (CQI) and reengineering involve gathering better evidence to improve operational processes in healthcare organizations, but this kind of analysis has not been widely applied to strategic decision making by healthcare organizations. As Berwick (1996) points out, measurement helps one know if a particular innovation should be kept, changed, or rejected; measurement can help understand causes; and measurement helps clarify aims. "When we try to improve a system we do not need perfect inference about a pre-existing hypothesis; we do not need randomization, power calculations, and large samples. We need just enough information to take a next step in learning." Encouraged by the Joint Commission, the CQI concepts are widespread among healthcare organizations. Berwick notes that most organizations leave too little time for reflection on work and that the immense authority of the status quo resists major change. This has serious consequences for strategic decision making in healthcare organizations. Information about CQI is not widely shared for competitive reasons, and is usually considered proprietary among management consulting firms.

Most CQI interventions in healthcare have been unit-based and clinically based rather than organization-focused or management-focused, and tactical rather than strategic. The authors believe that most CQI studies have not been published in peer-reviewed journals, indicating that the lessons learned have not been widely shared.

Another evidence-based approach to management that has been implemented by several large business firms, but not healthcare providers, is called "knowledge management." Davenport, DeLong, and Beers (1998) reviewed 31 knowledge-management projects at 24 business corporations. All projects studied had an individual responsible for the initiative and some commitment of human and capital resources, ranging from a chief knowledge officer with no formal budget to a consulting firm with more than 70 positions and a budget of more than $10 million annually.[4] They classified the objectives of these projects as to create knowledge repositories, improve knowledge access, enhance the knowledge environment, and obtain informal research knowledge. Examples of activities undertaken to meet these objectives include gaining competitive intelligence, establishing expert networks, making contributions to the firm's structured knowledge base a significant factor in compensation decisions, and managing knowledge-intensive assets, such as patents, to more effectively improve their return.

Hansen, Nohria, and Tierney (1999) contrast organizations that carefully codify and store knowledge in databases where it can be accessed and used easily by anyone in the company, with organizations where knowledge is closely tied to the persons who developed it and is shared mainly through person-to-person contacts. Both approaches are applicable to healthcare organizations that can compile yellow pages of on-call experts on their intranet, identify best practices that other units in the system may wish to replicate, and establish networks of experts in any given areas of operation and center-of-excellence sites.

Stewart (1999) describes British Petroleum's assembled portfolio of 15 projects where knowledge management has generated revenues by helping the company enter the Japanese retail market, reducing downtime at a polyethylene plant, and scheduling refinery shutdown and refurbishment. British Petroleum offers a web-based folder of artifacts, video clips, checklists, and e-mail hyperlinks to people who have stories to tell or who want access to such information.

Evidence-Based Management Decision Making

"Management" in healthcare organizations is defined here as strategy and implementation to accomplish a set of objectives. "Evidence" is defined as empirical data that is logically ordered and relates to specified assumptions. This evidence helps define a problem, diagnose its causes, or evaluate alternative interventions so that management action is judged as reasonably "accurate, precise, sufficient, representative, authoritative," (Booth, Colomb, and Williams 1995) and so perceived by stakeholders.

CQI and knowledge management projects depend upon collecting and assessing information. Our focus is directed toward improving strategic interventions by enhanced managerial support in generating and assessing data regarding best management practices and research. An evidence-based approach to health system management is the conscientious, explicit, and judicious use of current best reason and experience in making decisions about strategic interventions. The relevant skills include identifying emerging opportunities, precisely defining management challenges or opportunities, data collection, proficiently searching and critically appraising relevant information from published and non-published sources, and then deciding whether and how to use this information in practice. Also necessary is an understanding of the process of change, including an understanding of reliable information regarding stakeholder expectations and capacity, and the ability to conduct and evaluate natural experiments in which new methods are piloted or considered as pilot demonstrations.

Stewart (1998) and Axelsson (1998) argue that evidence-based management is primarily an attitude of mind that is necessary for a research culture to exist. Stewart suggests that a simple test for its existence is whether a questioning approach is accepted and encouraged. Axelsson cautions that in an evidence-based management environment, managers must be prepared to have their own decisions and actions systematically recorded and evaluated.

Managers should act based on information, keep track of the information they have, and measure how information makes a difference in considering and implementing strategic interventions. The manager requires information not only about what has occurred at other sites but also about the expectations of his own organization's stakeholders and the specific circumstances of the organization. Both the manager and the researcher seek better evidence, but for different purposes. The manager requires information to act, whereas the researcher often seeks information to construct a theory or to generate a set of hypotheses. Therefore, the manager focuses on the effect of a strategic intervention on the expectations of stakeholders, and the researcher focuses on constructing hypotheses and on the validity and reliability of conclusions. Such different purposes may constrain cooperative interaction, but to the extent that different aims are acknowledged, the articulation of such aims and their negotiation can allow the separate objectives to be attained.

Case Vignettes

Four vignettes were developed from our experience to make a case for the potential value of an evidence-based approach to healthcare management and the need for more investment in healthcare management research. The vignettes can be classified as follows: (1) where an evidence-based approach resulted in significant benefit ("Capital and Operating Budgeting Process at Partners Healthcare System"); (2) and (3) where results are not available but it is hypothesized that better evidence will result in a significant benefit ("Primary Care Management for Vulnerable Populations" and "Blended Payment Methods in Physician Organizations Under Managed Care"); and (4) where the failure to use available evidence resulted in significant costs, many of which could have been avoided ("The Merger of Two Academic Medical Centers"). Table I.2 demonstrates the different states of evidence's availability and use in the four scenarios.

TABLE I.2

Case Vignette Summaries

Vignette	Is Evidence Available?	Did Management Use the Available Evidence?
1. Capital Investment	Yes, in other industries	Yes
2. Primary care	No, or not shared	No, despite natural experiments
3. MD payment methods	Yes, in California IPAs	Not known
4. Merger	Yes, in healthcare	No

We do not regard these cases as proof of our assertions or suggestions, but merely as validation that pursuing a more evidence-based approach to strategic decision making may be a worthwhile investment by top management.

Vignette 1: Capital and Operating Budgeting Process at Partners Healthcare System

In 1997, Partners was a newly integrated delivery system comprising two tertiary academic medical centers, a rehabilitation hospital, and a psychiatric hospital. These organizations had no common hospital financial planning, no basis for making capital allocation decisions to meet system level strategic objectives, and no common performance metrics. Departments received allocations consistent with their historic levels, with adjustments for major asset replacements. This pattern sustained the current operating model but did not support the implementation of a new integrated system strategy.

The existing budgeting processes funded historic requirements of the individual operating entities and then added a "tax" to meet emerging system requirements. Degradation in individual operating entity performance, more aggressive reimbursement strategies by payers, and increasing system requirements all revealed that this approach was not sustainable.

Professor Simons of the Harvard Business School was engaged to define how other organizations had framed and solved this problem. He assured the executive group that although the problem may not be confronted by many academic health systems, it has been confronted by organizations operating in other industries. Capital ownership and management are essential to any corporate entity and define a critical area of management responsibility for any corporation made up of multiple operating entities in many lines of business. Capital management is the mechanism by which strategy is implemented and monitored, in which organizations declare where they are investing and where they are divesting. Professor Simons provided examples of several models at a working level and explained why those models were successful for their respective organizations (Simons 2000).

Based on the taxonomy of different models, the bases for their success, limits on their applicability, and the experiences of the organizations putting them into place, Partners Healthcare System translated their strategic objectives into capital resource requirements and defined key performance metrics for assessing where to invest and how to evaluate relative attractiveness of investments. The process involved the entire senior finance staff and all operating heads of the different care delivery operating entities. The new logic of the capital allocation models defined was tested by creating alternative investment "portfolios" that satisfied the constraints of implementing the corporate system strategy while meeting critical resource requirements of operating entities. The approach constructively forced a clearer articulation of which investments were attractive, why they were attractive, and how to gauge that the assumptions were, in fact, a sound base for future decision making.

This approach showed that capital allocation and operations budgeting were the primary core processes of the corporation, thus supporting a reallocation of funds from historic project categories by organizations to new ones more closely aligned to system strategy. In this way, Partners was able to avoid spending $650 million in long-term capital to fund projects that would have met historic approval criteria, but that were no longer in support of new strategy and care delivery objectives. Funding was instead provided for a common information system infrastructure; an integrated radiology service network; single "super" physician chiefs in orthopedics and psychiatry; and common clinical laboratory infrastructure and specialty labs. These patterns of resource allocations would not have been possible following the historic processes, decision criteria, or department-centric approach.

Vignette 2: Primary Care Management for Vulnerable Populations

Since the early 1990s, New York City has experienced an expansion of primary care services in many low-income neighborhoods with support from the state's Primary Care initiative and the city's Primary Care Development Corporation. Aid also came from hospital-sponsored organizations attempting to solidify their specialty and hospital referral base in anticipation of the growth of managed care, especially for Medicaid patients. In the 1970s and 1980s, the model for care delivery to urban low-income patients had been the 20-to-25-physician community health center clinic, often with a broad range of specialty and ancillary services. The 1990s model reflected a different philosophy: "Small is better." These care centers offer the look and feel of middle-class physicians' offices, often with only two to five physicians at the site and located in apartment buildings or near commercial areas. The rationale for the new model was generally either patient-based ("they will like it better") or provider-based ("it will be easier to manage").

A growing body of research (e.g., Bindman et al. 1995) documents shows how the lack of timely and effective primary care can result in increased utilization of other costly health services such as emergency room use and hospitalization. More than 43 million Americans lack insurance coverage, which often creates barriers to obtaining needed care. But even for low-income patients with coverage such as Medicaid or state child health insurance programs, primary care providers face a broad range of management issues that can affect how and whether patients use the care delivery system. Such management issues have become particularly acute as the pressures of funding cutbacks, growth of managed care, and rising levels of lack of insurance have forced the providers of these vulnerable populations to re-examine how they are delivering care and to develop more cost-effective approaches to patient management.

Some issues for primary care providers in urban areas are basic: Do patients prefer large, multispecialty practices with a broad range of services and one-stop shopping, or smaller neighborhood settings with three to five primary care providers? Other questions are more specific: Can a nurse telephone hotline be an important resource to a low-income parent trying to decide whether to take a wheezing child to the emergency department? How much capacity at a clinic should be set aside for walk-in patients without appointments? What is the most effective way to divert patients from the emergency department and encourage more timely use of primary care services? How do the answers to these questions differ depending on the culture, education, or social support of the patient? And once answers are known, what is the most effective way for providers to deliver needed services to help patients learn to use the healthcare system more effectively?

The ability of primary car providers of vulnerable populations to respond to these questions is likely to be critical to their survival. However, to date, most actions by providers have been informed to a large extent by anecdote, perceptions of providers in the trenches, or simply convenience for day-to-day operations, rather than by anything that might be considered even quasi–evidence based.

In the example of New York City's Primary Care initiative, neither the community health center model nor the career center model was based on much solid evidence about what patients wanted or what worked most efficiently. Little or no attempt was made to study how patients actually wanted care organized and delivered. Some patients, no doubt, have found the new, smaller settings to be an improvement over crowded, chaotic hospital outpatient departments or 100,000-visit-per-year community health centers. Others, however, might have expressed a preference for "one-stop shopping," more availability of translators, or the feeling of anonymity in a larger setting, especially for substance abuse, mental health, or AIDS-HIV services. No single answer exists for all patients; however, understanding the mix of patient preferences is critical for planning and marketing new facilities in an era of budget constraints and razor-thin margins. Many of the new sites have experienced significant problems in attracting a patient base and are operating well below capacity.

As to ease of management, little evidence may have been available to inform this intuitively based perspective in advance, but given the broad array of community-based facilities that has evolved, developing and tracking performance measures to test the hypothesis would seem essential. However, such an initiative would require cooperation among several primary organizations (since no single organization has a sufficient number or diversity of models to conduct the required analysis), and, not surprisingly, no attempt has been made to harvest evidence from this natural experiment.

Information is not available as to any studies conducted along these lines. However, numerous natural experiments are taking place that can be evaluated. Research can be conducted as student projects, doctoral dissertations, contracts let by government agencies, grants funded by foundations, or studies carried out as part of an evidence-based management cooperative.

Vignette 3: Blended Payment Methods in Physician Organizations Under Managed Care

Managers at a health plan and a large individual practice association (IPA) are trying to figure out better ways of paying primary and specialist physicians to maximize incentives for productivity and quality care.

Robinson's article "Blended Payment Methods in Physician Organizations Under Managed Care" (1999) shows the kind of evidence available to large health systems. His objective was to identify emerging payment methods within seven large IPA physician groups in the San Francisco metropolitan region that served 826,000 HMO patients during the summer and fall of 1998. The method of research chosen "emphasizes generalization from cases to underlying hypotheses rather than from samples to populations." Payment methods of IPAs were examined for primary care physicians, specialists, and physicians grouped by specialty department within the overall IPA structure.

Managers can learn several things from Robinson's article:

* IPAs have switched from fee-for-service and pure capitation to blended methods. Robinson also discusses the reasons blended methods were preferred.
* Several large IPAs in California have changed their methods of payment to physicians. Populations are specified by number of plan primary care and specialty care physicians, number of commercial and Medicare HMO patients, and MSO ownership and affiliation.
* IPAs did not rely on payment methods and financial incentives alone to influence physician behavior. Robinson refers to nonfinancial mechanisms for encouraging collegiality, skilled intervention, and commitment to patient interests. IPAs were simultaneously experimenting with administrative structures, membership criteria, ownership distributions, and governance mechanisms.
* IPAs moved to blended payment methods through a process of trial and error; they neither appeared to be familiar with nor directly influenced by the economic literature on optimal payment incentives. Robinson found this lack of influence as "sobering testimony to the limited impact of health services research on the real world of healthcare organization."

To what extent, and at what speed, is learning from such research as Robinson's taking place in healthcare organizations? What changes in payment methods are being implemented as a result, after considering the evidence? What are the costs and benefits for developing management support that is central to organizational mission and strategy, and is consistently brought to managers' attention?

Vignette 4: The Merger of Two Academic Medical Centers

Two academic medical centers in an urban area accounted for 11 percent of the market for complex care. Each percentage increase in market share would bring the enterprise an additional $50 million of revenue. The CEO of the then-merged academic medical center made the argument that it is best not to accept the conventional wisdom about integration, which emphasized benefits of global capitation, utilization efficiencies, and channeling through primary gatekeepers. He argued that merged institutions could better differentiate themselves marketing-wise (Van Etten 1999). He referred to growing evidence that patients would sometimes travel long distances for complex care. He added that as volume becomes a proxy for quality, payers would increasingly channel patients to larger programs, and that the merger reduced administrative overhead and increased organizational purchasing power that could result in ongoing capital savings.

Questions that top management might have raised and answered, either by considering evidence available in the literature or through contacting experts who had gone through the merger process either in or outside of healthcare include the following:

- What are the factors affecting demand for complex care at specific institutions?
- What is the likelihood of affecting any of these factors by relatively small investments?
- How does the level of expenditures in marketing affect the demand for complex care?
- Under what circumstances will patients travel long distances for complex care?
- To what extent are purchasers and payers willing to steer patients to larger centers for complex care?
- To what extent is a merger necessary to take advantage of savings in administrative overhead and increased organizational purchasing power?
- What information is it reasonable to assume should be provided to academic medical center boards to make this kind of merger decision?
- What amount of working capital is required to demonstrate the benefits of merger and to overcome short-term losses?

• As the merger is initiated, under what circumstances will which exit strategies be pursued?

Six months after the merger, a reporter (Rauber 1999) indicated that in the short term, the four hospitals that created the merged health system would have been better off if they had not merged, citing a report from the state auditor's office. Prior to the merger, the CEO had predicted that such consolidation would result in $65 million in profits in fiscal years 1998 and 1999. These anticipated profits never materialized, largely because the merged system failed to deliver on promises to eliminate duplication and cut costs. Rauber reported that the two top executives, including the CEO, had resigned. A month after the article appeared, the former CEO, in a speech to managers in another city, blamed poor results on a lack of trust between the two partners and the consequences of merging financial results into one bottom line, which meant losing hospital accountability for costs. In response to a question as to what he had learned about the strategic planning process that led to the merger, the former CEO replied "we didn't want to see the problems." The merger is being dissolved and many millions of dollars could have been saved if available evidence would have been gathered and acted upon.

Evidence-Based Management Cooperatives

Evidence-based management cooperatives (EBMCs) exist to create organizations at the health system level that bring together managers, consultants, and researchers with a common mission of improving healthcare management, databases, and organizational performance.[5,6] As Griffith (1999) suggests, an excellent place to start an EBMC is around noncompeting organizations and their existing alliances. A team of professionals is assembled to better understand the problems involved in effective healthcare management, to develop more effective approaches to managing health systems, and to create pathways to facilitate effective implementation of new knowledge and innovations.

EBMCs can be organized across several health systems or within one health system; but these two approaches are not mutually exclusive. A formidable constraint in organizing across systems is competition in specific markets among potential collaborators.

The same kind of constraint can be visualized with services or functions within a health system whose units compete for budgetary resources, but that also cooperate in competing with other health systems. The advantages of multiple EBMCs organized across health systems are obvious: more information can be shared across more organizational boundaries and EBMCs can specialize to become centers of excellence for given topics or methodologies.

The focus of EBMC activities will involve technical assistance, demonstration projects, and applied research efforts in four areas:

1. *Enhancing managerial skills and capacity.* Most healthcare managers and faculty teaching healthcare management acquired their skills and experience under drastically different circumstances—health systems were smaller and less complex and competitive environments were less threatening and organizational survival less risky. Through EBMC activities managers would gain skills and experience in generating and evaluating evidence regarding best management practices, and these practices can be successfully adapted to local circumstances.

2. *Improving information to support better strategic interventions.* Many strategic interventions chosen by healthcare managers are selected based on the recommendations of outside consultants, and EBMCs would enhance the manager's capacity to evaluate the evidence upon which the consultants base their decisions.[7] Follow-up can be conducted after interventions have been selected to learn whether the resulting benefits and costs were as forecasted, and to determine the soundness of underlying assumptions.[8]

3. *Understanding factors affecting implementation of strategic interventions.* A broad range of factors not directly related to healthcare management can influence the success of strategic interventions. In deciding why and how to implement some other organization's "successful" intervention, outcomes may be affected by contextual factors, state and local regulations, mission, workforce, and demographics. Learning about these factors will aid in developing strategies to customize strategic interventions to local organizational circumstances.

4. *Financing of strategic interventions.* Critical to the viability of effective strategic interventions in healthcare management is ensuring an adequate revenue stream for the costs of implementation. The role of EBMCs will involve technical assistance to prepare managers to develop more creative approaches to financing strategic interventions and to design business plans of greater sophistication, with more attention to managing risk.

How EBMCs Are Unique: Management-Based Research Networks Focusing on Evidence Concerning Best Practices

The EBMCs are modeled after practice-based research networks such as the Dartmouth Primary Care Research Cooperative in New England and the Ambulatory Sentinel Practice Network based in Colorado (Nutting, Beasley, and Werner 1999). Like those existing cooperative efforts, the proposed EBMCs will benefit from a linking of researchers, managers, and consultants to conduct a broad range of research, demonstration, and evaluation projects. Access to data and organizations from network partners will permit the pooling of numbers to conduct research, demonstrations, and evaluations that no single organization or research initiative alone could do. The involvement of organizations and managers in setting the agenda and in conducting the research will help ensure that these initiatives are directly related to practice and to the problems that are most pressing to managers, and that the findings of the research are translated into action quickly. The participation of researchers will help provide sufficient methodological rigor to permit managers, consultants, and board members to rely on the findings on EBMC initiatives. In several respects, however, EBMCs are distinct from other networks:

- The focus is on healthcare management. Other practice-based research networks focus on clinical content of care and quality improvement, or are based in large business corporations. The challenges of improving healthcare management are significant. Success is likely to be dependent on recognizing the special situations and opportunities of specific health systems and managers and will require designing strategies and gearing interventions that take these factors into account.
- Research/demonstration focuses on evidence and evaluation. Many strategic interventions would not have failed or may not have been undertaken if the available evidence had been rigorously reviewed, assumptions specified, financing alternatives known, and contingency plans and opportunities to manage risk identified. Organizational learning will take place when past interventions, both successful and unsuccessful, are carefully analyzed and experiences are shared with the managers accountable for the success of such future interventions.
- Management, management researchers, and consultants work together to improve practice within healthcare systems. Health systems have lacked the scale to finance research internally. However, just 10 percent of the annual consulting budget[9] for large health systems may be sufficient to finance enhanced capacity. This financing will serve to significantly expand the amount and quality of healthcare management research conducted.

How Will the EBMC Be Organized?

The EBMC is seen as a collaborating partnership of managers, consultants, and applied researchers. At the core of the cooperative is healthcare management to improve health system performance. The essential conditions of participation will be

1. A strong commitment to improvement of healthcare management through application of evidence;
2. A willingness to use and share management data from compatible management information systems to track and monitor strategic interventions and organizational performance;

3. An interest in participating in applied research projects (e.g., to obtain survey data from physicians on issues of interest to the EBMC); and

4. An interest in being involved in demonstration projects to improve health system performance. In return, these participants will receive comparative information on current ways of organizing services, access to the collective experiences of other cooperative members, results from applied research projects, and an array of technical assistance on statistical, management, financing, and marketing issues.

An important partner in the cooperative will be a research center, often university-based, with an interest and capacity in applied research on health systems and their performance, strategic interventions, and related management and finance issues. The academic partner will also provide expertise and experience in data analysis, survey design, program evaluation, and professional education. Although the goal of EBMCs will be to focus on issues of immediate interest to health system organizational performance, academic partners can offer technical and analytical skills to ensure that the information generated from this applied research is reliable, and to provide a vehicle for wider dissemination of findings through peer-reviewed journals and other communication approaches.

The university-based research center can assist with design and implementation of, for example, a "balanced scorecard" approach to the development of critical health system performance indicators. Such a strategy would allow units and divisions within health systems to compare performance with benchmarked peers (e.g., regarding market share and profitability of cancer centers).

The EBMC will require a core staff to administer the cooperative and coordinate its program of applied research, demonstration, and technical assistance. Some aspects of the EBMC are likely to be "virtual" in the sense that health system and academic partners may remain at their own institutions. But a central staff will also be required. In the early stages, the staff will help set the agenda, coordinate and conduct applied research, and arrange and supply technical assistance. As the EBMC matures, some amount of expertise is expected to evolve in-house, depending on the needs of the cooperative and the strengths and limitations of the partners.

Reaching Beyond the Members—Communication and Educational Missions

Although participating managers and their health systems will receive the most immediate benefits of the initiative, the EBMC will be committed to sharing research and findings. Accordingly, it will also serve as a resource center where other organizations and researchers can look to learn the latest news about effective healthcare management and health system organizational performance.

EBMC researchers (and their manager partners) will publish in peer-reviewed journals, but also will establish broader dissemination strategies (including a web site) to ensure that their work and findings reach all interested managers and researchers.

The EBMC also has another important educational mission: to help produce a cadre of new research, consultants, and management leaders interested in research on healthcare management and health system performance. The academic partners involved with the EBMC are expected to become nationally and internationally recognized centers of excellence on these issues, and will provide opportunities for students to gain knowledge and experience in a largely neglected field.

EBMC Budget Requirements

Two types of resources will be required for the success of the EBMC. The first is personnel, requiring a diverse array of expertise, including healthcare management, operations, governance, finance, marketing, research design, database analysis, and education. The distinctive strength of the EBMC is that the partnership brings together a critical mass of experience from all of these fields with a common mission: to take on the difficult issues that have precluded prior efforts targeted at only one aspect of healthcare management or a single dimension of the problems of financing strategic interventions. Many of the major participants will maintain their current roles in their respective organizations, with a portion of their time devoted to EBMC activities. However, the EBMC's agenda is a difficult and ambitious one, and will also require establishment of a strong core staff to provide leadership, administrative, and technical expertise.

The second resource requirement is funding for specific research and demonstration projects. Cooperation of providers and use of management databases can help reduce costs; however, the underlying research must be thorough and rigorous enough to be persuasive to managers and may often involve primary data collection. Some participating organizations may need financial assistance (or access to capital) to upgrade their management information systems to permit their involvement. Demonstration projects to test new approaches may also have significant implementation costs, as will the evaluations to assess the effect of these interventions.

As it matures, the EBMC is expected to rely primarily on internal financing, but also on a diverse combination of government and foundation grants to support much of its agenda. Demonstrating practical value will be a key criterion for attracting continuous funding. Although the healthcare management research area has been historically much neglected, the EBMC provides an attractive vehicle to support the research and demonstrations that are critical to improving health system performance. However, in its initial five-year start-up phase, the EBMC will require $4 to $5 million over a four-year period to launch the initiative and provide core support.

Complementary Initiatives Toward Improving Strategic Management

The following phenomena are assumed to be the results of ineffective managerial decision making in large nonprofit health systems[10]:

- The $200 million operating loss for the year ending June 30, 1999, of the University of Pennsylvania Medical Center (Freudenheim 1999);
- The bankruptcy of the Allegheny Health Education and Research Foundation;
- The bankruptcy of Health Insurance Plan of New Jersey;
- The failure of the UCSF/Stanford merger; and
- Hospital withdrawals from Medicare HMO markets with large operating losses (Kuttner 1999).

These situations are often characterized by the resignation or firing of CEOs, downsizing of thousands of employees, frustration and bitterness among hospitals and doctors who no longer are paid fair rates on time, plan members who are forced to seek new providers because their health plan has gone bankrupt, and lessened participation by hospital donors for a mission they see as attenuated and a community they see as no longer so adequately served.

Many complementary initiatives can be pursued by health systems in addition to forming evidence-based management cooperatives as suggested in this article. Most of the complementary initiatives cost money, and beleaguered managers will ask the authors, in the face of downsizing and capped salaries, where this money will come from. As suggested earlier, evidence-based management cooperatives can be financed by budgeting 10 percent of last year's management consultant fees.

Complementary initiatives, which may be informed by better evidence to improve strategic management, include improving the governance of nonprofit health systems, changing management incentives and organizational culture, better educating present and future managers, and improving the management of consultant contracts.

Improving Governance

Large health systems can be managed according to measurable goals and objectives set in advance, negotiated with stakeholders, and approved with oversight by the board. This is how successful large businesses are run. Large nonprofit health systems require more focus. They need to understand which businesses they are in and how well they are doing in each business, and to consider which businesses they wish to remain in. We are assuming that large product or service lines such as cancer, heart, women's health, and emergency services are characterized by different organizational competence and market share.

Offering Management Incentives and Changing Culture

Management salaries can be realigned with performance, and base salaries lowered and incentives primarily based on the organization or unit achieving measurable objectives, again negotiated with stakeholders and the board or owners. Knowledge management and management research will be encouraged to the extent that healthcare management markets work better. In that case, leaders who can better manage knowledge and learn from best practice and best experts are expected to be able to document better organizational performance, thereby further supporting improved health system processes of decision making.

Better Educating Present and Future Health Managers

Managers need to learn the skills and gain experience in managing knowledge and evaluating management research (as well as learn how to develop challenging but realistic performance objectives and effective implementation of the process of setting and monitoring these objectives). Nonprofits typically underinvest in education as well as in research. Graduate programs in health services management typically concern themselves more with educating entering managers (often with a gap between what they need to know and what they are taught) than managers who may already have master's degrees but who have been educated and have worked under drastically different circumstances.

Improving the Management of Consultant Contracts

Consultants complain that large health systems do not know how to properly use their services. This applies to managers specifying what they want from consultants, and then effectively following up with the recommended implementation after the consultant leaves. Managers typically do not do a sufficient job of managing contractors in terms of setting and monitoring performance. Managers should clarify the organizational mission, measure performance, specify strategies to attain objectives, and continuously monitor performance and results. Management consultants can have an important part to play in decision making, especially given the limited managerial support in many health systems. But the claims, evidence, and warrants of consultants must be carefully studied by managers and board members who have the skills, experience, and support to so consider the best evidence.

Conclusion

This article describes the benefits of using an evidence-based approach in considering and evaluating strategic organizational interventions. Before significant investments can be made, the practical benefits of an evidence-based approach have to be clearly documented and related to the costs involved and limitations in replication. We urge that such demonstrations be undertaken.

Acknowledgments

The authors gratefully acknowledge the research and editorial assistance of Melissa Robbins, and the thoughtful suggestions of Eran Bellin, Jo Ivey Boufford, Rob Burns, Alan Channing, Robert Curtis, Randi Feinstein, Steven Finkler, John Griffith, Sue Kaplan, Anna and Christine Kovner, Mary Stefl, Helen Smits, and Jacob Victory.

Notes

1. According to Bellin, "the notion that a leader might define both an objective and the way to measure its accomplishment is alien to this generation of managers. Their training sites are equally inept in bringing to the workforce managers with this notion of responsibility and the skill set necessary to accomplish this task. As a result, senior leaders rarely recognize the need for new creative descriptions to capture the human activity they manage, let alone find someone to do this and train their staff in the implementation of this style of management" (1999).
2. Analysis is limited to those articles within the journals' major article section (where main studies are presented) and studies section (if applicable). Articles were determined to be health management–related if they fell within the categories that are implicitly linked to the management of a healthcare organization. These categories include governance, professional integration (including job satisfaction, organizational commitment, teamwork), financing effect on the organization, internal systems (information systems, human resources, marketing, planning), financial management (cost containment, efficiency, technology), patient perspectives, organizational design (integration, networks, environment), quality and performance management, organizational staffing/training, managerial role (leadership, ethics, performance), and adaptation (strategies, community health, delivery).
3. For example, in "Research as a Foundation Strategy," by James Knickman, VP for Research and Evaluation of The Robert Wood

Johnson Foundation, the word "management" does not appear (Knickman 1999), although we listed this foundation as the second leading funder of healthcare management research.

4. According to Hansen, Nohria, and Tierney (1999), over the past few years Anderson Consulting and Ernst & Young have each spent more than $500 million on information technology (IT) and people to support their knowledge management strategies.

5. An example of an inter-organization focused on best practices and management research is the Center for Health Management Research, which is sponsored by the Universities of Washington and California, the Network for Healthcare Management, and the Washington Health Foundation. Founding members include Hospital of the Good Samaritan (LA), Intermountain Health Care (UT), Sisters of Providence (Seattle), Sisters of St. Joseph of Orange (CA), Tucson Medical Center (AZ), and Virginia Mason Medical Center (Seattle), and a variety of corporate and academic members. Goals of the center include research, development, and evaluation projects on behalf of corporate members and dissemination of health services research and best practices (Zuckerman 1999).

6. An example of an organized forum to encourage sharing of information as to best practices is the for-profit Health Care Advisory Board of Washington, D.C., which attempts to obtain data from many providers and share findings with its organizational subscribers.

7. Curtis (1999) suggests that the large consulting firms often base their recommendation on one or two experiences—often with the outcome still in doubt, the response outdated, and a "one-size-fits-all" solution.

8. Behavioral simulations are widely used by the Office of Public Management in London to learn whether proposed system changes will produce anticipated benefits (Parston 1999).

9. Typical consulting budgets for health system management have been estimated to range as follows: strategy and general management ($3 to $5 million), information systems and technology ($15 to $35 million), and clinical process improvement ($3 to $5 million) (Elton 1999).

10. Obviously, poor management decisions have also occurred in for-profit health systems such as Columbia/HCA and Oxford Health Plans (Kuttner 1999).

References

Axelsson, R. 1998. "Toward an Evidence-Based Health Care Management." *International Journal of Health Planning and Management* 13 (4): 307–17.

Bellin, E. 1999. Personal communication.

Berwick, D. M. 1996. "A Primer on Leading the Improvement of Systems." *British Medical Journal* 312 (6): 619–22.

Bindman, A., K. Grunbach, K. Osmond, D. Komaromy, M. Vranizan, K. Lurie, and J. Billings. 1995. "Preventable Hospitalizations and Access to Health Care." *Journal of the American Medical Association* 274 (4): 305–11.

Booth, W. C., G. G. Colomb, and J. M. Williams. 1995. *The Craft of Research*, 94–110. Chicago: The University of Chicago Press.

Curtis, R. 1999. Personal communication.

Davenport, T. H., D. W. DeLong, and M. C. Beers. 1998. "Successful Knowledge Management Projects." *Sloan Management Review* (Winter): 43–57.

Ellrodt, G., D. J. Cook, J. Lee, D. Hunt, and S. Weingarten. 1997. "Evidence-Based Disease Management." *Journal of the American Medical Association* 278 (20): 1687–92.

Elton, J. 1999. Personal communication.

Freudenheim, M. 1999. "Bitter Pills for Ailing Hospitals." *New York Times* Oct. 31 (Bus. Section): 1.

Griffith, J. R. 1999. Personal communication.

Hansen, M. T., N. Nohria, and T. Tierney. 1999. "What's Your Strategy for Managing Knowledge?" *Harvard Business Review* (Mar/Apr): 106–16.

Knickman, J. R. 1999. "Research as a Foundation Strategy." In *To Improve Health and Health Care 2000*, edited by S. Isaacs and J. Knickman. San Francisco: Jossey-Bass. 137–60.

Kuttner, R. 1999. "The American Health Care System." The *New England Journal of Medicine* 240 (8): 664–68.

Nutting, P. A., J. W. Beasley, and J. J. Werner. 1999. "Practice-Based Research Networks Answer Primary Care Questions." *Journal of the American Medical Association* 281 (8): 686–88.

Parston, G. 1999. Personal communication.

Rauber, C. 1999. "Audit: UCSF Stanford Deal Added to Losses." *Modern Healthcare* (Sept. 6): 20.

Robinson, J. C. 1999 "Blended Payment Methods in Physician Organizations Under Managed Care." *Journal of the American Medical Association* 282 (13): 1258–63.

Sackett, D. L., W. C. Rosenberg, J. A. Gray, R. B. Haynes, and W. S. Richardson. 1996. "Evidence-Based Medicine: What It Is and What It Isn't." *British Medical Journal* 312 (13): 71–2.

Simons, R. 2000. *Performance Measurement Control Systems for Implementing Strategy*. Saddle River, NJ: Prentice Hall.

Stewart, R. 1998. "More Art Than Science." *Health Service Journal* 108 (5597): 28–29.

Stewart, T. A. 1999. "Telling Tales at BP Amoco." *Fortune* 139 (11): 220.

Van Etten, P. 1999. "Camelot or Common Sense? The Logic Behind the UCSF/ Stanford Merger." *Health Affairs* (Mar/Apr): 143–48.

Zuckerman, H. 1999. Personal communication.

Discussion Questions

1. What is the management challenge for which evidence-based management is the solution?
2. How realistic are the authors' proposed solutions?
3. To what extent is education for healthcare management evidence-based?
4. What management competencies do entry-level managers require to practice in a way that is appropriately evidence-based?
5. How do the incentives under which healthcare managers function constrain implementation of a more evidence-based approach?

Required Supplementary Readings

Bigelow, B., and M. Arndt. "The More Things Change, the More They Stay the Same." *Health Care Management Review* 2000, 25 (1): 65–72.

Robbins, C. J., E. H. Bradley, and M. Spicer. "Developing Leadership in Health Care: A Competency Assessment Tool." *Journal of Health Care Management* May/June 2001, 46 (3): 188–202.

Strack, G., and M. D. Fottler. "Spirituality and Effective Leadership in Health Care: Is There a Connection?" *Frontiers of Health Services Management* Summer 2002, 18 (4): 3–18.

Warden, G. L., and J. R. Griffith. "Ensuring Management Excellence in the Health Care System." *Journal of Health Care Management* July–Aug 2001, 46 (4): 2001, 228–237.

Discussion Questions for the Required Supplementary Readings

1. What do healthcare managers do anyway?
2. Why don't healthcare management education programs measure the skills and experience of entering and graduating students to measure added value?
3. What is the value added to healthcare organizations of having a vital spiritual commitment?
4. Are "the best and the brightest" being attracted to healthcare management, and what difference does it make if they are not being attracted in sufficient numbers?

Recommended Supplementary Readings

Dreachslin, J. L. *Diversity Leadership*. Chicago: Health Administration Press, 1996.

Griffith, J. R. *The Moral Challenges of Health Care Management.* Chicago: Health Administration Press, 1993.

Griffith, J. R., and K. R. White. "The Executive Office." *The Well-Managed Health Care Organization,* 5th edition. Chicago: Health Administration Press, 2002, 113–144.

Kovner, A. R., A. Channing, M. Furlong, and J. Pollitz. "Management Development for Mid-Level Managers: Results of a Demonstration Project." *Hospital & Health Services Administration* 1996. 41 (4): 485–502.

Kovner, A. R. *Health Care Management in Mind: Eight Careers.* New York: Springer, 2000.

Pointer, D. D., and J. P. Sanchez. "Leadership: A Framework for Thinking and Acting." In S. Shortell and A. Kaluzny, *Health Care Management: Organization Design and Behavior,* 4th edition. Albany, NY: Delmar Thomson, 2000, pp. 106–127

Tyler, J. L. 1998. *Tyler's Guide: The Healthcare Executive's Job Search,* 2nd edition. Chicago: Health Administration Press.

Zuckerman, H. S., W. L. Dowling, and M. L. Richardson. "The Managerial Role." In *Health Care Management: Organization Design and Behavior,* 4th edition. Albany, NY: Delmar, Thomson, 2000, pp. 34–63.

THE CASES

Personnel decisions, critical to managerial effectiveness, are often postponed by healthcare managers or not handled with sufficient care. For example, considerably more time may be spent on the decision to purchase or lease a piece of valuable equipment costing $900,000 with a useful life of seven years than on the decision to hire a registered nurse earning $50,000 a year who may work for the organization for 20 years.

Even more important than the hiring decision is the continuous evaluation and motivation of subordinates and colleagues, many of whom may have been hired by a manager's predecessors. If the managers do not perform at an expected level of competence, what are the supervisor's options? What are the manager's options if she disagrees with her boss's expectations or evaluation? If the boss does not fire or transfer a manager being evaluated, her own effectiveness may suffer because she lacks a key aide to implement her strategy and support her politically. Ineffective managers may have been working loyally for an organization for many years. Searching for and training a new manager costs time and money; in addition, the risk exists that a new hire's performance will not be as anticipated.

Managerial personnel decisions become even more complicated when, as in "The Associate Director and the Controllers," the healthcare manager is dealing with a functional specialist who is line responsible to the top manager and staff responsible to the chief controller in a multi-unit medical center. The straight and dotted lines of authority on the organizational chart become fuzzy and difficult to agree upon in practice, especially when the associate director's boss and the medical center director of finance distrust each other. In this case study, key staff of the two recently merged units have different value orientations—the base hospital primarily serving attending physicians in their private practices, and the ambulatory health services program emphasizing the provision of respectful patient care to low-income patients residing in the local community.

The manager's job is often a lonely one. Important decisions are seldom made on an either-or basis, and often involve personal as well as organizational risks and benefits. In "A New Faculty Administrator for the Department of Medicine," the weighing of risks and benefits is different for Sam Bones, the chief of medicine, than it is for Sandra Compson, the group practice administrator, or for Compson's eventual successor. Similarly, in "The Associate

Director and the Controllers," the stakes of the game are higher for James Joel, the ambulatory health service program manager, and for Percy Oram, its controller, than for Milton Schlitz, the medical center director of finance, and for Miller Harrang, the chief executive officer of the ambulatory health services program.

Why must Joel decide to do anything at all? In "A New Faculty Practice Administrator," Bones must choose a new group practice administrator. But in "The Associate Director and the Controllers," Joel can decide not to get involved and allow Harrang and Schlitz to deal with the consequences of Oram's ineffectiveness. How much should it matter to Joel whether Oram remains on the job or not, so long as Joel can protect his own job? On the other hand, Joel is being paid to manage, not to observe or to protect himself. Good management generally makes a difference to the patient, as well as to an organization's ruling coalition. How much of a difference is open to question. But who will look after the manager's interest if she doesn't look after it herself? This is the first rule of managerial survival. Looking after one's own interest does not mean that the manager should lock her office door, read reports, and sit there telling subordinates what to do.

Healthcare managers often face tremendous pressures from government to move in certain directions and resistance from physicians who do not wish to move one step further than that required by law. How much value do managers add to organizational performance? Not much, according to Pfeffer and Salancik, who argue that the contribution of managers accounts for about 10 percent of the variance in organizational performance, and who agree with the sportscaster's cliché that "managers are hired to be fired."[1] An increasing amount of evidence, however, indicates that managers *do* make a difference in organizational performance, if only as they play a key role in obtaining the resources necessary for organizational survival and growth.

If the healthcare manager can never meet all the expectations of key organizational stakeholders, she can at least be seen as taking stakeholder interests into account in policy formulation and implementation. This requires regular communication, which takes valuable time. What makes for an effective healthcare manager? The answer depends on stakeholder perceptions as well as on any given manager's actual behavior or motivation. Sometimes—as in the short case of "Nowhere Job"—the right thing for the manager *is* to resign. Clearly healthcare managers must acquire information, learn skills, and have values consistent with an organizational context and its ruling coalition. It is not always easy to decide what actions to take after the manager receives disquieting information, such as that shown in the short case of "Manager Morale at Uptown Hospital."

Evaluating managerial effectiveness or contribution carries a cost. All pertinent information may not be available at a reasonable cost. Reliance on measurement may divert attention inappropriately away from what can be easily measured. Evaluating managers, like management itself, involves judgment, which in Ray Brown's phrase, is "knowledge ripened by experience."[2]

For management students, case discussions are an excellent way to get safe experience in forming managerial judgments.

Notes

1. J. Pfeffer and G. R. Salancik, *The External Control of Organizations* (New York: Harper & Row, 1978) p 17.
2. R. Brown, *Judgment in Administration* (New York: McGraw-Hill, 1969) p 9.

Case 1
A New Faculty Practice Administrator for the Department of Medicine

Anthony R. Kovner and David M. Kaplan

Sandra Compson was leaving her position as faculty practice administrator at Wise Medical Center to raise a family. Dr. Sam Bones, chief of medicine, asked Compson to become involved in the selection of her replacement before leaving.

Wise Medical Center is regarded as one of the largest and best-managed hospitals in Eastern City. The CEO, Dr. Worthy, was appointed in 1988. He has captained the dramatic growth of the medical center, its financial success, and the improvement of its medical teaching programs. Over the last five years, almost all the clinical chiefs have been replaced. Internal medicine is the largest department in the medical center. Dr. Bones is a specialist in cardiovascular disease and has an excellent reputation as a clinician.

His department has grown very large, and Bones has difficulty in staffing the large number of beds with medical residents. Bones is praised for his leadership skills, his intelligence, and his caring for those who work with him. He has been criticized for his unwillingness to make tough decisions regarding the economics of the department and for not getting rid of physicians who don't or won't meet his own and the department's high standards of quality. The medical center and the department face stiff financial pressures, and Dr. Worthy and others are trying to determine what the medical center's response to managed care should be. The medical center currently relies heavily upon referrals from its managed care panel, its network hospitals and clinics, and community physicians.

The faculty practice (FPP) in the department of medicine was formally launched three years ago in 2000, as were the faculty practices in various other departments. The FPP in the department consists of 16 subspecialties, and 100 providers who all share the faculty practice suite. The suite, which is 10,450 square feet, consists of 40 exam rooms, 10 consultation rooms, a reception and waiting area, a small laboratory, a technician's area, a billing office, and an office for the practice administrator.

The FPP staff for the department of medicine consists of six secretaries, two registered nurses, three midlevel providers, one medical technician, and one administrator. Larger physician practices including general internal medicine, neurology, and hematology/oncology bring additional staff with them when they are holding their sessions.

Compson, the practice administrator, is responsible for scheduling the subspecialty clinic sessions with each division within the department of medicine. Each provider is assigned a session with dedicated rooms. The medical center utilizes an electronic scheduling system, where all the providers have dedicated blocks of time to schedule patient appointments. It has been estimated that several of the physicians do not have enough volume to fill their sessions, while other physicians have a large backlog of patients and a long wait time to be seen.

The FPP suite currently operates from 9 a.m. to 5 p.m., Monday through Friday. Visits have increased by 15 percent over three years from 15,000 to 17,250. Demand is such that if more staff and space were available volume might be able to increase by an additional 7 percent with little or no additional investments.

Compson has very limited access to the financial information such as revenue, expense, and billing records for the faculty practice since an outsourced company performs all of the faculty practice outpatient billing. (It is important to note that the medical center's patient accounts department handles the inpatient billing.) The billing system ties directly into the scheduling system. Dr. Worthy and his leadership team previously selected both the billing/scheduling system and the billing company back in 1988. The systems are very outdated and the subspecialties have limited knowledge of their financial standing. Historically, this hasn't been a tremendous issue because all of the physicians are salaried and do not have any financial incentives to increase productivity.

The original operating concept of the faculty practice suite was to create a place with an upscale ambiance where physicians could see their patients. The purpose for creating the suite was to recover scattered examination space throughout the medical center and to take advantage of economies of shared space. Based on these concepts, decisions were made early to maximize treatment space at the expense of chart storage space, which is very limited. In fact, many providers are forced to bring their charts to and from other locations to each clinic session.

Recently, the division of cardiology wanted to create a Heart Failure program and approached both Dr. Worthy and Compson with a proposal that would have generated an additional 600 patients and 200 additional heart valve surgeries a year, bringing an additional $1.2 million in revenue to the medical center. But with no space available to accommodate this demand, and no capital to build a new facility, the proposal was denied.

Bones's final interview with Compson went as follows. . .

Bones: Sandra, as you know, you've done a splendid job here this past year and we'll be sorry to lose you. The situation of the departmental faculty practice as I see it is this: During the past few years the practice has been organized and it has grown dramatically. We seem to be having a lot of operating problems, such as space, poor support for the physicians, and antiquated billing and scheduling systems. The question now is, what kind of a job needs to be done by the group administrator and who should we look at? What do you think?

Compson: Well, Dr. Bones, as you know, I've enjoyed tremendously the opportunity to work with you and with the members of the department and I will be sorry to leave, although I am looking forward very much to raising a family. I think that the kind of person you need is not necessarily the type of person you needed three years ago. Then you needed someone who could "put out fires" and try to keep the place working. Now I think you need a systems person who can make the place run more effectively, at the same time keeping up the morale of the staff and working with the physicians.

Bones: I agree with you. I want someone personable and energetic, who isn't afraid of work, who can get along with the doctors and the hospital administration. I think the most important thing is getting our physicians the kind of support they need to run a first-class faculty practice. The systems aren't working down there. According to the reports I've seen (see Tables 1.1 and 1.2), the department isn't making the kind of money that it should be making, and we should be making it much more pleasant for our physicians to practice here.

Compson: As you know, per your instructions, I've started the interviewing process and will send you all the good candidates. I have spoken to several directors of programs of healthcare administration and to the hospital human resources department. There aren't a lot of good people available with systems and management experience in healthcare. I don't want someone who is strictly a systems person. The manager must be in touch with the needs, wants, requirements, and expectations of the customers. I see the customers of the faculty practice as both the physicians and the patients.

Bones: Sandra, I agree with you there. I know you'll excuse me, but I have to attend an important strategic planning meeting for the hospital. I still don't quite understand what they're going to do, but I wish they'd give more emphasis in the plan to building up the medical center's research capabilities.

Compson: All right. Then I'll be getting back to you soon. I will make appointments with Renee, your secretary, for all the promising candidates.

One month after Sandra Compson's interview with Bones, she has completed interviews with 11 candidates for the position. She has eliminated from consideration four graduates from health administration programs who lack appropriate work experience and three medical center employees in the finance department who she feels would not relate well to the physicians in the group. Compson has made tape recordings of all her interviews with the remaining four promising candidates and has had difficulty in choosing among them.

Compson's first interview was with David O'Brien, currently an assistant director for patient accounts in the finance department. The patient

TABLE 1.1

Faculty Practice Suite Billings and Collections, Fiscal Year 2000

Month	Billings	Collections	Contractual Allowances	Gross Collection Rate	Net Collection Rate
September	$ 3,241,151	$ 1,199,226	$ 1,296,460	37%	62%
October	$ 3,213,040	$ 1,349,477	$ 1,285,216	42%	70%
November	$ 2,864,251	$ 859,275	$ 1,145,700	30%	50%
December	$ 2,203,564	$ 1,013,639	$ 881,426	46%	77%
January	$ 3,514,687	$ 1,827,637	$ 1,405,875	52%	87%
February	$ 2,647,159	$ 952,977	$ 1,058,864	36%	60%
March	$ 3,268,573	$ 1,830,401	$ 1,307,429	56%	93%
April	$ 3,358,751	$ 1,612,200	$ 1,343,500	48%	80%
May	$ 3,046,892	$ 1,736,728	$ 1,218,757	57%	95%
June	$ 2,781,441	$ 1,668,865	$ 1,112,576	60%	100%
July	$ 2,813,332	$ 1,153,466	$ 1,125,333	41%	68%
August	$ 2,215,116	$ 863,895	$ 886,046	39%	65%
Total	**$35,167,957**	**$16,067,788**	**$14,067,183**	**46%**	**76%**

Item	Quarter 4 1999	Quarter 4 2000	YTD 1999	YTD 2000
Percent Utilization	72%	68%	69%	58%
Total Number Providers	80	100	80	100
Total Number of Provider Sessions	9,600	12,000	41,600	52,000
Visits	3,863	5,245	15,000	15,450
Revenue	$3,578,860	$3,686,226	$15,599,794	$16,067,788
Expenses	$3,175,864	$3,334,657	$12,703,456	$13,338,629
Net Profit/(Loss)	$ 402,996	$ 351,569	$ 2,896,338	$ 2,729,159

TABLE 1.2
Faculty Practice Suite Quarterly Statistics: Departmental Key Indicators June 1, 2000– August 31, 2000

accounts area is responsible for all inpatient billing within the medical center. The second interview was with Sal Sorrentino, a recent graduate from the City University program in health policy and management. Prior to attending the program Sal was the assistant director of a neighborhood health center. The third interview was with Marcia Rabin, a classmate of Sorrentino's at City University and director of human resources at a large multispecialty practice. The final candidate was Bonnie Goldsmith, who just recently completed two years with the U.S. Department of Health and Human Services (HHS) in Washington, DC, after graduating with a master in health administration (MHA) from City University. Compson has elected to review the tapes with Tim Brass, the senior vice-president of clinical operations before forwarding her recommendations to Dr. Bones.

David O'Brien

Compson (to Brass): The first interview is with David O'Brien who is approximately 25 years old, and dresses very conservatively. When I spoke with Barbara Karen, Wise Medical Center's senior vice-president of finance, she said that David was energetic and conscientious, and that he gets things accomplished. She gave him a very positive reference for this position. When asked about his weaknesses she did say that he was a bit intense, and sometimes intimidates and antagonizes others. She continued to say that David has no problems, it seems, in getting along with his superiors, but has limited experience in working with physicians. (Compson plays a tape of the interview.)

Compson: David, can you tell me in a few words something about your background and experience?

O'Brien: Sure, Ms. Compson. I attended Upstate College, where I was a business major. After graduation I started working in the hospital finance department, specifically patient accounts as a biller. Just last year I was promoted as the assistant director within patient accounts. My eventual goal is to receive my master's degree at City University, in their MHA program.

Compson: Going at night?

O'Brien: Well, I don't think there will be any problem. Others have done it here at the medical center, and I want to get out of finance and into management.

Compson: Dave, what would you say has been your greatest accomplishment in patient accounts?

O'Brien: I would say that I've really improved the system for inpatient billing and collections, starting with getting the bills out on time, all the way through to collections, and in refining and improving the data system that indicates how well we are performing. Performance has improved since I've taken the job—in speed, in accuracy, in the percentage collected, and in the time it takes for the hospital to get its money.

Compson: Dave, that does sound impressive. If you were faculty practice administrator, what would you consider to be your greatest asset?

O'Brien: I would say it's my ability to get a job done. There are too many people in this field who are just willing to go along with the way things have always been done until there's pressure from some quarter, and then it's often too late to do something, or to do it the right way.

Compson: And what would you say is your greatest liability?

O'Brien: Well, you know, in every organization some people are against change, because either it affects their own interest or because they just don't like change. After all, every change in somebody's department has to affect everyone involved in a relative, if not in an absolute, way. As my teacher used to say, "You don't make an omelet without breaking eggs." And I guess I must rub some people the wrong way who are against what I'm doing or about to do.

Compson: What aspect of the job in the faculty practice do you think is most important?

O'Brien: I think it's improving the net revenues. I've spoken with the billing clerk in the practice and she thinks the doctors could vastly improve utilization of the facility by making changes in the block scheduling, so that docs aren't allocated time slots if they're not using them effectively. Also, the reports generated by the practice could be greatly improved. I'd like to track physician productivity in dollars relative to the opportunity costs involved in their using examining room space.

Compson: Before you go, is there anything you would like to ask me about the job?

O'Brien: As a matter of fact there is. We've talked about the salary and the benefits, but if I perform as expected, what is the likelihood of a decent increase after the first year? You know I have a wife and two young children.

Compson: Well, I'd say the chances are pretty good. Dr. Bones is fair and I think he would be generous if the practice results improved significantly. (She turns off the tape recorder.)

Brass: He seems like a fine candidate.

Salvatore Sorrentino

Compson (to Brass): Sal Sorrentino is the next candidate. Sal is 27 years old. He is presentable, although he dresses a bit on the flashy side—fast talking and enthusiastic. When I spoke to his reference, Dr. Plotkin of the neighborhood health center, he highly recommended Sal for the position. He said that Sal was idealistic, energetic, and pleasant. If there was any weakness, Dr. Plotkin thought that Sal has a tendency to initiate or implement new policies and procedures without understanding the implications. I asked him to clarify, or to provide an example, and he said that Sal had decided to change the way patients were scheduled without getting any input from the physicians, nurses, or secretarial staff. The result was that patients were being triple booked, and having in some cases to wait for over two hours for their appointment. The issue was quickly resolved, and Dr. Plotkin believed that Sal had learned his lesson. Dr. Plotkin did reiterate that he highly recommends Sal for this position. (Compson plays a tape of the interview.)

Compson: Sal, can you tell me in a few words something about your background and experience?

Sorrentino: Yes, I can. I was a political science major at City University, then I got involved with various community and nonprofit groups. While working with St. Angelo's Church, I was active in trying to improve the availability of maternal and child health services to the Latino population; as a result, I met the assistant director for community relations at the neighborhood health center. It turns out that we were both vitally concerned with helping patients, and helping to provide needed services to the community. Before long I was offered a position as an administrative assistant at the health center. Shortly after starting this job, I was able to secure a scholarship to the City University graduate program in health policy and management.

Compson: And what would you say, Sal, was your greatest accomplishment at the neighborhood health center?

Sorrentino: Well, one of the things I am proudest of is the community health fair I planned and organized. We involved community groups of all ethnic and work-related backgrounds and got the health professionals to staff the booths at the fair. We worked with business corporations to get prizes and literature on, for example, proper nutrition. We conducted screening examinations for eye problems and provided tuberculosis and Pap tests. We followed up with all patients who needed help after the fair was over. The fair was well-attended and many people learned for the first time about the services the center had to offer. Of course, I accomplished a lot of other things, such as implementing a new billing system at the satellite of the neighborhood health center.

Compson: Tell me more about that.

Sorrentino: It wasn't so much really. But we needed to get more information than we were getting about patients coming for service. We had to make an effort to collect from those patients who could pay something and to have records that were suitable for reporting purposes. It was hard to implement because the staff was more interested in the patients getting service than in collecting the money.

Compson: I see. In the position we have been talking about, what do you think would be your greatest asset?

Sorrentino: Well, I see the highest priority for the group as that of attracting more patients. As my father told me, the way you make money in a business is primarily by increasing revenue rather than cutting back on expenses. I think the practice could improve rapport with patients and make changes in the suite so that the setting would be more attractive and comfortable for them. I think the practice would probably need an attractive brochure. The waiting area should be spruced up. I think the patient should know in advance how much services will cost. I'd like to devote part of my time to developing relationships with HMOs and managed care plans to increase referrals. I think the practice could benefit by extending the hours of operation. I think the suite should at least be open on Saturday mornings and one evening besides.

Compson: That sounds like an excellent idea. I've been pushing for Saturday hours also, but we aren't using our full capacity during the week as it is now. Another question, Sal, what do you think would be your greatest liability, if any, if you were chosen for the position?

Sorrentino: I don't know. I want to get things done in a hurry, I guess. I'm eager for results. Maybe I have a tendency to move a little too fast. Not really. It's hard to talk of one's faults. I really think that I can, would be able to do, the job perfectly well, and I'd like the opportunity to do so. I'm not always that good at following through on all the little details of an operation. But I'm excellent at working with people who will see to all the details.

Compson: I'm a little sorry to hear that because I think a lot of details are involved in this work.

Sorrentino: I didn't mean to say that I didn't like detail work or that I wasn't good at it. I would just say that it's a relative weakness—I really prefer the other kind of work I was describing rather than doing the billing clerk's work for her.

Compson: I see. What do you think is the most important aspect of the job we've been talking about in terms of the work that needs to be done?

Sorrentino: I guess first you have to get all your systems working properly, use of the suite, billing, and reporting; and I think next the most important thing is to increase your revenues. I think part of Dr. Bones's plan for the department is for the faculty practice to generate enough revenue to help support faculty member salaries.

Compson: You're right there. Is there anything now you want to ask me about the job, before you go up and talk to Dr. Bones?

Sorrentino: Two things really. First, what kind of person is Dr. Bones to work for? And, second, do you think there are good opportunities in management to further advance from this position?

Compson: In answer to your first question, I think Dr. Bones is an excellent person to work for, so long as you produce for him. He's loyal, gives you enough autonomy. Perhaps my only complaint is that it is sometimes difficult to see him, or rather that I have felt that he is such a busy man that I don't want to bother him with things I would like to discuss. I have recommended to him that he appoint another physician within the department as head of the faculty practice, at which time access to Dr. Bones will be less difficult. As to your second question, yes, I think the medical center is a large employer of people like yourself and that you can make a lot of useful contacts here. Also I feel that ambulatory care is the place to be in healthcare management in the future. (She turns off the tape.)

Brass: Well, these first two candidates have quite contrasting backgrounds. Yet it seems clear to me that either of them might do a perfectly respectable job, although of course the outcomes resulting from their work might be quite different.

Marcia Rabin

Compson (to Brass): Yes, that's so. The third candidate is Marcia Rabin. Marcia is 24 years old, attractive, and energetic. Les Carson, the CEO of Partner's Health Group, highly recommended her for the position. Ms. Rabin was the director of human resources for the Group, which consisted of 50 physicians and 20 support staff. Carson said she was hard working, gets along well with both professional and nonprofessional staff. If there is any fault to find with her, Carson said that Rabin takes her work too seriously, drives herself too hard, and as a result may be absent for a few days, largely because she has difficulty determining priorities. But Carson stressed that Rabin has performed very well on all the big jobs that he has given her to do, that she was reliable and competent. (Compson plays a tape of the interview.)

Compson: Ms. Rabin, can you tell me in a few words something about your background and experience?

Rabin: Certainly, I guess you don't want me to go back to high school, but I was president of my student government at Suburban High. In college I majored in psychology, and for a while I thought I would like to be a psychologist. But my father works in a hospital; he is director of housekeeping at Sisters Hospital, and encouraged me to go into healthcare management. After attending the City University masters program, I was hired as the director of human resources at Partner's. Previously they didn't have a department of human resources, but when the Group bought two additional practices and expanded from 10 to 50 physicians a department was established. While at Partner's I worked under the tutelage of Mr. Les Carson, the CEO.

Compson: What would you say was your greatest accomplishment as director of human resources?

Rabin: Really, I think it was my ability to fill all the entry-level jobs, or rather to keep filling them. Also, we started and finished a job classification system under my supervision, and inaugurated an annual pay increment schedule that I think worked more fairly than the previous system. I think my real accomplishment was in legitimating the department of human resources in the nursing home where such a department had never existed before. This meant being able to service other departments and to accomplish jobs for them that used to take up a lot of their time or that they couldn't do as well before.

Compson: That sounds interesting. In terms of the present position with Dr. Bones, what would you say was your greatest asset?

Rabin: I don't know exactly how to answer that question. My first response would be to say I like and am good at doing systems work—creating order out of chaos and working effectively with people so that they feel it is their system, not something that I pushed on them. Of course, this is difficult to do because, in my case, the departments had to accept the human resources system we established; it's the only way to do things as part of a large organization. But at least the pacing and some of the details were left to them, and first we proved that we really could be of help to them.

Compson: And what, if you'll pardon my asking, would you say is your greatest liability?

Rabin: Well, if you must know, Ms. Compson, I'm not aggressive enough. Sometimes I think my efforts aren't properly appreciated, and I don't push myself to the front the way some people do. I work hard and I work well and it annoys me, sometimes more than it should, that others who don't work so hard and do so well push themselves forward and move ahead faster.

Compson: What aspect of the job, as I have tried to outline it to you, would you say is the most important, I mean at this time in the history of the faculty practice?

Rabin: I think you have to set up more clearly defined ways of doing things, *systems* if you prefer the word. I noted in the materials that you shared with me that your collection rate isn't what it should be and that your utilization of examining rooms is well below capacity also. I don't think that this kind of systems work is so different from my work in human resources, plus I have taken a few courses in quantitative analysis and feel pretty comfortable with numbers.

Compson: Are there any questions that you would like to ask me?

Rabin: Well, one question is how have the physicians, most of them men, related to having a woman in this position? Second, when can you let me know if you are offering me the job? I have been offered a job as assistant director of human resources at King Hospitals, and although they aren't pressing me that hard, I would like to be able to tell them something soon.

Compson: With regard to the first question, sure, some of the physicians don't give you the respect as a manager that you would like to have, but I don't know to what extent this has to do with my being a woman. I think being a woman also has its advantages, with some of the docs. To answer your second question, I think it will take about a month for Dr. Bones to decide on a candidate. I can't tell you what you should say to the King people. You are one of the four candidates whom I am sending on to see Dr. Bones. (She turns off the tape.)

Bonnie Goldsmith

Compson (to Brass): Permit me to introduce our last candidate, Bonnie Goldsmith. She dresses conservatively and gives the impression of a modest, unassuming, kindly, young woman of 27. Her boss, Dr. Muldoon, who recently left the Centers for Medicare and Medicaid Services (CMS), recommended Bonnie as hard working, modest, and reliable. He said that Bonnie gets along with people, but tends to lack drive as well as the ability to think independently. However, Dr. Muldoon says that once a task is clearly outlined, Bonnie is thorough, dedicated, and relentless. As an example he praised Bonnie's work on a recent Task Force on the Aging Report. (She plays a tape of the interview.)

Compson: Bonnie, can you tell me a few words about your background and experience?

Goldsmith: Yes, I was a zoology major at City University. Originally I wanted to be a physician. In fact, I attended medical school for one year, then decided it just wasn't for me. I didn't know what I wanted to do. I don't know why but I thought that working in a hospital admitting department might be interesting, and I did that for a while. My father is a psychiatrist. The administrator is a good friend of my father's, and he talked to me and convinced me to apply to City University's graduate program in health policy and management. Back in school I really enjoyed the coursework related to quality improvement, information systems, and statistical analysis. A whole new world opened up to me, although I must confess I had a bit of difficulty with some of the heavy reading and writing courses. After graduation, I was fortunate to get a position with the CMS. Once again, my father's connections helped to open some doors for me. For the past two years at CMS I have been working to help complete a Task Force on the Aging Report, which was finally published 3 months ago.

Compson: What would you say has been your greatest accomplishment at CMS?

Goldsmith: I would say it was the staff work I did on the President's Task Force on the Aging. I went into a lot of nursing homes and other chronic care institutions and saw what a lousy deal most of our aged get. It isn't so much this way in Europe, which I visited a couple of years ago with my father. In Europe, the homes are more like residences and fewer people go into homes. When they do go, they can take their furniture with them, and it doesn't cost as much.

Compson: What kind of solutions did you come up with?

Goldsmith: Well, it's a pretty difficult problem. I mean the part about making it possible not to have to institutionalize the elderly. I guess there are tax incentives which could be passed to allow people to keep their relatives at home. Also, more people should be able to bring their relatives into homes for day care activities and to institutionalize them for a week or two each year if necessary, either because the aged member of the household is sick or because other members of the household want a rest. Of course, we need better regulation of nursing homes to set standards for care and to establish closer relations between homes and hospitals.

Compson: I see. What do you think would be your greatest asset in the position that exists here within the department of medicine?

Goldsmith: I don't know. Perhaps it's my ability to get along with and to understand the needs and problems of the medical profession. I don't have a big ego. I like analytical work, solving operations problems, and I think I'm pretty persistent in trying to solve them.

Compson: And your greatest liability?

Goldsmith: Well, some people think I'm not aggressive enough. I don't know what this means, really, unless it is forcing your opinions on others. I guess I'm not a great innovator, and I don't like to work that much. I mean I work hard, but I don't want work to be an obsession, like it is for my father. I mean that I'm married, with a nice husband and a young son, and I want to enjoy my work and do well, but I also want to enjoy my family. I guess you could call it a lack of ambition. But I think this country needs more people like me, people whose satisfaction comes from a job well done rather than striving for money, status, and power. I'm intellectually committed to group practice as a better way to deliver healthcare, and I'd like to do my part to see that primary care is improved in this country. So this may be a liability or an asset, I don't know.

Compson: I'm not sure either. But certainly if you do the job well, what you say makes sense. Well, enough of that. What aspects of the job strike you as most important?

Goldsmith: Well, I don't know. Certainly, the practice has to be organized systematically, and billing has to be improved. I'd like to track these processes scientifically, see what the standards are and should be, track the variance from standards by analyzing all the steps in these processes, and then work with all the individuals involved from physicians to receptionists in improving these systems. This might require a number of meetings, and I don't know how feasible such meetings would be because of people's time requirements. There are a few questions I would like to ask you.

Compson: Please go ahead.

Goldsmith: My first question is, do you think the faculty practice is going to grow? The second is incidental, but I would like to know more about the benefits, such as tuition remission, as I was thinking of furthering my education at City, perhaps taking some more courses in statistical analysis.

Compson: I think the faculty practice will continue to grow. Space is our key constraint now, and the medical center will have to figure out how we are going to better deal with managed care. Also, should we eventually combine the faculty practice plans in the various departments into one multidisciplinary group practice that is also in the managed care business? Of course this all has to be squared with the department's ambitious goals in teaching and research. Sometimes, despite the excellent reputation of the medical center and the quality of its leadership, I wonder if we can possibly excel in all these different areas as well as in all of the leading areas of clinical medicine. With respect to your second question, yes, I believe tuition remission for such purposes is available, although I don't see where you will have the time to fit everything in with the demands of this job, which are quite considerable, and with your family obligations. (She turns off the tape.)

Brass: Well, Sandy, now all you have to do is tell Dr. Bones whom you recommend for the job.

Compson: I need to sleep on it. This assignment has given me more problems than I bargained for, but that's the joy of working, isn't it, Tim, solving these problems?

Brass: I agree with you there. Sorry, but I've got to leave now. I want to think about this some more and I'll give you my opinion tomorrow.

Case Questions

1. What criteria would you use in evaluating the four candidates?
2. What are the strengths and weaknesses of each candidate?
3. What are Bones' criteria in evaluating the four candidates?
4. Whom would you recommend to Bones as your selection for the position?
5. What is the evidence that you used in making this recommendation?

Case 2
The Associate Director and the Controllers

Anthony R. Kovner

Fortunately for Jim Joel, he didn't lose his temper often. Otherwise, he might not have been able to function as associate director of the Morris Health Care Program of the Nathan D. Wise Medical Center (see Figure 2.1). But now, he had become so enraged at the Morris program controller, Percy Oram, that he had to concentrate hard to keep from yelling. Joel had just been informed by Felix Schwartzberg, an assistant director, that the accounting department was not collecting cash from the billing assistants in the family health units as previously agreed. Unfortunately, Oram did not usually keep Joel informed

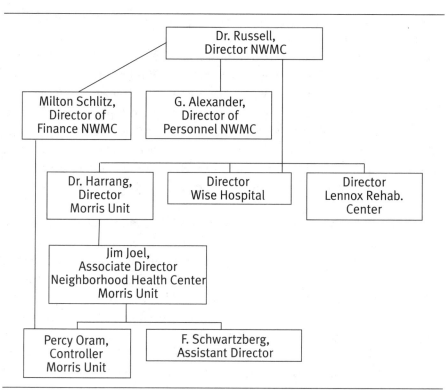

FIGURE 2.1

Organization Chart: Nathan D. Wise Medical Center

of his actions. But in any case, Joel knew his own reaction was excessive—an aspiring health services executive did not throw a tantrum, which is what he now felt like doing.

Joel was 30 years old, ambitious, and a recent graduate from Ivy University's master in healthcare administration program. Before returning to school, he had worked as a registered representative on Wall Street, where he had found the work remunerative but uninteresting. The director of the Ivy program, Dr. Leon Russell, assumed the post of director of the Nathan D. Wise Medical Center three years ago. Joel, one of his best students, asked to join Russell toward the end of that year, and he was hired shortly thereafter as an assistant hospital administrator. The Nathan D. Wise Medical Center is located in New York City and comprises three large programs: the Nathan D. Wise Hospital, the Lennox Rehabilitation Center, and the Morris Health Care Program. The hospital and the rehabilitation center are owned by the Wise Medical Center, but the Morris Health Care Program is operated by the Wise Medical Center under contract with the City of New York and is located in a city-owned facility.

Russell had been impressed with his former student's drive and promise and had originally created a job for Joel. This included half-time as a staff assistant at Wise Hospital and half-time as an evaluator at the Morris Unit, where new methods of delivering ambulatory medical care were being developed and demonstrated. However, the director of the Morris Unit, Dr. Lawrence White, had resigned to become commissioner of health of a Midwestern city, and six months later, his associate director, Mr. Phillip Bright, had announced his intention to resign to join White. Two years ago, Russell had hired a replacement for White, Dr. Miller Harrang, a 45-year old physician, who had previously been medical director of the Ochs Ambulatory Care Unit in another part of New York state. Since Joel was not being fully utilized at Wise Hospital, although he had performed capably whatever he had been asked to do, Russell decided to offer him the position of associate director of the Morris Unit.

Joel felt ambivalent regarding Russell's offer. He knew he would take the position, even before requesting a night to think it over, but at the same time he had certain reservations. Joel was enjoying his work at the hospital. He had submitted an in-depth plan for increasing efficiency of the operating room, which had been enthusiastically accepted by the medical staff executive committee, and he was just starting an evaluation of patient transport in the hospital. His key interest was implementation of his master's thesis on nurse staffing. Joel believed that by assigning rooms to patients on the basis of their nursing needs, one-third fewer registered nurses would be required. Joel wished to be director of a large general hospital within ten years. He wasn't sure how working at the Morris Unit would advance him toward that goal, nor how comfortable he would feel working in a facility serving the poor in a slum section of the city.

However, after taking the job, Joel found before long that he liked working at the Morris Unit immensely. Morris was rapidly expanding—in the last year, the number of physician visits had increased 25 percent to 215,000. Through a generous grant from the Office of Economic Opportunity (OEO), the budget had increased from $1.5 million to $2.5 million. Joel worked 65 to 70 hours a week. There was so much to do. He liked Harrang, his present boss, and he liked the people who worked at Morris. The atmosphere was busy and informal, a nice change of pace from the Wise Hospital where things happened more slowly. Dramatic change was the norm at Morris, whether this was conversion of the medical and pediatric clinics to family health units, or confrontations with a community health council resulting in increased participation in policymaking by the poor. There was no formal division of responsibility between Harrang and Joel. Harrang spent most of his time in community relations (time-consuming and frustrating), in individual conversations with members of the medical staff at Morris, and in working out problems with the Wise Hospital. Harrang also took responsibility for certain medical units such as the emergency room, obstetrics-gynecology (ob-gyn), and psychiatry. Joel's primary responsibility lay in the area of staff activities such as finance, personnel, and purchasing. He also supervised several departments or units, including laboratory, x-ray, pharmacy, dental, housekeeping, and maintenance. Responsibility for the family health units was shared by the two top administrators.

Under the former top administrators, White and Bright, the Morris Unit had been run as a unit independent from the Wise Hospital. The unit was decentralized, with departments such as laboratory and internal medicine handling their own personnel and often their own purchasing. It was Russell's wish to create a more integrated medical center, and Joel saw an important part of his job as creating staff departments (such as personnel and purchasing) and upgrading these functions with the help of medical center experts.

When Joel arrived, the controller's department consisted of four individuals: Bill Connor, the controller, who promptly resigned (Joel never met this individual whom he was told had personal problems of an unspecified nature); Peter Stavrogin, an industrious bookkeeper, who was a 55-year-old East European refugee with a limited knowledge of English; a payroll clerk; and a secretary. This was the staff for an organization of more than 400 employees that was funded by five different agencies under five different contracts. The accounting department had heavy personnel responsibilities as well, at least so far as payroll was concerned, because no personnel department as such existed. One of the first things Joel did was to hire Connor's replacement. In doing so—and to conform with Russell's policy of an integrated medical center—Joel enlisted the help of the medical center staff: Milton Schlitz, the director of financial affairs, and Grover Alexander, the director of personnel. Alexander volunteered to place the ads and check the references of applicants for the controller position, and Schlitz suggested that he screen the applicants. The best three or four would then be reviewed by Joel and Harrang who, between them, would select the new controller. Joel was pleased with this arrangement, although he thought the recommended salary for the position was too low. He agreed to go along, however, based on the recommendations of Alexander and Schlitz, who had considerably more experience in these matters.

However, because of what Schlitz and Alexander believed to be a shortage of qualified accountants, and the undesirable location of Morris, they found only two prospective applicants. Albert Fodor, a 55-year-old certified public accountant (CPA), with no hospital experience but good references, was the obvious first choice to be Morris's new controller. Fodor was pleasant and industrious. It took him six months to learn the job. Fodor then resigned, citing that the tremendous pressure and workload were too great for a man of his years. The payroll clerk also resigned at this time for a higher-paying job at another hospital.

During the next three months, Joel employed three new billing clerks as well as a personnel assistant and a purchasing agent. Most of the accounting department's work, which would have been done by the controller, was performed by Joel, who handled the budgetary aspects, while Stavrogin covered the accounting aspects. This system was unsatisfactory, however, because both felt Joel should spend less time troubleshooting financial problems and more time on the programmatic aspects of the job. Also, Joel wanted to conduct and supervise a variety of special studies for contract purposes and cost comparisons, an undertaking hardly feasible under the present setup.

So Joel went back to Schlitz and Alexander, insisting that the salary for the controller job be raised $3,000 per year because of the complexity of the job and the distance from Schlitz's direct supervision. Schlitz agreed reluctantly; he knew he would have to raise salaries or face morale problems in the accounting department at Wise Hospital.

After an intensive advertising program, eight to ten candidates had been screened by Schlitz, and three candidates were sent to Joel and Harrang, of whom Perry Oram seemed the best. Oram was 40 years old, without a CPA but with solid accounting experience in a medium-sized business firm. Oram had no hospital or healthcare experience. Schlitz and Joel did not feel that such experience was necessary for the job, although, of course, they would have preferred it. Oram was physically attractive, well-dressed, and married with no children. He said he was interested in advancing himself in the expanding hospital field. Joel went over the Fodor experience with Oram, stressing the work pressures. Oram responded that he was looking for a job where he would have more autonomy, where he was in charge and responsible, and where he knew he would be rewarded (or blamed) based on his performance. Of course, he would like to spend a lot of time at first learning the ropes with Schlitz. Joel told Oram he would let him know later that week if the job was his. Afterward, Joel and Harrang agreed that Oram was the best of the three candidates. However, Harrang had a vague feeling of unease—Oram seemed too good, too qualified for the job. Independently, Schlitz also agreed that Oram was the best of the three candidates. Alexander checked Oram's reference which confirmed the high opinion of Schlitz and Joel. Oram was then offered the job as controller of the Morris Unit, which he accepted.

From Joel's point of view, things went fairly well at first, perhaps because Joel was busy with other matters and because Oram was spending a lot of time at Wise Hospital with Schlitz. The first sign of trouble was the lateness of the monthly statement that Joel had instituted and required. The statement included detailed categories of departmental costs, comparing costs (Joel hoped eventually to compare costs with performance as well) for this month, last month, and this month last year, as well as cumulative totals for this year. Joel had reviewed with Oram how he wanted the statement done (in what categories), with a cover sheet that would suggest the reasons for any large variances. Oram agreed to furnish such a report, but one month after the month in question, Joel still hadn't received it. When asked, Oram said that he was too busy, and that he was working on it. When the statement finally did arrive on Joel's desk, there was no cover letter about variances, and there were large variances caused by sloppy accounting (items in one category last year, for instance, that were in another this year, causing large discrepancies). Even some of the amounts were incorrect, where salaries of certain individuals had not been counted in the proper categories. Joel, patiently but with irritation, explained that this was not what he wanted. He told Oram why he wanted what he wanted, and when he wanted the report—15 days after the end of the month. Timeliness, he emphasized, was especially important because, although the city contract remained at the same sum every year, changes in the OEO budget had to be individually approved by Washington, and OEO funds had to be spent by the year's end. This meant that a lot of shuffling had to be done (e.g., transfer of city positions because of increased salary costs to the OEO budget) based on correct information. Oram apologized and agreed to improve performance.

At the same time, Joel had begun to hear complaints about Oram from other staff members. Linda Lee, the personnel assistant, and Felix Schwartzberg, the assistant director, complained about his rudeness, arrogance, and insensitivity to the poor—like his repeated statements about "welfare chiselers." Such terminology was at odds with the philosophy of the unit. When changes in employee paychecks had to be made because of supervisory mistakes or because of inadequate notice concerning an employee's vacation, Oram reluctantly did the extra work. He warned those involved, without clearing it with Joel, that eventually checks would not be issued on this basis.

Joel had been approached by Oram two weeks previously about a personal matter. Oram explained that he had to come to work an hour and a half late twice a week because of an appointment with his psychiatrist. The psychiatrist couldn't see him before or after work, and he hoped Joel would be sympathetic. Oram was willing to stay late to make up the time. Joel said he wanted to think it over before responding, and then discussed Oram's situation with Schlitz and Harrang. They all agreed that they would have liked to have known this before Oram was hired, but that if the work was done and he made up the time, it would be permitted. It was agreed that Joel would check occasionally in the accounting office, which was located in a separate building a block away from the health services facility, to see if Oram was indeed putting in the extra time.

For about the next six months, Oram's performance remained essentially the same. The cover letter was superficial and the statements were late and often contained mistakes. (The statements did, however, eventually arrive and were eventually corrected.) The special studies requested of Oram were done late and Joel often had to redo them. In checking on Oram, Joel never found him in the office after 5:00 p.m., but he did not check every day. The routine work of the accounting department was being done effectively, but this had been the case before the current situation with Oram, when no controller had been present. Oram had added another clerk, and Joel suspected that Stavrogin was still performing much of the supervisory work as he had been previous to Oram's arrival. Joel was not happy. He discussed the situation with Harrang, who agreed that the statements were less than acceptable. Harrang told Joel to do as he liked, but to clear it first with Schlitz.

Soon after, Joel went to Wise Hospital to discuss Oram with Schlitz. Schlitz, a CPA, had been controller of Wise Hospital, now Wise Medical Center, for 27 years. Schlitz was talkative but often vague, hard-working, basically conservative, and oriented primarily to the needs of Wise Hospital (at least in Joel's opinion) rather than to the Medical Center at large. This was reflected in the allocation of overhead in the Morris contracts (e.g., administrative time allocated was greater than that actually provided) and in the high price of direct services, such as laboratory, performed for Morris by the hospital. More important, Schlitz saw his job almost exclusively as worrying about "the bottom line"—whether the hospital or the Morris Unit ran a deficit or broke even—rather than in terms of performance relative to costs. Nevertheless, Joel thought he had established a cordial relationship with Schlitz, and their discussion about Oram was indeed cordial for the most part. Schlitz agreed that Oram's performance left something to be desired. He was particularly unhappy about the time Oram put in. On the other hand, Schlitz felt that the Morris Unit was in good financial shape and that there was nothing to worry about. In view of the experience with the previous controller, Fodor, Schlitz wondered if indeed they could find a better man for the salary. Schlitz urged that they talk to Oram together but said that he would go along with whatever Joel wanted to do.

Acting on Schlitz's recommendation, Joel set up a meeting with Schlitz, Oram, and Harrang to discuss his dissatisfactions. During the course of the meeting Joel did admit that the monthly statements were improving, but only after extensive prodding. Oram remarked that the reason for this meeting surprised him; he had thought, on the basis of previous meetings with Joel and Schlitz, that they were pleased with his work. He then asked, in fact, to be included in more top-level policy meetings, as he felt that controllers should be part of the top management group. Oram said he felt isolated, which resulted in part from the location of the accounting department in a separate building. Joel responded that he would welcome Oram's participation in policy meetings after the work of the accounting department had been sufficiently upgraded, and that Oram would be kept informed of and invited to all meetings that concerned his department.

Returning to the Morris facility, Joel discussed his perplexity with Harrang. Actually, he asserted, he did not understand what was going on here. Oram never gave him what he wanted. He had no way of knowing how busy Oram actually was. Lately, Oram had said that he couldn't produce certain studies by the stipulated dates because he was busy doing work for Schlitz or attending meetings at the hospital with Schlitz and the controllers of the other units of the medical center.

Harrang replied that he believed that Schlitz was indeed responsible in part for Oram's lack of responsiveness. Schlitz had probably told Oram not to listen to Joel but to do what he, Schlitz, recommended, because Oram's salary and benefits were largely determined by Schlitz rather than by Joel. Schlitz didn't want the accounting department at Morris to use more sophisticated techniques than the hospital because this would reflect badly on Schlitz. Moreover, Schlitz wanted his "own man" at the Morris Unit so that the hospital benefited in all transactions with Morris (e.g., there should be enough slack in the city budget to meet any contingency, with as many staff as possible switched to the OEO budget).

Joel had to agree with Harrang's observation. But on the other hand, Harrang had become increasingly bitter toward Russell over the last six months. This concerned a variety of matters, most specifically Harrang's salary. Harrang was working much harder than he had bargained for at Morris, and he didn't feel he was getting the money or the credit he deserved. Nevertheless, Joel did think that Schlitz might be part of the problem; he had never been particularly impressed with Schlitz.

Several weeks later, a new state regulation was passed stating that for city agencies to collect under Medicaid, all efforts must be made to collect from those who, by state edict, could afford to pay. This was in conflict with Morris's philosophy of providing free service to all who said they couldn't pay, and there was much opposition to implementation of the policy by the professionals at Morris. The professional staff felt that no special effort should be made to collect from those who had formerly received free services. Oram disagreed with this philosophy and said that Morris should make every effort to collect.

When it came to implementing collections, Oram requested that the registration staff who were to collect the money should be part of his department, or that a separate cashier's office should be set up on the first floor of the health facility. Otherwise his department didn't wish to be involved. Schwartzberg, the assistant director in charge of registration, argued that the registration staff should continue as part of the family health units because of other duties, that no space was available on the first floor for a cashier's office, and that it was not fair to patients to make them stand in two lines, as they would have to under Oram's arrangement, before seeing a health professional. Joel and Harrang sided with Schwartzberg and discussed with Oram a plan under which he would be responsible for the cash collection aspects of the registrar's work. It was agreed that Oram would devise, within a week, a plan for implementation. After two weeks, Schwartzberg reported to Joel that Oram had not devised a plan and was unwilling to cooperate with the plan Schwartzberg and the chief registrar had devised.

Joel pounded his desk. What concerned him was not so much this specific matter, which he knew he would resolve, but what to do in general with Oram. Joel was working Saturday mornings with a militant community group over next year's OEO budget and was still working 60 to 65 hours per week. He didn't think Oram's performance would improve unless Schlitz agreed with Joel's priorities and, even in that event, sufficient improvement was unlikely. On the other hand, Joel did not look forward to hiring a fourth controller in the two years he had worked at Morris. Moreover, the routine work of the accounting department was being performed to the satisfaction of Schlitz. Joel decided to go for a walk by the river and make his decision.

Case Questions

1. What is the problem from Joel's point of view? From Oram's point of view? From Schlitz's point of view? From Harrang's?
2. In what ways should Oram be accountable to Joel and Schlitz?
3. Given that Oram's performance is not acceptable to Joel, what options does Joel have to affect Oram's performance?
4. What do you recommend that Joel do now? Why?
5. What is the evidence that you used in making the above recommendation?

Short Case A
Nowhere Job

David Melman

John Ernest works for a young and growing healthcare company. The company has been successfully developing a market niche by contracting with colleges and universities to manage and operate their campus health centers. Ernest has been hired to develop the operational structure of a new product that will connect the managed care health insurance coverage of the students with their campus health center. This new product will result in cost savings and superior service delivery. It is a new concept in the industry and, while

Ernest does not have significant healthcare experience, he does have a great deal of energy and enthusiasm and is expected to learn on the job.

Ernest is not given a formal job description. He is verbally given a list of performance objectives, but these objectives are changed without his input and without detailed new objectives put in their place. Ernest's work environment is unusual in that he mostly works out of a home office, with occasional trips to the corporate office 70 miles away. Ernest is told that he will report to the corporate medical director, who is located in Miami, 1,200 miles away. Communication is made by telephone, fax, and e-mail.

Ernest makes progress in achieving organizational objectives but is facing obstacles in terms of his isolation from others in the company. He is not informed of changes in project objectives, or of the underlying reasons for these changes. Ernest finds that this isolation limits his ability to grow and contribute because he is unable to describe his company's needs accurately to outside vendors without being so informed himself.

Ernest asks to have a formal job description and stated performance objectives based on the format suggested by a human resources consultant hired by the company. He receives no response. He is asked to complete the contracts with several outside vendors he has negotiated. Ernest is told he now reports to an outside consultant who has been hired to help coordinate technical operations, including information systems. This outside consultant tells Ernest not to proceed with these contracts the very day after the CEO has told him to complete them.

Ernest attempts to contribute to the sales and marketing efforts of his company by proposing that the company sponsor an institute at a prestigious university, and he wants to contribute his time and energy to make this project a success. He is told it is a good idea, but the vice president of sales and marketing does not keep his commitment to respond to Ernest's proposal. Ernest sends reminders and continues to develop the idea with the university. He is trying to expand his job responsibilities to include business development but needs the support of others in his organization to make a meaningful contribution.

Case Questions

1. What should Ernest do?
2. What are the risks to Ernest?
3. How could Ernest have anticipated these problems before accepting his current position?
4. What should be Ernest's priorities in evaluating an alternative career opportunity? Why?

Short Case B
Manager Morale at Uptown Hospital

Anthony R. Kovner

Date: April 1995
To: Martin Dexter, CEO
From: Paula Long, Director of Human Resources

In talking about our management development program with several participants, I received the following feedback, which I think is serious and urgent enough to bring to your attention:

1. Morale is very low because of delayed program development, no allowance for overtime or per diems, and the resultant squeeze on management.
2. The hospital suffers from lack of supervisory staff, inadequate systems support, lack of trust among employees and managers, and a lack of a forum for communication upward.
3. The hospital provides a lot of substandard care, doesn't look nice, and is not "user-friendly." There are too many employees who don't "carry their load" and who are nasty.
4. The "word" for many potential users in the minority community we serve is to not use Uptown but rather to go to St. Stephen or Washington Hospitals.
5. Top management has not communicated to middle managers the strategic plan. There are no open lines of communication nor is there any shared management philosophy.
6. Good things and accomplishments by small groups aren't recognized or appreciated.
7. There is no feeling that morale will improve if financial performance improves.
8. Managers and department heads are afraid to fire someone they can't replace.
9. People are worried about their jobs.
10. No one trusts the message of the relationship with our teaching affiliate.

I have several ideas about what we should do about this, but I wanted to send this off to you right away while I continue to consider the situation.

Case Questions

1. What should CEO Dexter do in receiving Paula Long's memo?
2. How could such conditions have occurred at Uptown Hospital?
3. What constraints and opportunities does CEO Dexter face in implementing these recommendations?
4. How can CEO Dexter overcome constraints and take advantage of the opportunities?

CONTROL

You may regard as a Utopian dream my hope to see all our hospitals
devoting a reasonable portion of their funds to tracing the results of the
treatment of their patients and analyzing these results with a view to
improving them. You may prefer to ponder over the voluminous discussions
now appearing in our journals and in the lay press about the pros and cons
for state medicine and who is to pay the cost of medical care. I read these
discussions, but they seem to be futile, until our hospitals begin to trace
their results.
—E. A. Codman, 1935

I envision a system in which we promise those who depend on us total
access to the help they need, in the form they need, when they need it. Our
system will promise freedom from the tyranny of individual visits with
overburdened professional as the only way to find a healing relationship; will
promise excellence as the standard, valuing such excellence over
ill-considered autonomy; will promise safety; and will be capable of
nourishing interactions in which information is central, quality is individually
defined, control resides with patients, and trust blooms in an open
environment.
—Donald Berwick, *Escape Fire: Lessons for the Future of Health Care*, 2002

COMMENTARY

Hospital cafeteria manager to counter staff before the start of the work day: "Give our customers what they want from our daily menu and kitchen selections."

First customer to counter staff: "I want a hot dog with mustard and relish." Counter staff hands out a hot dog with mustard.

Customer: "There is no relish on my hot dog."

Staff: "Sorry." Takes back the hot dog and adds relish.

Customer: "Thanks." Proceeds down the cafeteria line to the cashier at the end.

This simple example raises a lot of the concepts related to control in healthcare or in any organization for that matter. Let us set this example into the context of a hospital's mission, vision, and values.

The *mission* of the hospital in this case is to provide the finest care by skilled and pleasant staff. The *vision* is that care will always meet best-practice standards, be timely, error free, appropriate, and provided at a reasonable cost. The key *values* are that patients come first and employee satisfaction is valued. The cafeteria fits into these goals by providing hospital workers a meal they want at a reasonable price. The hospital leadership is pleased that staff brag about working at the hospital and this includes the good food in the cafeteria. The cafeteria manager sets rules for appropriate work for the counter staff, leaving it up to them to match food to customer request. There are clear limits to what the staff can do. The price of one hot dog does not buy two. Chocolate sauce is not offered for your hot dog. These rules are not burdensome because the customers are socialized to know the first rule and don't ever ask for chocolate sauce on their hot dogs.

From an organizational point of view, this example is similar to the nursing supervisor saying to the staff nurse: "These are your patients. With your good skills and education I am confident you can care for them. Call me if you need help."

Management in healthcare means creating the space and support systems so that skilled people can meet the needs of the people they serve. If the relish jar is empty, the best counter staff cannot meet their customer's wishes. If the procedure kit is not in the examining room ready to use, the patient may not get a Pap smear test.

In our cafeteria example, an *error* was made and because of the customer's rapid *feedback*, it was corrected. If the quality is measured by the end result of this transaction (a hot dog with mustard and relish) the quality score was perfect, the transaction a success, and the customer was satisfied. The error was recognized—"Sorry"—and corrected: "Thanks."

Using a more accurate measure of quality, this transaction did not get a perfect score. Ideally, the error should not have occurred. There is a *cost of poor quality* here in the fraction of a minute used by staff, this customer, and other customers backed up in line, while the error was corrected.

It is worth noting that this quality problem was observed in time and corrected by the customer. Patients are usually unable to provide such a corrective feedback to caregivers. Professional caregivers—not the patient—are expected to define appropriate care. Therefore, caregivers carry a greater burden and responsibility for avoiding errors.

The theory of errors says that human beings are bound to make mistakes and errors will occur. The goal of error reduction is to create systems that stop errors. For example, a self-serve condiment station can be placed beyond the cashier so customers can help themselves. This needs a system for regularly replenishing the supply. This kind of system redesign is sometimes called *reengineering* the process.

Did this employee make a mistake due to lack of *motivation*? The vast numbers of workers want to do a good job and not make mistakes. In this example, most likely the employee simply forgot. It may do more harm to criticize this employee for negligence and more good to create a system so that the right decisions are always made.

The genius of the McDonald's franchise is a system designed to produce the identical package of french fries in thousands of locations using relatively unskilled employees. Such a system starts with working with farmers to produce the right kind of potato, creating a standardized package, and using a metal scoop for filling the package. By such attention to the details of its system design, McDonald's can convince millions of people that they make the best french fries, which gives them a great market advantage. Healthcare has a long way to go to create such systems to reduce error.

Standardization and Variation

A hundred years ago, the hot dog might have been handmade and no two were exactly alike. Shopping then was a more complicated process: "I want the fifth hot dog from the left, it looks bigger." Now that hot dogs are standardized and identical, there should be no reason to choose one from the next. Although variation is still possible—how well cooked, how hot, how much relish, what kind of mustard—we do not expect this kind of customer-driven variation in a hospital cafeteria line. Hospital care is a combination of standardized activities (hernia surgery) with variation (left or right side). Both best-practice standards combined with appropriate variation are required without error for good quality of care.

Standardization Can Be Cheaper and Variation Expensive

Back to our cafeteria: What about the attractiveness of the plate and napkin? What about the interpersonal relationship between the server and the customer? Does the server smile? Here quality is in the mind of the customer.

Quality in healthcare is not defined by the customer alone. The hospital nutritionist might say that the hot dogs have too much cholesterol and it would be healthier to replace them with meatless "veggie" dogs, and that the employees should set an example of healthy eating. Note that this changes the definition of quality from customer preference to expert knowledge about nutrition and health. This role of such professional criteria of quality is a distinctive feature of healthcare. Healthcare organizations must sometimes balance both patient satisfaction and adherences to expert definitions of quality.

A System of Control

Healthcare where professional judgment, cost, and the patient's perceptions all matter have led to the concept of the "value compass" and "balanced score card." Outcomes are measured in terms of patient satisfaction, cost of care, physical functioning (e.g., less pain, the ability to climb stairs) and physiological measures such as blood pressure and cholesterol levels (issues the patient may be unaware of, but the clinical research literature tells us are key indicators for a future healthy life).

A system of control comprises five elements:

1. *Goals and objectives* (in our example, this is meeting customer needs).
2. *Information* used to measure performance.
3. *Evaluation of performance in relation to goals and objectives.* Did the customer get what she wanted?
4. *Expectations.* Two levels of expectation were described in our cafeteria example. Did the customer eventually get what she wanted? Is this good enough? Or do we have a higher expectation of getting it right the first time? In this case, this transaction fell short.
5. *Incentives.* These can be based on an internalized desire to do a good job or on external rewards. The desire to make the customer happy and the desire to please the supervisor in hopes of a merit raise ideally go together without a conflict. The manager is delighted when good care is

given. Problems start where there is a disconnect between satisfying the customer or the manager.

Goals and Objectives

Mission, vision, values, goals, and objectives are widely used concepts (see Table II.1). Our mission may be to meet the needs of our customers, our vision is to be the best, the values we live by are our religious beliefs, our goal is to survive this year, and our objective is to break even.

A goal is a broadly stated intention or direction—to improve the quality, for example, by lowering the infection rate. Organizational goals are determined by the preferences of individuals with power. Organizations are collectives of people and things brought together to achieve a common purpose. Individuals with similar goals create the organization. Goals are important because they provide organizational focus. They provide a long-term framework for dealing with conflict and they encourage commitment from those who work in an organization. Goals are implemented by individuals working together on budgets, allocation of functions, and the authority structure.

The individual wants housing and food and health and entertainment. This person decides they can do this best by working for pay as a nurse in a clinic. Nursing can be both a means (paycheck) and an end in itself (the satisfaction of helping people in a friendly work environment). The clinic's goal of good quality and reasonable cost assumes that this nurse continues to have an enjoyable job and a paycheck. It is the role of the manager to make this happen.

TABLE II.1
Organizational
Directions

Concept	Definition	Example	Requirement
Mission	Reason for existing	To meet the primary healthcare needs in our town	System maintenance
Vision	What we hope to do	People will move to our town because our care is so good	Adaptive capability
Values	The philosophy that guides behavior	Mutual respect for both caregivers and care receivers	Values integration
Goals	An intention or direction	To open a new clinic this year	Goal attainment
Objectives	A measurable intention	The new clinic will see 100 patients a week by the end of the year	

Organizations may have objectives to measure production, sales, profit, quality, and to reduce inventory. An observation can determine unit or organizational objectives by reading formal official goal statements or by observing what is happening in an organization. These observations may reveal shifts in resources or decision-making power among units or individuals, what types of individuals are leaving or being recruited to the organization, and what the organization is not doing and which population it is not serving. Many large corporations expend a lot of effort in goal specification.

What happens if healthcare organizations do not specify objectives? Organizations may lack focus in their programs and may be less likely to abandon products and services that are neither effective nor efficient. The powerful and their short-term interests will tend to be favored over the weak and the long-term; there will be less adaptation to the environment; and there will be a greater tendency to retain the status quo.

Healthcare managers should determine their organization's operative objectives. Official goals may not always provide reliable guidelines for managerial behavior. When those in power go against what a manager sees as the long-range interests of an organization, the manager should be careful, speaking out only if he or she is willing to pay the price and is certain about the facts.

Information

Healthcare managers must obtain information for key product lines about volume of services, the quality of care, service and production efficiency, market share, system maintenance, and the health status of the population served. They may use the following measures to assess performance: cost per case, cost per visit, cost per day, profit, fixed and variable costs, market share, capital expenditures as a percent of sales, days of receivables and payables, top admitting physicians and their characteristics, staff turnover and overtime, sick time, and disability and fringe benefits costs. In addition, healthcare information systems are being expanded to include revenue by service line, budgeting and variance reporting, and clinical performance review. Computerized medical records are linked to cost and revenue data, concurrent review for quality of care, and to final-product cost accounting for groups of similar patients at alternative levels of demand. Risk management relies on incident reports of untoward events, which are then aggregated and analyzed.

Performance Evaluation

One of the problems with control systems is that they may measure the wrong thing. They can also measure the right thing inaccurately. These issues are particularly relevant for outcomes-of-care measurement. The easiest response to information we do not like is to say the data are wrong. There is no information accurate enough to be accepted in a hostile, fearful environment. One of the important aspects of continuous quality improvement (CQI) is to create a climate "free from fear," where data can be accepted for what they are despite their inaccuracies and still be used to make improvements.

Increasingly, healthcare managers have access to performance data comparing their organizations to other similar ones. In the past, a nursing home board of directors may have simply believed that their care was outstanding without question. The first step, then, was to measure their care; for example, the frequency of bed sores or the percent of patients under physical restraint. The next step was to have comparative measures and ask questions. Why are 15 percent of our patients under restraint while the statewide average is 8 percent? The third step is to make this information public on accessible websites. This is being done by third-party payers such as Medicaid for nursing homes. Concurrent with these steps is a change from denial (our patients are sicker) and fear to a desire to improve. Managers can visit another similar nursing home with a very low restraint rate to learn how to improve their own situation. This requires collecting performance data over time to track improvements. This process of systematic comparison to best-practice organizations is called "bench-marking."

Expectations

It is well documented that medication errors occur frequently in hospitals. The wrong medicine, the wrong dose, and the wrong time are all parts of this problem. Although no clinic wants medication errors, there are different ways to respond to this problem. What is the level of expectation for good performance? It could be "zero tolerance for error." It could be that "we will make yearly improvements to continuously reduce out error rate." It could be "Everyone has this problem and we are no different" or "We have the best nurses and physicians so I am sure our error rates are lower than anyone else." One's performance expectations make a difference.

Incentive Systems

How does the manager transform the individual worker's desire for a paycheck into a pursuit of organizational goals so that both are achieved exactly together? Incentives are stimuli to affect performance. Adoption of incentives is usually based on the answers to the following questions: Does the incentive contribute to the desired results? Is the incentive acceptable to those workers whose behavior managers wish to affect? Could implementation of the incentives produce other dysfunctional consequences (e.g., rewards for cutting costs might lead inadvertently to reduced quality of care).

Organizations use both positive and negative incentives. Incentives can be monetary or not. One of the underlying ideas of CQI is that monetary incentives are often actually disruptive. The assumption is that people want to do a good job and that the systems within which they work all too often frustrate their good intentions. How can the admissions clerk rapidly process an admission when the computer has crashed? How can the dietary department provide hot food at the bedside when the patient is waiting in the x-ray department? CQI calls for management to lead the effort in improving these systems, whereas rewarding individuals may create rivalry rather than teamwork.

THE READINGS

The reading in this section by Sahney and Warden, "The Quest for Quality and Productivity in Health Services," describes the core concepts of quality improvement as applied to healthcare. These concepts have transformed the way health managers think about the work of their organization.

Quality improvement (QI), quality management (QM), continuous quality improvement (CQI), and total quality management (TQM) are all words used for this way of thinking. Some argue about the subtle differences in the meaning of these words. Others use them interchangeably. More recently, these ideas have merged with concerns about safety and error reduction in healthcare.

There is fad and fashion related to quality improvement methods. Consultants sell their own special flavor of QI, but at the core it has some good basic ideas. The organization that is enthusiastically and persistently focused on meeting the needs of the people it serves, tracks its progress in doing so, and organizes to best meet these needs has a better chance of success.

The Quest for Quality and Productivity in Health Services

Vinod K. Sahney and Gail L. Warden
Excerpted from *Frontiers of Health Services Management* 7 (4), Summer 1991.

Implementation of TQM at Henry Ford Health System

Henry Ford Health System is a vertically integrated regional health system. It has an annual operating expense budget of over $1 billion and a workforce of over 15,000 employees. It consists of a teaching hospital, three community hospitals, two multispecialty group practices with over 1,000 physicians, 35 ambulatory care centers, two nursing homes, an HMO with over 400,000 members, and multiple other health-related businesses.

Initiating the TQM Process

Henry Ford Health System (HFHS) initiated the TQM process in October 1988. A task force was formed by the CEO under the leadership of the Corporate Vice President of Planning and Marketing, to study and recommend how to launch TQM within Henry Ford Health System. The first three months were spent reading and discussing the concepts of Deming, Juran, and Crosby. The task force visited several corporations and hospitals.

The task force prepared a document, outlining the key concepts of TQM and keys for successful implementation. The findings of the task force were presented to the CEO and at a later date to senior management at the Management Policy Committee. The CEO was committed to implementing TQM, but it would be fair to say that there were many skeptics. Some of the senior management questioned the necessity of such an initiative; others questioned whether we could afford a new initiative and its cost; some felt that they were already practicing it; some suggested that we wait until the budget planning cycle, which would occupy management for the next three months, was over. Some were unable to find the time to read material that was circulated, but those that did became more and more convinced. A decision was made to proceed further. Some of the reasons for TQM implementation were to

- Develop a quality culture throughout HFHS with a focus on continuous quality improvement
- Improve services to our patients
- Increase value for our customers
- Improve productivity and control increases in the cost of healthcare
- Improve work environment in order to maintain and attract qualified workforce
- Improve organizational understanding of practice pattern variations
- Use benchmarking to compare performance and learn from the best practices.

Selection of a Consultant

A request for proposal (RFP) was developed with the help of the management engineering group and sent to 15 consulting organizations. The RFP requested detailed philosophies of implementation and the fee structure for different packages. The task force developed criteria for evaluating vendor proposals (see Table II.2). Twelve organizations responded with detailed proposals. Paul Batalden, M.D., and his Quality Resource Group at HCA was

TABLE II.2

Henry Ford
Health System
Quality
Management
Process: Criteria
for Evaluating
Vendor
Proposals

1. Depth/breadth of experience with quality improvement engagements, and specific improvement experience in healthcare: including inpatient and outpatient; service and clinical components
2. Willingness and ability to modify approach for healthcare, particularly training materials
3. Improvement process structure and plan, consistent with HFHS requirements
4. Type and degree of support provided in addition to basic implementation plan:
   - Willingness to assist HFHS in education program development
   - Willingness to provide service on-site
5. Professional level of consultant resources proposed:
   - Style, experience, sophistication, and credibility of proposed project team
   - Intensity of resource to be provided (i.e., consultant time and skill mix)
6. Pricing
7. Established, proven history
8. Exclusions and restrictions

selected as the external consultant to guide the TQM implementation process in its early stages. Batalden's background as a physician, the depth of his understanding, past experience in a group practice, experience of implementation in hospitals, and the proposed fee structure were important factors in his selection as the HFHS consultant. It was felt that he was genuinely interested in changing the healthcare industry through TQM.

Henry Ford Health System's Total Quality Management initiative was named "Henry Ford Quality Management Process." This was done to clearly convey the idea that it was a process and not a program. The objective was stated:

> To develop and implement a total quality management process that can be followed throughout the organization to improve the quality of healthcare services provided to our customers. The goal of the process is to retain market leadership in healthcare delivery through quality.

Initial Implementation Steps

A two-day orientation was held for the top 70 executives of Henry Ford Health System with Donald Berwick and Batalden as external facilitators. The evaluations were mixed. Many felt that TQM was the greatest thing since sliced bread and others thought it was a waste of their time—they already knew this stuff. Some commented that this would be the next program of the year and hoped that it would die a quick death. At the end of the two-day orientation, every participant was given a copy of *The Deming Management Method* (Walton 1986) with a personal message from the CEO. This book presents Deming's management method in an easy-to-read style. It has numerous case studies from industry. The author is a journalist who followed Deming for over two years, attended his lectures, and interviewed him on multiple occasions. It was felt to be a good introduction for people beginning to grapple with TQM issues and principles. A small group of internal staff called the Corporate Quality Resource Group (2 FTEs) was created and spent the summer of 1989 with the consultants developing an implementation plan and customizing the HCA material for HFHS training. Each of the operating entities and staff groups was asked to select two individuals who would guide the process within the group. This group was called the Quality Technology Council (QTC) and consisted of approximately 30 members. The QTC began meeting twice a month and began improving its own understanding and learning the concepts of TQM. One of Deming's 14 points was discussed in detail at each meeting. External speakers were invited to share with the group their experiences with TQM.

In fall 1989, all QTC members were trained by external consultants for six days on key concepts of TQM. These courses were called Q101 and Q102. Based on the comments of QTC members, course material was revised. In October 1989, a three-day course that combined Q101 and Q102 and compressed the material from six days to three days was offered to the members of the Management Policy Committee (MPC). Management Policy Committee members for the most part report directly to the CEO and constitute the policymaking and resource allocation body of the system. In retrospect, this was a big mistake. Prior to training, MPC members felt that since they were extremely busy and quick studies, they should be able to absorb the concepts quickly. However, in actual experience, the members of the group realized that they did not have enough time to finish the exercises and fully grasp the concepts. Since that time nine of the 13 MPC members have gone back and retaken the full six-day course. Their unanimous advice is that we should not have shortened senior management training. During the past year MPC has discussed each of Deming's 14 points in detail, with each discussion being led by a different member. The MPC also has had several half-day and three one-day retreats to develop the Henry Ford Health System Quality Framework. This framework includes the system mission, vision, quality definition, and quality guidelines (see Appendix II.1).

A significant factor in the rollout of the Quality Management Process at Henry Ford Health System was to establish Quality Steering Committees at the system level as well as at each operating group level. The job of the quality steering committee is to guide the implementation of the quality management process within its operating group. The steering committees consist of senior managers who make resource allocation decisions within the group.

A second important step is to anchor the quality management concepts at higher levels before moving it one step lower in the organization. Chief executive officer learning and practice was followed by top management learning and practice followed by middle management learning and practice.

Each of the operating entities and the staff groups was then charged with developing a Quality Framework within its own entity or division. The sequence of the Quality Management Process rollout is described below.

A. *Quality Management Awareness and Learning.* This is the first step during which each operating group formed its own quality steering committee and identified its coach (a member of QTC). In weekly sessions, Deming's 14 points were discussed in detail. The Quality Steering Committee, including the CEO and the coach, participated in the six days of formal training. This step took approximately the first six months.

B. *Quality Management Framework Development.* Each entity worked on developing its quality framework. This included mission, vision, quality definition, and quality guidelines. This process was a slow and tedious one and is still in progress in many divisions. It took longer to accomplish because it took senior management and the Board of Trustees nine months to finalize the System Quality Framework.

C. *Quality Management Practice.* The concepts taught in Q1011 and Q1012 started being used. The meeting skills and participation skills had an immediate impact. Soon meetings had agendas and time frames, and participants began using such processes as brainstorming, nominal group techniques, and multiple voting to assist in decision making. Practice teams were formed to enable newly trained managers to further strengthen their understanding of the concepts. Each MPC member participated on a team. The CEO is a member of a team that flow-charted the Policy Making Process. Other senior management members worked on such processes as the capital budgeting and mergers and acquisitions.

D. *Customer Awareness Development.* Each entity or division was asked to review the current mechanisms for customer feedback and to identify its customers. A systemwide customer feedback questionnaire was implemented for all inpatients. Similarly, an ambulatory care feedback mechanism is being used on a sampling basis for all medical centers. A number of focus groups have been conducted in addition to community surveys. A systemwide team is working on developing a System Quality Report.

E. *Organization Quality Awareness Building.* Organization-wide awareness building has been initiated through the use of multiple presentations ranging from two hours to one full day. Board presentations have been made. The Henry Ford Health System Board of Trustees has appointed a Quality Committee that has met four times. A charge of this committee is to guide the Henry Ford Quality Management Process. All of the other entities have conducted board, as well as, management retreats on quality. At these meetings trustees have been asked to define the role they should play in quality improvement.

The focus of the activities during the first year of TQM, viewed as the initiation phase, was geared to learning and building quality management awareness throughout the system (see Table II.3). During the first year of implementation ending on October 1, 1990, over 350 senior managers and physicians were trained in formal six-day training sessions. Over 60 physician members of the Henry Ford and Metro Medical Groups have undergone this extensive training. Quality Steering Committees have been formed in every operating group, and coaches have been assigned. Managers within each operating group have developed their preliminary rollout plan for 1991. These plans were presented to the System Quality Steering Committee in its preliminary format. Currently, each operating group is finalizing its Quality rollout plan. This plan addresses how the entity plans to roll out the Quality Management Process, needs for formal training, facilitator training, key projects it plans to initiate, and plans for further employee involvement to solidify the

TABLE II.3
Henry Ford Health System Quality Management Transformation

PHASE I	PHASE II	PHASE III
Initiation	Transformation	Integration
• Learning	• Chartered teams	• Quality management way of life
• Practice	• Recognition	
• Framework	• Customer measurement	
• Customer awareness	• Cross-organizational	
• Organizational awareness	• Outcome measure link	
	• Human Resource policies	
	• Process design	

commitment and to move the Quality Management Process implementation. These plans were reviewed in December 1990 by the System Quality Steering Committee and will form key parts of the system plan.

Ongoing Training

Approximately one year after initiating the process, the internal Quality Resource Group took over the training function from the external consultants. A team was formed consisting of senior managers and quality coaches who took responsibility for different sections of the teaching material. Each section leader taught the material at least once. The presentation was videotaped. Each section leader then selected management volunteers from within the HFHS to teach the material. It was the section leader's responsibility to go over the material with and prepare the individual who was next in line to teach the section. Teaching notes and the videotapes have been extremely helpful in preparing new teachers. In addition, external consultants observed and critiqued the initial teaching by the HFHS staff. To date, over 50 managers and physicians have participated as instructors and facilitators in the training program.

A decision was made early to keep the training systemwide and invite participants for each training session from across the system. In a class of 36 participants, no more than nine participants were from any one operating entity or staff group. This decision was made to further the notion of systemness among the participants. Participant evaluations of the training sessions have almost unanimously singled out this strategy as a good one. Participants have enjoyed interacting with other system members. Each training class is six days in length and taught in two three-day sessions approximately six weeks apart. Participants include a complete cross section of physicians, nurses, and managers.

Department of Quality Improvement Education and Resources

In order to further accelerate progress within the system, the CEO in October 1990 announced the formation of a new Department of Quality Improvement Education and Resources. The mission of this new department is to promote, guide, and support the organization-wide quality transformation of the Henry Ford Health System. In addition, the department is charged with developing new theory and applications of modern quality improvement technology for use in healthcare. A chair with an endowment of $1 million was established for the chairman of the department. This department consists of a professional and administrative staff of 10 FTEs, and is a major commitment of the system toward the development and application of TQM.

Management Evaluation

To further solidify the implementation of TQM within the organization, the CEO indicated that one of the four dimensions on which each individual reporting to him would be evaluated in 1990, was progress made as a role model based on TQM principles as well as the progress made in the implementation of TQM by the areas reporting to the individual.

Strategic Plan

Henry Ford Health System has just completed a year-long process to develop a 10-year strategic plan for the system. This plan was developed by the Futures Committee of the Board of Trustees. One of the six system requirements identified was to: "Develop a cohesive, vertically integrated healthcare system which demonstrates a commitment to excellence and the process of continuous quality improvement."

During November 1990, the next step in TQM began with the introduction of the first steps of Hoshin planning within the organization. The senior managers reporting to the CEO were each asked to develop their 1991 objectives and plans in support of the six key requirements of the system developed by the Futures Committee of the Board of Trustees. For 1991, plans are in place to further integrate strategic planning and the TQM process within the organization.

Lessons

The involvement and the commitment of the CEO is crucial in implementing a TQM process within any organization. Early in the process, senior managers must spend sufficient time learning and practicing key concepts and methods. There is a tremendous temptation to take short cuts or avoid training sessions to save time, but experience shows that it slows the process at later stages. It is important that senior management develop a conceptual framework for quality and discuss it with employees. This framework must be developed through a participatory process by management and not delegated to staff or consultants.

As the TQM process takes root in the organization, process improvement teams will be formed. In the early stages, it is important to manage this process and to form only a few teams. Each team should have a trained facilitator who acts as a coach for the team. It is critical to develop trained facilitators before teams get formed.

The TQM process offers a great opportunity for management to communicate organization mission and vision for the future. It offers an opportunity to listen to the concerns of the employees. It provides management with a powerful tool to motivate employees and change the culture of the organization. In the early stages, TQM may be perceived as an add-on activity by managers. It is important that leaders continue to emphasize that TQM concepts need to be practiced in everything that managers do, and that quality improvement is a fundamental business strategy of the organization. In addition, TQM is the basis for productivity improvement as well as cost reduction within the organization.

It is important not to equate symbolism with real progress. It is easy to put out slogans, pins, and fliers. It is much more difficult to change management behavior. It is also important not to equate progress with the number of teams formed, or with holding meetings using newly acquired meeting skills or the number of surveys done. Real progress will be made when TQM concepts are incorporated in daily ways of doing work, and when management focuses its attention on the process of everything it does.

TQM and Clinical Applications

A question often asked is "can TQM be applied to clinical care or is it applicable to administrative functions only?" Brent James (1989) has addressed this question. He says, "The roots of continuous quality improvement are the same quality principles that medical practice has taught since its inception. The major difference is that the continuous quality improvement theory uses those principles in a formal, explicit fashion. It rigorously applies scientific methods to organized medicine's commitment to learn from every patient, so that the next patient will receive better treatment."

Recently, many case studies have appeared in which the formal TQM process has been used by clinicians to improve the process of clinical care to the patients. We cite a few examples. The first example is from Latter Day Saints Hospital in Salt Lake City. The process studied was "post-operative deep wound infection" (James 1989). A team from the hospital studied prophylactic antibiotic usage for all inpatient elective surgeries performed and related the outcome to the process of care. Based on the study, the process was modified and the outcome improved significantly. The deep-wound postoperative infection rate was cut by 50 percent. Laffel and Blumenthal (1989) have also given several examples of the application of TQM in clinical settings. They state, "The elimination of unnecessary variation in clinical practice may similarly improve the quality of care . . . should physicians choose to follow similar procedures for determining the sources of infection and for selecting and modifying antibiotic coverage, it is likely that the hospital would be able to implement their care plans more efficiently and accurately."

Caldwell, McEachern, and Davis (1990) describe the implementation of continuous quality improvement in clinical areas at West Paces Ferry Hospital in Atlanta. Following the TQM process, the team reported a 44.5 percent decrease in antibiotic costs due to elimination of waste. Another team at West Paces Ferry Hospital examined the birthing process with a focus on reducing c-section rate (McEachern, Schiff, and Hallium 1991). The team consisted of physicians, nurses, and administrators. The c-section team developed a flow chart and collected data on c-section rates over two years. A run chart was developed. The team then brainstormed causes of c-section and developed a cause-effect diagram. Systematic process improvements were introduced and results monitored. The authors report decline in c-section rates from 21.0 to 17.8 percent.

The application of TQM to clinical processes offers an excellent communication tool for physicians, nurses, and other professional caregivers to communicate with each other. Documenting the care process and systematically introducing change to improve the process will allow the teams to see the impact of the changes. In addition, the documented care processes become an excellent tool for new employee orientation as well as for communicating with other departments. As clinical processes are documented, opportunities will be identified for improvement of hotel and administrative services being provided to patients and physicians in relation to the clinical care. This coordination of care will allow for reduction of length of stay, unnecessary tests, and patient stays (Coffey et al. 1990). Finally, one of the central themes of TQM is understanding variation in a process and reducing of variation. The concepts of TQM can be applied to understanding clinical practice variations among physicians. This is a key activity at Henry Ford Health System. A number of physician teams are using TQM concepts to study clinical processes. Total Quality Management provides common language for all healthcare providers to effectively communicate with each other.

Evidence of Impact

Total Quality Management principles have only recently been applied in healthcare. Most hospitals are in the first or second year of the implementation process. Although a number of case studies have been reported (Society for

Health Systems and Health Care Information and Management Systems Society 1990) at national meetings showing the positive impact of the approach, it is premature to use them to declare that TQM has been successful in healthcare.

What about other industries? Here there are many successful implementation cases (Spechler 1989). Xerox Corporation by its own admission was in trouble in 1982. The Japanese had made significant inroads into the copy machine business. A benchmarking study conducted by Xerox showed that its unit manufacturing cost equaled the Japanese selling price and defects per machine were sevenfold compared to Japanese products. In 1983, Xerox launched its total quality management process. In 1984, Xerox did not have a single copier rated as "best" in any of the seven categories of copiers. By 1986, Xerox had leadership in two of the classes and by 1988 Xerox was rated the best in six out of seven classes in consumer ratings. During the same period, Xerox experienced a 38 percent improvement in customer satisfaction. In 1989, Xerox was awarded the Malcolm Baldrige National Quality Award (Riddle 1990).

Similar testimonials have been given by numerous companies including Ford Motor Company, General Motors, Motorola, and Hewlett Packard. One thing is clear with TQM—not only does quality improve, but productivity improves and the work environment and employee morale also improve significantly.

Sahney's First Law of Quality

The quality progress accomplished by any organization is directly proportional to the degree of cultural change congruent with the philosophies of TQM within the organization and the degree of use of tools and techniques of process improvement.

Experience indicates that methods and process improvement do not last unless the cultural change process is anchored in the organization. Similarly, if the organization spends its resources in motivational talks to the employees but does not follow up with a methodology and education for process improvement, very little is gained. This is why programs such as guest relations programs do not have a lasting impact. Resources are best used when work proceeds simultaneously on both the cultural change and the application of tools and techniques.

Sahney's Second Law of Quality Progress

The quality progress accomplished in any organization is directly proportional to the (a) square of (degree of senior management commitment in using the principles of TQM) and (b) the degree of all employees actually using the principles of TQM.

Benefit accrues much slower in the beginning because efforts of the few practicing TQM are countered by others who stick to old ways. As more and more senior managers commit to TQM, the progress accelerates.

Success in the final analysis depends on the ability of management to be able to execute the TQM process in a consistent fashion, with determination, single-minded focus, and energy.

Visible Actions by Senior Management in Successful Implementation of TQM

If TQM is to be successful, management must take active leadership in each and every area of the process as it is being implemented. Batalden et al. (1989) has outlined his prescription for a successful launch of TQM process:

- Management must learn the meaning of quality, including an understanding of the importance of the customer, and that there are multiple customers in the production process.
- Top management must sponsor and encourage the continuous improvement of quality, including the wise use of teams that can work effectively together to improve the system and other processes, including group processes and organization and system change skills. .
- Management must learn the meaning of statistical thinking: how to speak with data and manage with facts; how to take the guess work out of decision making; how to reduce variation and unnecessary complexity through the use of seven standard tools of data analysis and display (e.g., cause and effect diagrams, Pareto charts, histograms, scatter diagrams, flow charts, run or trend charts, and control charts); and how to link the results of the use of these tools with the appropriate management action.

There are many visible actions senior management can take to reinforce the implementation of the TQM process within the organization. These actions are categorized under the 12 key concepts of TQM, which have guided the TQM implementation at HFHS.

Discussion

Total Quality Management is a possible answer to the problems besetting healthcare. It is a new paradigm in healthcare management. It is a new way of looking at the delivery of healthcare. This change, like all other changes, will not be easy. Healthcare managers and supervisors are entrenched in their jobs. Change can be threatening. Therefore, TQM needs to be introduced with great care. Anchoring the TQM process at the top management level and rolling it out from top to bottom slowly and deliberately is the answer. Changing the culture of the organization cannot be accomplished quickly— managers must learn to view their jobs differently. Instead of telling employees what to do and when to do it, and inspecting employee performance, managers should be more like coaches. Their job is to guide and lead by example— to detect the need for training and retraining and where barriers need to be systematically brought down. Persistence and patience is essential for successful implementation. In addition, healthcare providers must work with payers and insurance companies jointly to study the current healthcare payment and delivery process. Opportunities to improve the process must be identified followed by pilot implementation. The FOCUS-PDCA [Plan-Do-Check-Act] method can be applied and systematic changes made in the process. Only by examining this process in light of customer-supplier relationships can we make progress that is beneficial to all. TQM holds great promise for healthcare organizations. Total Quality Management implementation will fail if

- Management separates TQM activities from daily work
- It is viewed as a project by employees with a start and finish date
- It is delegated by senior management to a staff function
- It is viewed as activities done in quality committee meetings.

Many of us are now learning that the traditional approaches to quality assurance and cost containment are not the answer; instead we must seek an organizational and cultural transformation committed to improving the quality of everything we do, and through that, enhancing productivity. One learns very quickly that just another program that is designed to be a quick fix is not the answer. Instead, one learns that embarking on total quality management has great potential but that it will only be achieved through the direct involvement of senior managers and their commitment to it.

We found that establishing a Total Quality Management Initiative must begin with CEO curiosity and trustee involvement, followed by the development of a quality framework and a process that involves every major entity in the system.

Special attention must be paid to the introduction of Total Quality Management to senior managers. We found that it needed to begin with in-depth discussions about Deming's 14 points followed by several days in the classroom. At the end of that period, our managers were asked to practice and to begin to facilitate and teach the concepts to others. It is at that point that they begin to internalize the knowledge that they have been exposed to and begin to apply what they have learned, in their day-to-day management practice.

Beyond the senior managers' introduction to the process there must also be the development of individuals at the next level of the organization who have the curiosity, interest, and commitment to become coaches and teachers. In our organization we found that such an approach has allowed us to roll out the program much more quickly, and to create an upward pressure on senior management to maintain its commitment and demonstrate it to the organization.

The development of Total Quality Management Teams has also had a special impact on the organization. Despite the natural tendency to form a team for every problem that surfaces, we found that it is more important to have fewer teams but to have as many people as possible given the opportunity to participate in the process. An example of one team that has demonstrated this is a team that has been trying to define an ideal process for an ambulatory care patient encounter.

It is also desirable to create employee awareness about Total Quality Management through a planned process. This can be accomplished through presentations, employee orientation, corporate newsletters, and external speakers. As the employees learn more about and have an opportunity to participate in the process, a natural curiosity begins to evolve that facilitates the development of the initiative. The greatest benefit we have observed is a boost in morale and pride in the organization.

It is important, however, to recognize that there will be resistance at every level partially because it is a change, partially because of the time that such an initiative takes away from the employee's ordinary duties, and the cost that is associated with it with initially no visible financial return. Finally, it is important to reinforce the fact that cultural transformation requires not only the support of management and its participation, but also requires management to take the time and patience to let it evolve. Anyone becoming interested in Total Quality Management needs to recognize that it is a long journey and that the transformation is not going to happen overnight.

Healthcare leaders have the opportunity to use TQM to cut waste and improve quality of the services provided and in the process keep the healthcare system in the private sector. Can it be done? We think so. It depends on how successful we are in implementing TQM concepts in the healthcare industry.

Henry Ford Health System is dedicated to developing and providing the highest quality, compassionate healthcare to serve the needs of the southeastern Michigan community. The System's services will be the most comprehensive, efficient, and clinically effective in the region, supported by nationally recognized Henry Ford education and research programs.

Vision

Henry Ford Health System will:

- Evolve into the highest quality, most comprehensive and integrated health system in the region.
- Develop a Center for Health Sciences to be engaged in leading edge tertiary care, research and education.
- Provide virtually all of the healthcare needs of the population served, from primary care to highly specialized tertiary care.
- Offer a range of health insurance and managed care programs which meet the diverse needs of the population and payers.
- Think of itself as an entity to which the users of its services belong. Administrative systems will emphasize ease and convenience of use by the members.
- Be a responsible member of the community and assume leadership in developing sound healthcare policies at the local, state and national level.

Quality Definition

Quality is continuous improvement in patient care and service, education and research, and all other activities in which we are involved, in order to make the System a leading standard of excellence within the healthcare industry.

Corporate Values and Quality Guidances

Henry Ford Health System embraces these basic values and quality guidelines and recognizes their role in its continued success.

1. *Customer Focus*
   - Quality patient care and service is a key principle for HFHS.
   - HFHS is committed to continuously improving the quality of services to its internal and external customers, and to giving priority attention to their concerns.
   - Communication with customers is key to better understanding their needs and expectations, continuously improving processes, and building their trust.

2. *Management and Clinical Leadership*
   - Leadership demonstrates commitment and behaves in a manner consistent with quality management concepts, including: team work; continuous improvement; process focus; and statistical thinking.

(continued on next page)

- Leadership accepts principal responsibility for creating an environment that encourages the involvement of all System employees and medical staff in continuous quality improvement.

3. *Employee Focus*
   - HFHS employees are an important asset and resource, and will be treated fairly, with dignity, and respect.
   - Employees will be given an opportunity to develop their potential through education and training, including the use of tools and techniques of quality improvement.
   - Communication with all employees about the System's mission, strategy, plans and objectives is key to building their understanding and trust.
   - Employees are an important source of knowledge about current processes and ideas for improvement.
   - Employees at every level will be active members of quality improvement teams.

4. *Measurement*
   - All work units within the System are committed to using customer and process knowledge as an input to identify key quality indicators.
   - All work units will develop quality reports using key quality indicators to monitor progress and to identify areas for improvement.
   - The System is committed to the process of competitive benchmarking as a means of improving its services.

5. *Community Focus*
   - HFHS will continue to improve the health status of the population it serves.
   - HFHS will volunteer its expertise, time and facilities to meet civic and professional needs; participate in advocacy for healthcare; and be a responsible corporate citizen and neighbor.

6. *Systemness*
   - To deliver quality products and services to our customers, all components of the System must collaborate and work in concert and harmony. The achievement of systemness is essential for consistent quality and service in meeting both internal and external customer expectations.

7. *Recognition and Reward*
   - HFHS leadership will create an environment that encourages people to practice, participate, and teach the principles of quality improvement. Groups and individuals will be recognized for quality improvement practices.

Acknowledgment

The authors wish to acknowledge the helpful comments of many colleagues who read the first draft of this article and gave us many helpful suggestions. Special thanks go to Paul Batalden, M.D., Lauretta Fortune, Linda Taylor, Anita Fennessey Watson, and Richard Wittrup.

References

Batalden, P., D. Smith, J. Bovender, and D. Hardison. 1989. "Quality Improvement: The Role and Application of Research Methods." *Journal of Health Administration Education* 7 (3): 577–83.

Berwick, D. M. 1990. "Commentary: Peer Review and Quality Management—Are They Compatible?" *Quality Review Bulletin. Journal of Quality Assurance* July 16 (7): 246–51.

Caldwell, C., J. E. McEachern, and V. Davis. 1990. "Measurement Tools Eliminate Guesswork." *Healthcare Forum Journal* July–August 33 (4): 23–27.

Coffey, R. J., K. B. Brewer, M. Becker-Staples, and H. L. Hodgson. 1990. "Reduction of Unnecessary Patient Days Through a Total Quality Approach to Improve Discharge Planning." *Proceedings of the Quest for Quality and Productivity Conference*. Norcross, GA: Institute of Industrial Engineers.

James, B. C. 1989. *Quality Management for Health Care Delivery*. Chicago: Hospital Research and Educational Trust, American Hospital Association.

Laffel, G., and D. Blumenthal. 1989. "The Case for Using Industrial Quality Management Science in Health Care Organizations." *Journal of the American Medical Association* November 262 (24): 2869–73.

McEachern, J., L. Schiff, and A. Hallium. 1991. "A Quality Improvement Approach with a Cross Function Team to Lower C-Section Rates." *Proceedings of the Quest for Quality and Productivity Conference*. Norcross, GA: Institute of Industrial Engineers.

Riddle, E. 1990. "Xerox Leadership Through Quality." Presentation made to Henry Ford Health System executive management staff.

Sahney, V. K., J. I. Dutkewych, and W. R. Schramm. 1989. "Quality Improvement Process: The Foundation for Excellence in Health Care." *Journal of the Society for Health Systems* 1 (1): 17–30.

Society for Health Systems and Health Care Information and Management Systems Society. 1990. *Proceedings of the Quest for Quality Conference*. Norcross, GA: Industrial Engineering and Management Press.

Spechler, J. W. 1989. *When America Does It Right: Case Studies in Service Quality*. Norcross, GA: Industrial Engineering and Management Press.

Walton, M. 1986. *The Deming Management Method*. New York: Dodd, Mead & Company.

Discussion Questions

1. What are the central ideas behind quality improvement?
2. What would you look for and expect to see in a healthcare organization which is actively working on quality improvement?
3. Why do quality improvement efforts fail and why do they succeed?
4. If you are the new the head of a healthcare organization and you wanted to strengthen its quality improvement efforts, what would you do?

Required Supplementary Readings

Batalden, P., and P. Stoltz. "Performance Improvement in Healthcare Organizations: A Framework for the Continued Improvement of Health Care." *The Joint Commission Journal of Quality Improvement* October 1993, 19 (10): 424–452.

Bradley, E. H., E. S. Holmboe, J. A. Mattera, S. A. Roumanis, M. J. Radford, and H. M. Krumholz. "The Roles of Senior Management in Quality Improvement Efforts: What Are the Key Components?" *Journal of Healthcare Management* Jan/Feb 2003, 48 (1): 15–28.

Finkler, S. A. "Measuring the Cost of Quality." *Hospital Cost Management and Accounting* February 1996, 7 (4).

Leape, L. "Error in Medicine." *Journal of the American Medical Association* 1994, 272 (23): 1851–57.

Discussion Questions for the Required Supplementary Readings

1. What are the most important things for a health services information system to measure?
2. Errors are frequent in healthcare. They often have serious consequences. What would you do to reduce them?
3. What is the role of senior management in promoting QI?

Recommended Supplementary Readings

Arrington, B., K. Gautman, and W. J. McCabe. "Continually Improving Governance." *Hospital & Health Service Administration* Spring 1995, 40 (1): 95–110.

Austin, C. J., and S. B. Boxerman. *Information Systems for Health and Management*, 6th edition. Chicago: Health Administration Press, 2003.

Batalden, P., E. Nelson, and J. Roberts. "Linking Outcome Measurement to Continual Improvement: The Serial 'V' Way of Thinking About Improving Clinical Care." *Journal of Quality Improvement* April 1994, 20 (4): 167–80.

Batalden, P. B., and P. K. Stoltz. "Performance Improvement in Health Care Organizations: A Framework for the Continual Improvement of Health Care." *The Joint Commission Journal of Quality Improvement* October 1993, 19 (10): 424–52.

Berwick, D. M. "Continuous Improvement as an Ideal in Health Care." *New England Journal of Medicine* 1989, 320 (1): 53–56.

———. "Controlling Variation in Health Care: A Consultation from Walter Shewhart." *Medical Care* December 1991, 29 (12): 1212–25.

———. "The Toxicity of Pay for Performance." *Quality Management in Health Care* 1995, 9 (1): 27–33.

———. *Escape Fire: Lessons for the Future of Health Care.* New York: Commonwealth Fund, 2002.

Carey, R. G., and R. C. Lloyd. *Measuring Quality Improvement in Health Care.* New York: Quality Resources (Division of the Kraus Organizations Limited), 1995.

Codman, E. A. *A Study in Hospital Efficiency* (1917). Oakbrook Terrance, IL: Joint Commission on Accreditation of Health Care Organizations, 1996.

Donabedian, A. *Explorations in Quality Assessment and Monitoring.* 4 vols. Chicago: Health Administration Press, 1980–82.

———. "The End Results of Health Care: Ernest Codman's Contribution to Quality Assessment and Beyond." *The Milbank Quarterly* 1990, 67 (2): 2433–56.

Eisenberg, J. M. *Doctor's Decisions and the Cost of Medical Care.* Chicago: Health Administration Press, 1986.

Finkler, S.A. "Control Aspects of Financial Variance Analysis." In *Health Systems Management Readings and Commentary*, 5th edition, edited by A. Kovner and D. Neuhauser, 171–88. Chicago: Health Administration Press, 1994.

Flood, A. B., J. S Zinn, S. M. Shortell, and W. R. Scott. "Organizational Performance: Managing for Efficiency and Effectiveness." In S. Shortell and A. Kaluzny, *Health Care Management: Organization Death and Behavior*, 4th edition, Albany NY: Delmar Publishers, 2000.

Griffith, J. R., and K. R. White. *The Well-Managed Healthcare Organization*, 5th edition. Chicago: Health Administration Press, 2002.

Griffith, J. R., V. K. Sahney, and R. A. Mohr. *Reengineering Health Care, Building on CQI.* Chicago: Health Administration Press, 1995.

Holland, T. P., R. A. Ritvo, and A. R. Kovner. *Improving Board Effectiveness: Practical Lessons for Nonprofit Health Care Organizations.* Chicago: American Hospital Publishing, 1997.

Huntington, J., and F. A. Connell. "For Every Dollar Spent—The Cost Savings Argument for Prenatal Care." *New England Journal of Medicine* Nov. 10, 1994, 31 (19): 1303–07.

Institute of Medicine. *Crossing the Quality Chasm.* Washington, DC: National Academy Press, 2001.

Juran, D. "It's Not My Problem: The CT Nursing Transport Team." *Quality Connection* Winter 1993, 2 (2): 8–9. Reprinted in *Health Services Management: A Book of Readings,* 6th edition, edited by A. Kovner and D. Neuhauser, 140–145. Chicago: Health Administration Press, 1997.

Kindig, D. *Purchasing Population Health.* Ann Arbor, MI: University of Michigan Press, 1997.

Kovner, A. R., Guest Editor. (Special Issue): "Community Benefit Programs for Health Care Organizations." *The Journal of Health Administration Education* Summer 1994, 12 (13): 253–387.

Leape, L. L. "Practice Guidelines and Standard: An Overview." *Quality Review Bulletin* February 1999: 42–48.

Lewis, L. E. "Improving Productivity: The Ongoing Experience of an Academic Department of Medicine." *Academic Medicine* April 1996, 71 (4): 317–28.

McLachlin, C. and A. Kaluzny. *Continuous Quality Improvement in Health Care,* 2nd edition. Gaithersburg, MD: Aspen, 1999.

Milio, N. *Engines of Empowerment: Using Information Technology to Create Healthy Communities and Challenge Public Policy.* Chicago: Health Administration Press, 1996.

Morrissey, J. "Stocking Up on Savings." *Modern Health Care* June 24, 2002, 32 (25): 28–33.

Mottaz, C. J. "Work Satisfaction among Hospital Nurses." *Hospital & Health Service Administration* Spring 1988, 33 (2): 57–74.

Mutter, M. "One Hospital's Journey Toward Reducing Medication Errors." *Joint Commission Journal in Quality & Safety* June 2003, 29 (6): 279–288.

Neuhauser, D. "The Qualify of Medical Care and the 14 Points of Edwards Deming." *Health Matrix* Summer 1988, 6: 7–10. Reprinted in *Health Services Management: Readings and Commentary,* 4th edition, edited by A. Kovner and D. Neuhauser, 180–86. Chicago: Health Administration Press, 1990.

Neuhauser, D., L. Headrick, and D. M. Miller. "The Best Asthma Care: A Case in Continuous Quality Improvement." *Quality Assurance and Utilization Review* Fall 1992, 7 (3): 76–80.

Pointer, D. D., and J. E. Orlikoff. *Getting to Great: Principles of Health Care Organization Governance*. San Francisco: Jossey-Bass, 2002.

Roovers, T. K. "Improving the Operating Budget Process at Abbott Northwestern Hospital." *The Quality Letter*. Alexandria, VA: Capital Publishing. Reprinted in *Health Services Management: A Book of Readings*, 6th edition, edited by A. Kovner and D. Neuhauser, 146–51. Chicago: Health Administration Press, 1997.

Trabin, T. (ed). *The Computerization of Behavioral Healthcare: How to Enhance Clinical Practice, Management, and Communications*. San Francisco: Jossey-Bass Publishers, 1986.

Tarquinio, G. T., R. S. Dittus, D. W. Dyrue, A. Kaiser, and E. G. Neilson. "Effects of Performance-based Activity, Research Portfolio, and Teaching Mission of the Department of Medicine." *Academic Medicine* July 2003, 78 (7): 690–701.

Umbdenstock, R. J., and W. M. Hageman. "The Five Critical Areas for Effective Governance of Non-For-Profit Hospital." *Hospital and Health Services Administration* Winter 1990, 35 (4): 481–92.

Zelman, W. N., D. Blazer, J. M. Gower, P. O. Bumgarner, and L. M. Cancilla. "Issues for Academic Health Centers to Consider Before Implementing a Balanced Scorecard Effort." *Academic Medicine* 74 (12): 1269–77.

THE CASES

If, as Peter Drucker says, "the basic problem of service institutions is not high cost, but lack of effectiveness,"[1] performance expectations in health services organizations must be defined in terms of goal attainment instead of increased budget allocations. The traditional approach to control when output measures are available, as in automobile production, is to relate capital and operational costs to unit of production. In healthcare, costs are usually related to process activities; therefore, a control system sensitive to cost must include some assurance of quality because cost control does not inherently consider output quality.

The three cases here present very different problems of control. Twin Falls has been recognized as a leader in applying the concepts of continuous quality improvement (CQI) both within their hospital and in the community they serve. Three pillars of CQI are customer-mindedness, statistical-mindedness, and organizational transformation. These pillars relate to the three questions that underlie their goal to make Twin Falls the healthiest community in the country. Why do we do what we do? (Does this meet customer needs?) How do we know it works? (How do we understand and measure the process and the outcomes of care?)[2] How can we do it better? (How do we go about creating a learning organization?)

The cases "The Primary Care Instrument Panel at Central Community Health Plan" and "Memo to the Chief of Pediatrics" both examine the need for information organized in a way to improve quality and manage costs. The first is for a primary care practice in a managed care context. The second is for a hospital-based clinical department.

Notes

1. Peter Drucker, "Managing the Public Service Institution," *The Public Interest* 33 (Fall 1973): 43–60
2. E. J. McEachern, D. Neuhauser, P. Miles, and J. Bingham, "Managing Rural Health Care Reform," in *Health Systems Management: Readings and Commentary*, 7th Edition, edited by Anthony R. Kovner and Duncan Neuhauser, (Chicago: Health Administration Press, 2000), chap. 8.

Case 3
Healthier Babies in Twin Falls, Idaho

Dorothy Shaffer

Emily Blackwell is spending a summer in Twin Falls, Idaho, learning about continuous quality improvement. She has been providing staff support for Paul Miles, M.D., who chairs the hospital's project to make the area the healthiest place in America to have a baby.

Idaho, the seventh most sparsely populated state, has the lowest physician-to-population ratio in the nation (114 physicians per 100,000 people versus a national average of 184 per 100,000).[1] The state's population is one million, with 145,000 people living in Magic Valley, an agricultural-based community in south central Idaho (11,000 square miles). The Valley, composed of eight counties, has a population density of 12.2 persons per square mile (PPSM) compared to the national average of 69.4 PPSM, and two of the counties are classified as "frontier."[1] This area of Idaho is unique with its low population, lack of public transportation, and the worst low-birthweight and perinatal mortality rates in the state. In 1988, Magic Valley's low-birthweight rate was 6.6 percent with a state average of 5.1 percent. Concurrently, the perinatal mortality rate was 10.7 per 1,000 for Magic Valley and 9.2 per 1,000 for the state.[1]

Twin Falls, population 29,000, is the largest town in this eight-county region, and the city is home to the two largest hospitals in Magic Valley. The Southcentral Public Health Department is also located here. There is no managed care in the area or in the state. One of the hospitals, Twin Falls Clinic, with a 44-bed capacity, is under private ownership and is the only hospital in Idaho that is not a member of the Idaho Hospital Association. The facility provides limited services with no general pediatrics or ob-gyn, but it does have some subspecialties unique to the area, including plastic surgery, rheumatology, and endocrinology.[2] The other hospital in Twin Falls is Magic Valley Regional Medical Center (MVRMC), a not-for-profit, county-owned hospital that serves as a secondary care institution for the eight-county region and is designated as the Medicare regional referral center. The hospital is managed by Quorum Health Resources, has a $55 million revenue, and a 165-bed capacity. There are 123 physicians with privileges at MVRMC, 80 of whom are very active. Their patient population is made up of 50 percent Medicare and 14 percent Medicaid patients.[3] Four smaller rural hospitals are also located within this region; they are staffed by family practitioners and all are under different ownership and funding. The Department of Public Health is run by the district and serves this same eight-county region. The department has a number of outlying facilities and multiple specialty and preventive health clinics within its Twin Falls office. All of the hospitals and health services have separate visions, separate patient registrations, and separate databases. Communication between these facilities is poor, and care is often duplicated. Within this environment, healthcare resources are scarce, difficult to access, and disjointed. This is a condition not uncommon to much of America, but because Idaho has an inadequate supply of physicians and resources, the status of its healthcare cannot continue to be ignored. In 1987, the hospital board at MVRMC revised its vision statement to read, "MVRMC will be a standard of excellence and cooperation in making Magic Valley the healthiest place in America." With this change, John Bingham, the hospital administrator, introduced a new way to approach healthcare to achieve this vision. His interests were based on the Deming Management Method,[4] but he was also influenced by both Bronowski[5] and Senge.[6] The process, labeled continuous quality improvement (CQI), emphasizes cooperation, systems thinking, and an understanding of statistical variation and human interactions within a given system. This model involves a strict reliance on data collection and analysis, while using the scientific method to institute change and improvement. Deming, an American statistician whose work was closely linked to Japan's postwar economic growth, used the above ideas to transform business management and production.[4] Bingham wanted to attempt the same transformation in healthcare.

Bingham was aware that many of these ideas were broad and difficult to initiate. Nevertheless, he was driven by two fundamental questions: "Why do we do what we do? And how do we know that what we do works?" which led him to a third question: "How can we make what we do better?"[7] His shift to quality improvement and a systems view of healthcare (see Figure 3.1) was supported by the Hospital Corporation of America (HCA), the hospital's

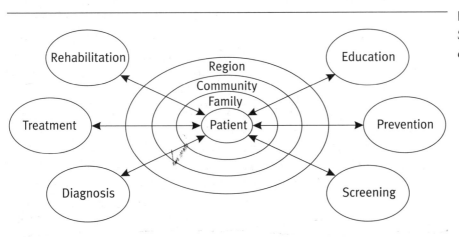

FIGURE 3.1
Systems View of Healthcare

former management group before Quorum. Magic Valley Regional Medical Center became a pilot hospital of HCA for implementing quality improvement. However, even with this support, Bingham had reservations about the change in thinking because the new approach could be perceived as another fad in healthcare reform and the question still persisted of whether Deming's theories could be effective or not in the healthcare industry. Regardless, he started at the top, with the hospital board, as a way to anchor these ideas first and then incorporate them into the daily functioning of the hospitals and the surrounding community.[7] He and the hospital began accomplishing this vision by addressing parts of the system, with the continual focus on restoring and improving the community's health.

During the time of this transition, the state was involved in the Idaho Perinatal Project and had been working for eight years to address the issues of perinatal morbidity and mortality. In an effort to decrease this problem, the project's goal was to standardize the equipment and training for neonatal resuscitation across the state. They successfully improved the facilities and staff training without improving the process, and the mortality rates did not improve. As mentioned, by 1988 the state's perinatal mortality rate was 9.2 per 1,000 and the low-birthweight percentage, an indicator of neonatal morbidity, was 5.1 percent, which still left Idaho with the same problem it had attempted to fix.[1]

Dr. Paul Miles, a pediatrician in Twin Falls and member of the hospital board at MVRMC, was working with the Idaho Perinatal Project. Because of his close connection to Mr. Bingham and the MVRMC, he decided to apply the quality improvement theories to the ongoing perinatal project. Thirty-three physicians in Magic Valley provide obstetrics care, and 20 percent of the MVRMC admissions are pregnancy related. Approximately 50 percent of the total deliveries in the area were performed at MVRMC, with the majority of high-risk newborns treated in their neonatal intensive care unit (NICU).[8]

The very high-risk newborns are transferred to tertiary care centers in Boise, Idaho (130 miles west) or Salt Lake City, Utah (200 miles southeast). This eight-county district, although fully up-to-date with its equipment, still had some of the worst outcome data, mentioned earlier, in one of the worst states. Within this region and using quality improvement guidelines, Miles realized the great opportunity that existed to better the health of pregnant women, newborns, and the community as a whole.

In Miles's thinking, the next step to take in solving the problem of perinatal morbidity and mortality in Idaho centered on the vision of making Magic Valley the healthiest place in America to have a baby and to cooperate with all of the care providers in the area. To achieve this goal, a systems approach was adopted, keeping in mind the strengths and weaknesses of the community while always keeping the patient at the focal point of care. Magic

Valley Regional Medical Center, along with the Public Health Department and a few physicians, began looking at prevention and improvement along with treatment. They wanted to become proactive in their problem solving with an emphasis on continual learning and improving on the existing model.

Formally, the CQI plan contains a step-by-step approach in applying the scientific method to problem solving. Initially, a problem is identified and a plan for improvement is made (the hypothesis). Then, the plan is executed (testing the hypothesis). Next, the results are checked (data analysis). Finally, the results are acted upon (rethinking the hypothesis).[9] And so, once the change has been made, its effectiveness is documented, with the aim to decrease variation within the entire system, thus making the community a healthier place in which to live. While this formal approach to problem solving provides an excellent structure to create positive changes and growth, the initial attempts at applying CQI to the perinatal project were much less formalized. Instead, a few individuals concentrated on the philosophy behind the new approach and used those theories as a guide with the hope that this type of problem solving could help the status of healthcare.

Within this structure, Miles felt that an initial step to improve perinatal morbidity and mortality was to look upstream and concentrate on prenatal care itself, and so his hypothesis—that women who do not receive prenatal care are more likely to have high-risk infants—was tested. This statement is based on the fact that prenatal care is associated with improved perinatal morbidity, but it is unclear what aspects of prenatal care account for this association.[10] By focusing on the area of prenatal care, those involved in the project hoped to see a decrease in neonatal intensive care admissions, a decrease in long-term morbidity of children, and an increase in the overall health of the community. The team that was organized to approach this problem was not an official quality improvement team of the hospital, and its members changed as new areas were addressed. Miles initiated and led many of the efforts of the group and was aided by Bingham of MVRMC; Cheryl Juntensen, director of Public Health District V; Maggi Machala, pregnancy program coordinator for Public Health District V; and the ob-gyn physicians in Twin Falls. The group was organized to meet as a whole in making major decisions, but otherwise individuals would carry out their own projects.

In an attempt to clarify the process of prenatal care current at the time, the group tried to use the perspective of the consumer—the patient—to see how the process worked from that viewpoint. Flowcharts were used in attempting to identify obstacles to care. An informal analysis of access to prenatal care was performed by Machala, and a questionnaire was given to mothers who had delivered at MVRMC in an attempt to identify any complaints and concerns they had about their care. Once all of this information was gathered, the group was able to name some areas for improvement. These areas included

FIGURE 3.2

Obstacles to
Prenatal Care

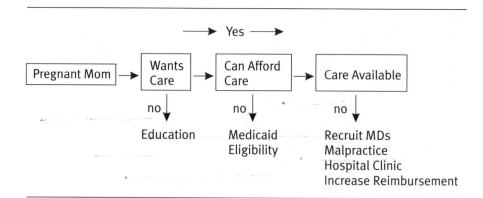

educating the patient about the hospital before she arrived in labor, improving time delays once in the hospital, and ensuring prenatal care to avoid drop-in deliveries. Within the community, improvement areas focused on access, efficiency, and affordability of care. It was clear to Miles that any efforts at improving the current process could greatly benefit the patient population, but the process of this improvement could be time-consuming and difficult.

As a means of reducing the variation of care within the system, the group tried to identify the main problem areas (see Figure 3.2). With respect to access to prenatal care, multiple factors from financial to psychosocial were impeding the process. In 1988, Medicaid eligibility was set at 43 percent of the federal poverty level, which gave insurance to a small number of people in need. However, even for those who were fortunate enough to receive Medicaid, the reimbursement for prenatal care and delivery was only $400, an amount that did not cover the physician's overhead. Also, from the delivering physician's point of view, many of these patients who could not afford their care were also high-liability concerns with multiple, time-consuming psychosocial issues. The availability of physicians was also a problem. In the area were five obstetricians, located in Twin Falls, with all other deliveries performed by family practitioners. However, if a family practitioner performed more than 40 deliveries per year, then his or her malpractice insurance greatly increased.[11] And so, in an area lacking adequate numbers of physicians, not all patients could receive care, and those cut out of the system were the ones who could not pay or were difficult to manage.

With respect to the efficiency of the system, the obstacles to improvement were identified by Machala.[11] She revealed the difficulty that patients were experiencing because of having to make multiple visits to multiple care sites with numerous delays. A patient making different visits to different sites, for pregnancy testing as well as for Women, Infants, and Children (WIC) and Medicaid reimbursement, would increase the physician-to-patient ratio. Also, the group saw the need to improve the efficiency of clinic visits for the public health patient population. And last, they saw patient education as a necessary component of improving the patient's and community's health while preventing future problems.

Instituting these improvement goals was a long process, and at times different members of the group led the effort. In an attempt to increase the affordability of care by increasing Medicaid eligibility, a group effort was made at the state level to lobby for change. In January 1989, the Medicaid eligibility increased from 43 percent to 67 percent of federal poverty level. In August 1989, the federal Office of Budget Reconciliation Act increased eligibility to 75 percent, and later, in April 1990, the level increased to 133 percent of poverty level.[11] These efforts allowed for many more patients to have insurance and seek care.

However, this increase in Medicaid eligibility did not affect physician reimbursement or physicians' desire to take on new patients. So an eight-member committee, supported by the Idaho Medical Association and the Maternal and Child Health Committee, consisting of obstetricians, family practitioners, and pediatricians, lobbied for a change in the reimbursement policy. By 1990, a change was made that decreased pediatric hospital reimbursement to allow for an increase in obstetrical reimbursement. This effort resulted in an increase of prenatal care and delivery reimbursement from $400 to $1,200.[12]

In the area of improving access to care, MVRMC, the Public Health Department, Family Health Services (a community health clinic), and the obstetricians worked together to ensure availability and efficiency of services. At first, the health department created four decentralized area sites and incorporated "one-stop shopping" at each of these sites.[11] The health department also received a federal Maternal and Child Health grant for all women with income below the 185 percent of poverty level. This block grant ensured comprehensive and efficient prenatal care, including one-stop shopping for pregnancy testing and education, smoking cessation, applying for WIC, Medicaid screening and receipt of a temporary card, nutrition counseling, and social work intervention. This program expanded services to many women previously uninsured and enabled the patient to be seen promptly by her physician. Timely obstetrical care could now be provided without the physician being concerned with payment or multiple psychosocial issues. Magic Valley Regional Medical Center also established an obstetrical clinic, staffed by the obstetricians in the community, to ensure that any woman wanting care could receive it if she was not able to be seen at a private office.

Another factor of access to care, the low physician-to-patient ratio, has been a problem well known to the people of Idaho, and any previous effort to improve this condition was encouraged again. However, the group was not successful with recruiting efforts, and some of the obstetricians were not willing to make recruitment a priority, concentrating instead on the other improvement areas. However, the family practitioners, who were limited because of malpractice quotas, were soon able to see more patients because the additional malpractice insurance was being paid for by the county hospitals.[11]

In an attempt to improve the patients' education and perceived need for prenatal care, the Public Health Department, through the block grant, began classes, "Baby Your Baby," to educate future mothers about pregnancy, birthing, child rearing, and contraception. The department identified the women who were smoking and tagged their charts so that all healthcare workers could encourage the patients to stop smoking. These women were also enrolled in smoking cessation classes. The health department worked to ensure that all of their patients were thus educated and informed about their healthcare.

From 1988 to 1991 all of these changes were being instituted in an attempt to test the program's hypothesis, and by the end of 1991 the group was ready to begin data analysis and to see if the expected outcome was accurate. The results would help them answer the questions: "How do we know that pregnant women are getting the best prenatal care that they can, and how do we know that the care we give works?"

With respect to affordability, the number of Medicaid deliveries increased dramatically from 123 in 1988 to 231 in 1990, the year reimbursement fees increased to $1,200, and Medicaid eligibility increased to 133 percent of the poverty level. At the same time, the number of drop-in deliveries, those women receiving no prenatal care, declined (see Figure 3.3).

FIGURE 3.3
Number of Drop-In Deliveries

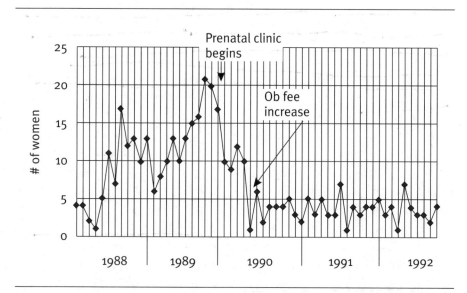

FIGURE 3.4

Number of Low-Birthweight Infants

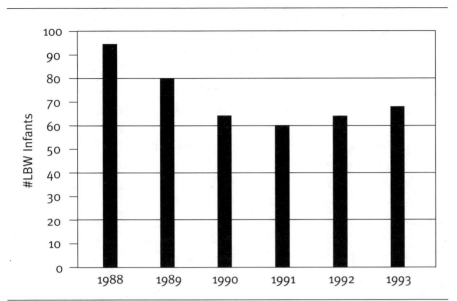

The group also looked at NICU admissions as another indicator of perinatal morbidity, and again they saw a dramatic decline from 184 admissions in 1988 to 137 admissions in 1991. During this decrease in admissions the total number of deliveries at the hospital had increased. The number of NICU patient days, which gives a better indication of how sick the admissions are, showed a steady decline from 1,726 days in 1988 to 974 days in 1990. However, in 1991, the figure increased to 1,162 days. Along with this indicator, low-birthweight figures were analyzed. As hoped for, the incidence of low birth weight decreased along with the increase in prenatal care, but then increased in 1991 (see Figure 3.4).

·With respect to patient education, results were not available for review. The Baby Your Baby classes were well attended, but it was difficult to assess the direct effectiveness of these sessions. Similarly, the results of the smoking cessation program are still being studied and follow-up data are being accumulated.

Financially, both increases and decreases occurred in healthcare costs. Because of the expanded eligibility rules, the number of women receiving Medicaid increased. Approximately 200 more women were enrolled, each costing an average of $2,000 per pregnancy. This increase created an additional cost of $400,000. However, along with this increased expenditure for prenatal care came a decrease in NICU patient days. One day in the NICU costs an average of $1,000. In 1988, the total was 1,726 patient days, while in 1990, it decreased to 974 patient days. This change created a savings of $750,000. During 1991, when the total number of days increased to 1,162 days, the savings as compared to 1988 was still $564,000.[12]

Having found these results, the group concluded that their efforts not only had increased the number of pregnant women receiving care but also had improved the health status of their babies, directly contributing to the overall health of the community. The general agreement was to continue the current care they developed, but from their data they were able to identify some problem areas that still needed improvement. One of these areas was the increase in NICU patient days for 1991. Miles was uncertain whether this figure was part of normal variation or something that could be improved. In attempting to explain the NICU data, he discovered that the twinning rate in Twin Falls for that year had increased compared to past years. Twins are at a 50 percent higher risk for low birth weight and at a five times higher risk for mortality than are single births.[10] Miles discovered that in 1991 the twinning rate in the area was double the national average.[8] This increase was most likely the major cause for the increase in NICU patient days.

However, that odd variation of the twinning rate did not satisfy the group. Some members looked at the issue of prenatal care—its definition and implementation. Different aspects of care vary from physician to physician and, interestingly, since 1988 the rate of women beginning prenatal care within the first trimester has been steady at 60 to 63 percent.[1] The significance of this finding is unclear, but the group is curious to see if increasing that percentage could influence perinatal morbidity and mortality.

These areas, along with programs to improve data collection and to make better use of statistics, are some of the projects that are being considered for the group's next improvement undertaking. However, members are also aware of some inevitable roadblocks. One of the other community obstetricians has increased his prenatal care fees to $2,000, which is above the current Medicaid reimbursement amount of $1,200. It is feared that others might follow his move, possibly leading to a significant decrease in affordability and access to care. Also, five family practitioners in Twin Falls are going to stop their obstetrics service. And the hospital clinic closed with the verbal agreement that the obstetricians in town would care for anyone who needed prenatal care—but that outcome has been difficult to track. The Maternal and Child Health Block grant was discontinued in January 1992, leaving many women without access to comprehensive care, and there still remains for all patients a one-month waiting period for the first obstetrical visit. Further, the Hispanic population in the area is growing, but there are no translation services available within the healthcare system. Finally, Medicaid has stated that it will stop all payment from April 1993 to the beginning of its next fiscal year, July 1, 1993. The obstetricians and family practitioners are unsure if they will take on new patients who will be delivering and not paying for their care during the months from April to July 1993.

Miles is concerned about the course that prenatal care could take and would like to readdress the issues of providers, access, and payment as soon as possible. He would also like to have a better understanding of what specific factors in prenatal care truly affect outcome. He has applied for a grant to develop an interactive video to educate future mothers and to develop a systems approach to prenatal care by creating a uniform database and vision within the entire region.[12] However, the views of the group are varied. Juntensen and Machala, in agreement but aware of their decreased funding, continue to follow the health department's pregnancy program annual plan that highlights the community need for prenatal care as well as the strategies to follow in continuing to improve early access and comprehensive care.[13] But because of the anticipated problems for the future of prenatal care, Machala has distributed a pregnancy program progress report (1989–1991) that emphasizes the need to increase the number of women receiving care in the first trimester. There is also concern about the appropriateness of the current content and amount of patient education and whether or not a need exists for specific education before women actually become pregnant. Mr. Bingham continues to support the efforts of the group and the mission of the hospital, but he has become aware that with this initial improvement in the health of the community, the NICU appears to be becoming underused, overstaffed, and less profitable.[7] This financial reality, while not changing Bingham's vision to improve the health of the community, is a factor that is requiring some of his attention. The obstetricians are not interested in recruiting more physicians; they want to see if there is a problem first before making any further efforts to improve prenatal care. The group plans to meet next month to decide what to do next.

Miles has asked Blackwell to plan the agenda for the next meeting and to give him her priority list for the next steps to take. Blackwell knows that Miles expects three questions to be answered: Why do we do what we do, how do we know what we do works, and how can we make what we do better?

Acknowledgement

The author wishes to thank Paul Miles, M.D., Duncan Neuhauser, Ph.D., and Linda Headrick, M.D., for their teaching and guidance.

Notes

1. Idaho Department of Health and Welfare, *Annual Summary of Vital Statistics* (Boise: IDHW, 1988, 1989, 1990).
2. Conversation with Jodi Craig, August 1992.
3. Magic Valley Regional Medical Center, *MVRMC Current State* (Twin Falls, ID: MVRMC 1989).

4. M. Walton, *The Deming Management Method* (New York: Putnam Publishing Group, 1986).
5. J. Bronowski, *Science and Human Values* (New York: Harper and Row, Publishers, Inc., 1965).
6. P. M. Senge, *The Fifth Discipline* (New York: Doubleday/Currency, 1990).
7. Conversation with John Bingham, July 1992.
8. Perinatal Data Bank (Magic Valley Regional Medical Center, Twin Falls, ID, 1988).
9. Joint Commission on Accreditation of Healthcare Organizations, *Striving Toward Improvement: Six Hospitals in Search of Quality* (Oakbrook Terrace, IL: JCAHO, 1992).
10. N. F. Hacker and M. Moore, *Essentials of Obstetrics and Gynecology* (Philadelphia, PA: W. B. Saunders Company, 1986).
11. M. Machala and M. Miner, "Piecing Together the Crazy Quilt of Prenatal Care," *Public Health Reports* 106 (July–August 1991): 53–60.
12. P. Miles, *A Systems Approach to Rural Prenatal Care*, Unpublished grant proposal.
13. Idaho Department of Health and Welfare, *Pregnancy Program Annual Plan* (Boise: IDHW, 1992).

Case Questions

1. What is the process that leads to healthy babies as viewed by the Twin Falls team?
2. Who is served by this process?
3. How would one measure improvement in the process and outcome?
4. What needs to be done to change the organization of care to keep improving this process?
5. What should the team do next?

Case 4
The Primary Care Instrument Panel at Central Community Health Plan

Duncan Neuhauser

Two student teams are doing a field elective project under the supervision of Peter Alexander, M.D., who is chief medical officer and chief operating officer of Central Community Health Plan (CCHP). Central Community is a managed care plan with 500,000 enrollees in an area with a population of 2.5 million people and is by far the largest health plan in the area.

The teams each include a medical student, nursing student, and health management student, all of whom are enrolled in an interdisciplinary course on continuous quality improvement (CQI) in healthcare. The teams are expected to work on a problem assigned to them: to understand the process and causes of variation, and to plan an improvement to this process.

Dr. Alexander finished his residency in general internal medicine the week before he started this job at Central Community Health Plan (CCHP), turning down several similar positions to accept this one. Before starting his residency, he worked for the Hospital Corporation of America. He did his residency on a half-time basis. While doing so, he developed a successful consulting company advising physician groups about managed care.

Peter: CCHP now contracts with 3,000 independent providers who are mostly physicians in our service area. We have contracts with 22 hospitals in the area, which account for about a third of the total in the area. These contracted hospitals agree to provide care at low prices and to participate in utilization review, and have reputations for good care. The physicians also have contracts defining the prices they charge for services and agreeing to utilization review. CCHP has revenue and expenses of about $2 billion a year.

Student: All over town, hospitals and physician groups are being purchased and grouped together as systems of care competing with each other. Do you plan to do this?

Peter: We have three choices. First, we could buy hospitals, group practices, nursing homes, pharmacies, home care organizations, and such. A lot of capital would be tied up in this approach, but we would have more direct control.

Our second choice is to buy nothing, but contract with independent physicians, hospitals, and other providers. In this case, our organization will be small in staff. I envision a corporate headquarters of about 50 people for this $2 billion to $3 billion corporation. Our corporate staff will consist of physicians, practice management consultants, management information system managers, quality improvement coaches, and people who write contracts with providers and employer groups. The value added, based on the relatively small capital invested (compared to owning hospitals), would be great.

The third choice would be a mix of one and two. If the opportunity or need arose to own a provider corporation, we could buy it. We would take a mixed approach, depending on the circumstances. Of these three, we are taking the second approach for now.

[handwritten annotations:]

→ No objective → What will we measure & how

* PRO-ACT good analytical tool

* keys to understand the organization as is b/f we make changes   Peter Alexander is the control system

> Design a control system → Hard to look @ alternatives

Student: Is this wise? Why wouldn't the providers create their own managed care plan and go directly to the payers, thereby passing CCHP entirely? In a sense, HMOs like Kaiser Permanente do this.

Peter: HMOs like Kaiser Permanente have a different set of strengths and weaknesses and a role to play. We think there is a larger role for a plan like CCHP.

We are planning to select about 800 primary care providers out of our 3,000 providers and to work with them closely. We call this core group our "platinum providers." The 800 physicians are members of 90 group practices. They will have an opportunity to own part of CCHP. We will provide them with expert advice on improving their practice. We will provide an information system in support of their practice, which will have several components. It will eliminate their back office paperwork related to billing. The patient's credit card or CCHP member card "swiped" by a machine reader will bring up the patient's record, record the care provider, and make billing from plan to provider automatic. The patient's self-pay component will be taken care of before the patient leaves the office.

We plan to have a council of expert medical advisers to bring the latest knowledge to our partnership. Our staff is prepared to assess the group's readiness for managed care and to give advice on improving market share, improving office practice, analyzing competitors, and planning. We plan to be able to provide these groups with accounting support, information systems, and group purchasing with the goal of reducing the percentage of the group's income that goes to office expense from the current 55 percent to 35 percent. We plan to have the capacity to develop "clinical profiling" for individual physicians and groups and for all our plan members. These include

1. pathophysiological outcomes (for example, average blood-sugar level for your diabetics);
2. patient satisfaction;
3. functional health status (for example, sickness days);
4. future patient health risk (for example, percent of appropriate patients who have had mammography); and
5. costs to payer of plan—both direct and indirect (for the XYZ corporation, the costs per employee and family member, both medical care costs and other company costs such as sick leave days).

These measures will be the basis for data displayed on our physician instrument panel.

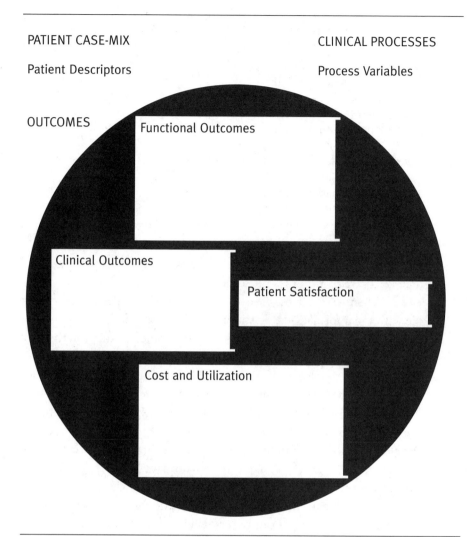

PATIENT CASE-MIX

Patient Descriptors

CLINICAL PROCESSES

Process Variables

OUTCOMES

Functional Outcomes

Clinical Outcomes

Patient Satisfaction

Cost and Utilization

FIGURE 4.1

Template for an Instrument Panel Displaying Inputs (Patient Case-Mix Variables), Clinical Process Variables, and Outputs (Clinical Outcomes, Functional Outcomes, Patient Satisfaction, and Cost and Utilization)

Student: What is an instrument panel?

Peter: It's like flying an airplane. What "real time" information should a primary care provider have to be able to manage his or her practice superbly? Our goal is to have ready access to the information needed to measure costs, quality, and satisfaction for the physician's panel of providers at CCHP. Here is an outline of one (see Figure 4.1).

Student: Will you pay the doctors more if they have better satisfaction scores than others? Will you punish those with worse scores? I know of a managed care plan where doctors get $10,000 end-of-year bonuses for very satisfied patients and lose $10,000 if their patients are dissatisfied.

Peter: What would be Dr. Edward Deming's answer to that question? Our whole idea is to be partners with physicians, not to punish them and

TABLE 4.1
Basic Statistics for the Total Health Insurance Product (HMO, Managed Care, Medicaid HMO, Individual Company Plan, etc.)

Per Member per Month (PMPM); Statistics by Each Provider
• Inpatient days PMPM • Outpatient days PMPM • Specialty services PMPM • Total care PMPM • Inpatient admissions per 1,000 members • Inpatient average length of stay • Paid by plan per inpatient admission • Paid by plan per inpatient day • Paid outpatient care claim • Paid specialty care claim

not to own them. They have suffered too much from unthinking, venal managed care plans. We want to be different.

When we meet next week, I want one student team to present me with the information that should be in our primary care instrument panel. Here are some ideas. Table 4.1 shows some information that will help us track our comparative costs.

You might also think about the HEDIS measures. As you know, these are the performance measures that employer-payers judge us on. They expect us to have this information. The HEDIS data are changing but will continue to include such measures as (1) the percentage of the elderly who've had influenza immunizations; (2) the percentage of women of the appropriate age ranges who have had a Pap smear and mammography; (3) the percentage of our children who are up-to-date on their immunizations; and (4) how we are doing on our prenatal and well-child visits. Many of our payers will insist on seeing these data.

Here is an example of a reporting form about patient satisfaction generated by a national healthcare marketing research corporation (see Figure 4.2). The bar graph shows the results of three yearly surveys of member satisfaction for the Alpha Health Plan. Their satisfaction is improving, but tracks at below the average for all plans and is significantly below the best HMO in their market. Perceptions about access to specialty care are going down over time for Alpha Health Plan and are now significantly below the average of all HMOs and worse than the top HMO.

We're also thinking about generating another kind of report from information we can get now from our insurance information system. This physician report would give average information for all the members of the group and for the individual physician. It would show for Dr. Athens' patients their average age, utilization by age, case

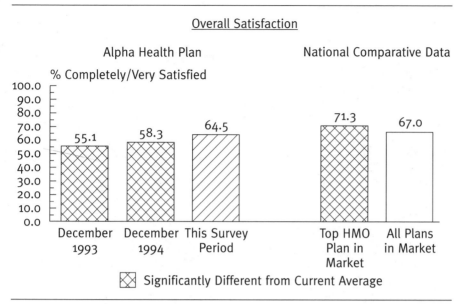

Overall Satisfaction

FIGURE 4.2
Alpha Health Plan—Health Plan Report of General Member Satisfaction, December 1995 (Total Sample N=384)

severity, future risk, payments by diagnostic codes, and utilization over time compared to all the members in our HMO. A map would show the residence of patients coming to the group practice of Dr. Athens. A third report would list procedure codes and her charges to our health plan (see Table 4.2). If you look closely, you will see that these numbers are made up, but they give you an idea of what they could look like.

Student: It looks like the doctors are being paid on a fee-for-service basis now rather than capitation. Can you lower costs that way?

Peter: Good question. There are several possibilities. Good physicians are ready to adjust their practice patterns to fit the partnership goals. We can change the payment methods and we would do this in cooperation with our platinum provider partners. With 90 practices, we can do cooperative experimental changes by inviting some groups to change, measuring the results, and then watching to see what happens. The bottom line is that it is in all our interests to prosper and not go out of business.

However, our fee-for-service process is now the way our data are generated. We know who our enrollees are, where they live, and some basic demographics (age, sex, family size). We know the charges sent in by doctors, x-ray, labs, pharmacy, and hospitals linked to the patient and to the patient's primary doctor.

Student: What is a value compass?

Peter: Think of a regular compass. Patient satisfaction is measured in the northern direction, functional status (like average activities of daily

TABLE 4.2
A. R. Athens,
M.D.: Procedure
Codes
Submitted
to CCHP,
1/1/96–
11/15/96

Description	Number	Total Charges	Average
Office/out PT visit (E&M) estab PT: moderate complexity, 25 min.	187	$12,903	$69
Office consultation new/estab PT: high complexity, 80 min.	55	$11,660	$212
Office/out PT visit (E&M) estab PT: low complexity, 15 min.	222	$11,100	$500
Inj., tendon sheath, ligament/ trigger points/ganglion cyst	43	$3,080	$71
Arthrocentesis, aspiration and/or injection; major joint	25	$1,950	$78
Arthrocentesis, aspiration and/or injection; small joint, bursa/ ganglion	25	$1,550	$62
Office consultation new/estab PT: moderate complexity, 60 min.	7	$1,246	$178
Office consultation new/estab PT: low complexity, 40 min.	5	$780	$156
Arthrocentesis, aspiration and/or injection; intermed. joint	10	$670	$67
Office/out PT visit (E&M) estab PT: high complexity, 40 min.	5	$640	$128
Office consultation new/estab PT: low severity, 30 min.	5	$580	$116
Injection triamcinolone acetonide, per 10 mg	31	$465	$15
Office/out PT visit (E&M) estab PT: problem/minor 10 min.	7	$287	$41
Immunization, active influenza virus vaccine	12	$180	$15
Administration of influenza virus vaccine	9	$90	$10
Incision & drainage of abscess; simple or single	1	$70	$70
Office/out PT visit (E&M) estab PT: minimal, 5 min.	2	$68	$34
Methotrexate sodium, 50 mg	1	$23	$23
Injection, vitamin B-12 cyanocobalamin, up to 1000 mcg	2	$22	$11

living score) is to the west, costs per members per month to the south, and physiologic status to the east. Each of these is scored along each direction. The goal is to be farthest away from the center on all four directions. This form of presentation allows for comparisons with the previous level or with others.

I want one student team to present to me what you think should be the core information for the physician's instrument panel. Be prepared to tell me how it will be collected, how it should be used, and how useful it will be for achieving our goal of excellent care at a reasonable and competitive price.

Here are two more reporting forms I want you to look at. The first is a "spider web diagram" (see Figure 4.3). Such diagrams can show many performance measures. In this example, each measure is based on a target that becomes 100 percent and the points indicate how closely the group has achieved each goal. In this case, 85 percent of employees are satisfied with their work while 98 percent of outpatients and plan members are satisfied. This example of a spider diagram comes from a large hospital-based system.

The other performance report is from a regional hospital. One of its quality indicators is readmission within 14 days after a prior discharge. This is reported monthly over three years with three sigma upper and lower control limits. If a point is outside these control limits, this would be "out of control." As you can see, the percentage of readmissions is stable at 3 percent over this time with random fluctuation (see Figure 4.4). The control limits vary with each measure as a result of small changes in the number of admissions per month. What tools would you recommend we use and why?

I have a task for the other student team. As you know, we can't just give out this information and expect it to be used. We are planning an ongoing, continuing medical (and nursing) education program using the method of academic detailing. To start, when a group practice is ready to have a third individual and comparative practice data printout, one of our central office physicians and administrative staff will visit their plan to review their own information. We expect they will be interested in learning and improving in one or more of their care dimensions. We must be prepared to respond "just in time" to this perceived need with a package of learning material (articles, audiotapes, videotapes, special consultation, seminars, or whatever learning modality they prefer). If they want to improve patient satisfaction, we need to be ready with immediate practical answers.

Student: What is academic detailing?

Peter: It's the same idea as a drug company detail selling, where a representative goes to the doctor's office to educate the physician about the

FIGURE 4.3
Lutheran
Medical Center
Performance
Report

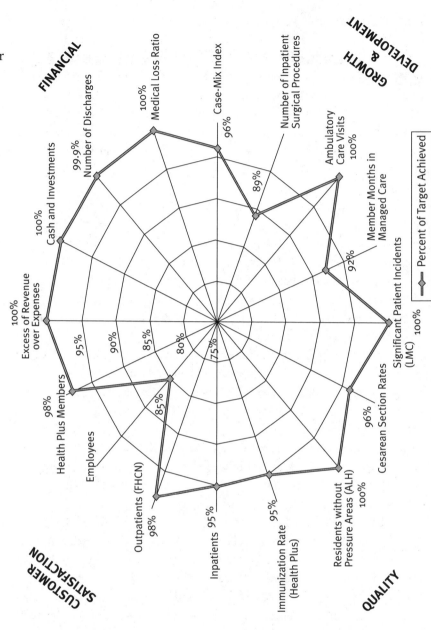

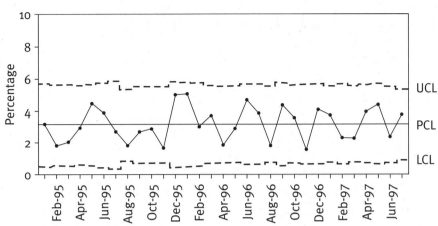

FIGURE 4.4
Readmissions
Within 14 Days
of Prior
Discharge,
1995–1996

UCL = Upper Control Limit (+3 Sigma), LCL = Lower Control Limit (0)
Indicator: Readmissions within 14 days of prior discharge
Numerator: The number of patients readmitted
Denominator: Patients admitted to ANMC
Dimension(s) of Performance: Appropriateness, Continuity, Effectiveness, Efficacy
Analysis: Chart displays normal variation. Control limits recalculated as of June 1997.

benefits of his or her company's product. Academic detailing uses the same method, but sends out academic health center staff to provide education about good care practices.

I want the second student team to report back next week on the educational topics we need to have ready to go. Bring me a list and be prepared to explain the reasons for inclusion. You might even draft a full outline of a top-priority topic.

See you next week.

Case Questions

1. Design the physician "instrument panel." What should be in it?
2. Justify your rationale for these components. How costly would it be to obtain this information?
3. What is needed to implement your goal of an appropriate instrument panel? (Just defining the ideal does not get you there.)
4. Compare the spider diagram and control chart approaches. Which would you recommend and why?
5. Design a "just-in-time" education program to respond to requests from physician groups. What topics should be covered?
6. For a high priority topic, outline the content of the educational module.

Case 5
Memo to the Chief of Pediatrics

David Valacer and Jeanne Weber

MEMORANDUM

To: Chief, Department of Pediatrics
From: David Valacer and Jeanne Weber
Date: October 29, 2001
Re: Control Systems for the Department of Pediatrics, Eastern Shore Medical Center

As the new Chief of Pediatrics, you have an opportunity to establish an environment that will align with the Medical Center administration's vision of developing Eastern Shore Medical Center (ESMC) into a medical facility with clinical centers of excellence, higher ranking residency programs, and a center of clinical research. With that in mind, we present the following recommendations to you as you plan the restructuring of the Department of Pediatrics, its operations, and departmental policy.

Pediatrics: Performance, Objectives, and Accountability

Pediatrics is one of 12 clinical departments at ESMC, a member hospital of the Alliance Health System of Central New Jersey (see Figure 5.1). The work of the unit can be divided into three primary service areas: Clinical, Educational and Research. The Clinical Service provides general and specialty medical services to infants, children, and adolescents hospitalized at ESMC or through the hospital-based pediatric ambulatory service. The inpatient unit has 27 beds for general and specialty Pediatric medical and surgical services, a 21-bassinet Level III Regional Perinatal Center with a Neonatal Intensive Care Unit, a 6-bed Pediatric ICU (PICU), and a same-day surgical recovery stay area. The 27-bed inpatient unit has an average daily census of 13 to 15 children, and the PICU has an average daily census of three to four patients. Comprehensive outpatient care is provided through the Family Health Center's Pediatric Clinic located on the hospital campus. The hospital is currently completing arrangements to set up satellite Pediatric subspecialty ambulatory consultation services at Brookside Medical Center, another Alliance Health System hospital located about 30 minutes from ESMC. The Educational Service supports Accreditation Council for Graduate Medical Education (ACGME) residency training in general pediatrics and pediatric clinical rotations for students for

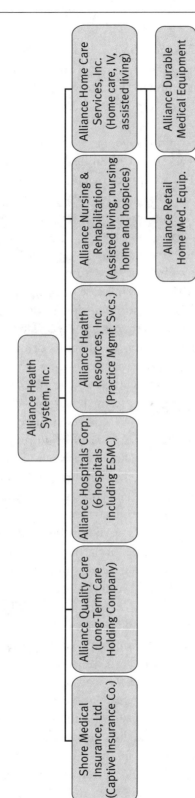

FIGURE 5.1
Current
Corporate
Structure

1. Joint Ventures between Alliance Health System, Inc. and other third parties are not reflected above.
2. Alliance Health Resources, Inc. is owned equally by Alliance Health System, Inc. and Alliance Hospitals Corporation.

the South State Medical College (SSMC). Individual faculty currently participate in limited industry-sponsored, contract-funded clinical research trials. Investigator-initiated, grant-funded clinical research has occurred rarely over the past five years, and there are no basic science research programs at the ESMC campus.

Pediatrics provides comprehensive care to newborns, infants, children, and adolescents with a broad range of healthcare issues. The service seeks to improve the care provided to patients by making the transition from inpatient to outpatient care seamless. The Department has initiated a five-year strategic plan to further develop the continuum of services provided by expanding subspecialty clinical services on-site and to expand community outreach by increasing full-time equivalent (FTE), hospital-supported, subspecialty faculty. The objective is to double ambulatory pediatric specialty patient visit volume by the fourth quarter of 2004, and to increase subspecialty pediatric staff from 9.0 FTEs to 13.5 FTEs. This increase in full-time faculty also will facilitate the Department's immediate goal of attracting higher quality clinical interns and residents by improving the reputation and status of its residency program. In the past five years, we have received very few residency applicants from the U.S.-based medical school graduate pool. Our objective is to increase the number of these applicants to 25 percent of our applicant pool by the end of 2006. Finally, the hospital and the Department have identified expansion of clinical research activities by Pediatric faculty and residents. To foster development, ESMC is organizing a Clinical Research Center (CRC) that will support both inpatient and outpatient clinical research activities. The immediate objective is for each full-time Pediatric faculty member to initiate one clinical research trial (funded or unfunded) using the CRC resources within the next 24 months. Within five years, each full-time Pediatric faculty member is expected to be the on-site principal or participating investigator of at least one contract or grant-funded clinical research project.

The Chief is responsible for directing all administrative and clinical aspects of Pediatrics. You are accountable for organizing full-time and voluntary faculty to realize current objectives and to develop short-term and long-range strategies for unit growth and development. You will lead the planning and expansion of the pediatric ambulatory center and oversee the operation of its clinical services. Additionally, you will lead the development of the faculty practice expansion strategy, and be responsible for negotiating agreements for satellite services and forging alliances with voluntary faculty. Other responsibilities include organizing and directing the residency training program, crafting the training experience of interns and residents, and planning the development and securing grant funding for the Pediatric arm of the CRC. Assessment of your performance is complex and will include attaining or making significant progress toward achieving Departmental objectives in the core competency areas of clinical and educational services as well as making significant advances in the development of a clinical research program. As with all other full-time faculty, you are expected to increase admission and ambulatory visit volume in your subspecialty area as well.

Measures of Performance

In order to determine whether we meet the objective of increasing specialty patient volume, methods must be developed to track and measure a variety of patient data. For the Departmental clinical service component of the unit, desired data includes hospital discharges, daily inpatient census, length of stay by admitting diagnoses, and ambulatory visits including the number and source of new referrals. Additionally, it is important to track payer mix, case mix by diagnosis, and geographic home residence location. Equally important is the need to develop a system to accurately assess patient satisfaction, staff satisfaction, and changing community needs.

To benchmark our Pediatric residency training program, we need to begin by reviewing the residency applications for the past five years to extract data regarding undergraduate and graduate training, ethnic and geographic origin, and stated long-term career and life goals. An anecdotal assessment of how the hospital and its residency program are viewed by medical students would also be beneficial in order to address the hospital's reputation to would-be applicants. Prospective applicant tracking will be necessary to maintain an applicant information database capable of identifying changes in applicant demographics. Going forward, annual review of where those candidates ranked highly by us in the residency match end up (if they do not come to ESMC) will provide us with a list of our nearest "competitor programs" against which we can compare our relative strengths, weaknesses, and opportunities for improvement.

The creation of an institutional CRC at ESMC is central to the development of a clinical research program in Pediatrics. A CRC capable of supporting adult and pediatric clinical research for both hospitalized and ambulatory based protocols will require a substantial investment by the hospital in space and trained personnel capable of supporting clinicians as they develop clinical research skills, implement protocols, and market ESMC CRC opportunities to potential industry partners. Tracking available grant opportunities and appropriate physician response is important. Time and effort spent on grant submissions, fund seeking, and physician effort in this activity must be recognized, perhaps by the development of some sort of relative value unit system. An outside development consultant might be considered to provide important insight and advice in developing this new core competency.

Incentives to Affect Attainment of Objectives

Clinical Service

Full-time faculty members do not have incentives to attain the Department's objective to increase pediatric specialty patient volume. While staff physicians must generate a minimum faculty practice income to ensure their contract salary, exceeding minimum target volume does not result in additional income. Failure to achieve target practice levels results in dollar-for-dollar loss of individual income, but there is no other immediate consequence to falling short of volume targets. Repeated failures to build volume might eventually result in loss of reappointment; however, there is no recent precedent for this response from administration. An additional disincentive to increasing faculty practice volume is the current collection ratio of less than 50 percent for private practice billing. Currently clinical faculty staff are likely to realize a very poor return on any increase in clinical effort even if an incentive plan were put in place.

There are no direct financial incentives to increasing inpatient or outpatient Medicaid or indigent patient care services. The ambulatory Medicaid fee schedule and collection ratio is far worse than that of private payers (including managed care organizations) and the patient population is very often far more demanding. The disincentives for full-time faculty who cover the ward service are similar. Medicaid reimbursement rates for in-hospital physician services are not competitive with the inpatient or outpatient fees of private insurers. The faculty perceives that they are better off focusing their clinical efforts on their private practice patients to meet their revenue targets rather than pursuing excellence in clinical ward service.

That said, there are non-financial incentives to full-time faculty for both ambulatory and ward service activity including recognition of professional expertise amongst community, peers, and staff; personal gratification (so-called "psycho-dollars"); and access to potential future clinical research subjects. Voluntary staff may respond to similar non-financial incentives of recognition and personal gratification.

Educational Service

Voluntary faculty is required to perform clinical service in return for active admitting privileges to the Pediatric inpatient service, and many voluntary faculty gain personal and professional satisfaction from academic clinical service. There is a relative disincentive to participation for some voluntary faculty members in that opportunities for clinical service are limited to rotations as voluntary ward attendings requiring one to two hours daily to supervise residents and medical students. This single option for participation prevents some private practitioners, who are more distantly located from the hospital, from taking a more active role in the clinical teaching service.

There are negative financial incentives for full-time faculty to increase participation in resident and medical student education beyond the department's required minimum. Additional time spent in teaching activities reduces time available to pursue revenue-producing activities. Currently there is no relative value unit system by which teaching quality and/or effort can be translated into financial or non-financial rewards for voluntary or full-time faculty.

As with clinical practice, both voluntary and full-time faculty may be inspired by recognition and/or personal gratification. Continued designation as a major teaching hospital of the State Medical College is an important non-financial incentive to the full-time faculty, especially in maintaining an academic appointment and furthering their own career aspirations.

Research

While occasional private practitioners (usually subspecialists) do participate in industry-sponsored clinical research, the department's research focus is centered on full-time faculty. There are short- and long-term financial incentives to engaging in funded clinical research. Short-term incentives include a potentially substantial revenue stream to support service expansion and development and professional recognition at local, national and perhaps international levels. Long-term incentives are the multiple career opportunities that result from professional development. Also, there are important non-financial incentives similar to those discussed in the Educational section above. The Medical Center has no core research laboratory space to promote bench research, although collaboration with the State Medical College is possible.

Strengths and Weaknesses of the Control System

The Department is organized in a classic vertical hierarchy. All full-time staff physicians are employees of ESMC. The Chief of Pediatrics, a newly created full-time position, is elected by the voluntary faculty for a three-year term and must be reappointed through this process. The Chief reports directly to the hospital CEO. The Chief is director of the ACGME-accredited General Pediatric residency program, and along with the Director of Housestaff Education coordinates all Pediatric resident and medical student rotations and academic programs. Currently, in most Pediatric subspecialties, there is one full-time faculty member. There is an approved plan to recruit second members into each subspecialty area. All of the current full-time faculty report directly to the Chief of Pediatrics. With the introduction of additional faculty members into each subspecialty division, staff will report through Section Chiefs to the Department Chief. There is very little ongoing quality assessment in the Department. Monthly Morbidity and Mortality Rounds report and record adverse events on hospitalized patients and nursing incident reports document less serious patient accidents. There is no systematic evaluation of even simple quality measures, such as length of stay, which could be benchmarked across physician staff or to other similar hospitals.

As is true in most U.S. hospitals, all inpatient and outpatient pediatric nursing personnel report to the appropriate director within the Department of Nursing. Similar reporting lines exist for Pediatric Social Workers, faculty practice support staff and administrators through the Departments of Social Work Services or Clinical Business Administrative Services. There is no official cross accountability between these different service lines.

The current top-down departmental management system facilitates crafting and clearly stating a cohesive vision for the Pediatrics Department and developing a strategic plan for implementation. There are clear lines of responsibility for decision making which can expedite realization of interim objectives and long-term goals. This system also supports a more consistent and coordinated public representation of the department. The difficulty with this system is that it fails to fully engage several groups of important stakeholders, including the full-time and voluntary faculty, pediatric allied health workers, and consumers in defining a common vision or planning short- and long-term strategies to move the department toward vision-oriented goals. The lack of democratic process fails to fully engage physicians and gain their complete and long-term investment in pursuing goals and objectives. This system also fails to recognize the role of the consumers and the purchasers of pediatric healthcare, as important stakeholders deserving input into the planning process.

The most serious weakness in the current control system is the lack of a comprehensive clinical information system capable of providing any measure of quality. There is an electronic scheduling system that physicians can use to track simple targets like practice volume and payer mix. Private ambulatory practice activity can be tracked through outsourced billing records that provide some simple financial measures. Hospital discharge data provide rough estimates of inpatient service quantity and market share, but neither efficiency or productivity for inpatient or outpatient services is measured or tracked.

Recommendations to Improve the Control System

Hospital by-laws require that there be a single Chairman of each clinical department with ultimate responsibility for departmental functions and public representation. While the new full-time Chairman's role in the public pronouncement of the Pediatric Department's mission and vision is of pivotal importance, it is recommended that the department's administration reorganize overall into a less vertical, more horizontal hierarchy. Greater input from full-time subspecialty faculty is key to proposing and refining mutually agreed upon goals and objectives, and in developing and implementing strategic plans to achieve them. Ownership is crucial if the department is to focus the entire physician staff's energy into the timely realization of objectives in clinical, educational, and research arenas simultaneously. Specifically, it is recommended that subspecialty section representatives be assembled into a Faculty Executive Committee responsible for developing well-articulated and reasonably achievable objectives that can move the department forward in its two core competencies of clinical and educational services while developing increasing competency in clinical research. Recognizing that voluntary private physician staff are also important stakeholders in the future growth and development of Pediatrics, it is recommended that a parallel, democratically chosen Voluntary Faculty Executive Committee be assembled. This committee could work with the new Chief to clearly define unmet needs of the voluntary staff, prioritize them, and recommend action plans by which hospital administration might address these needs. Most notably, recognizing that healthcare consumers are important stakeholders in the future of the department, it is recommended that a working pediatric community advisor board be assembled. Members should be prepared to sit as representatives on one of the two proposed physician committees as well as meet together with the two committees regularly.

In the short term, the opportunity to shift non-physician staff (nurses, aides, secretaries, billers) out of their traditional departmental reporting hierarchies is not feasible. Early attempts to do so may impede the Department's ability to achieve initial and necessary successes, especially in financially important areas. It is, however, vital that the new Chief of Pediatrics include integrated hospital services in the strategic planning process from the outset. We recommend that the Directors of Nursing, Clinical Business Administrative Services, and Social Work Services be invited to sit on the two physician executive committees. These three directors should appoint representatives from their respective departments to work with one or two physician staff members in cross-service, goal-oriented task forces assembled to address specific objectives. These task forces will present recommendations to the appropriate physician executive committee including the pediatric community board representatives, these three key Directors, and the Departmental Chief. The inclusive nature of these committees should encourage cooperation across traditionally separate hospital services and promote implementation of mutually agreed upon operational and policy changes without disturbing the present hospital organizational structure.

We recommend that you identify the development of a comprehensive electronic information system as an early strategic priority for the envisioned growth and development of the department. Timely access to clinical and financial data will be essential to evaluating productivity, efficiency, and population outcomes. Opportunities for accurately measuring, tracking, and benchmarking performance at many levels are dependent upon comprehensive information systems. We suggest that you immediately join with other Clinical Chiefs and key hospital administrators to address this serious, hospital-wide administrative deficiency. Information services are not only necessary to support the desired development of clinical services, but are essential to the development of clinical research programs as they provide the necessary electronic patient databases. Implementation of comprehensive information systems also will support and enhance medical student and residency education programs by teaching new physicians how to use such systems to implement quality assessment and improvement programs in both the inpatient and outpatient settings.

While initiatives to improve clinical service and financial management for the department will be seriously impaired in the scope and rate of progress without the installation of adequate information services, this may be the hardest recommendation to implement in the short term. The hardware, software, and human resources required to start up and maintain the necessary system will require a significant financial investment from the hospital.

Case Questions

1. What information should be collected? How often?
2. How should the information system be aligned to the organization of the department? Of the Alliance Health System?
3. How would you introduce this system so the people who need to use it will:
   a. understand it, and
   b. use it correctly (entry of data, interpretation of the results)?
4. How will you know if the system is a success?

Short Case C
CQI at Suburban Hospital

Larry K. McReynolds

Clara Maass Health System is composed of a 475-bed community hospital, a 120-bed long-term facility, a 10-bed subacute unit, and a visiting nurse agency located in north Newark, New Jersey. The hospital is the largest entity of the health system, having been in existence for 125 years. As a community-based nonteaching hospital, the medical staff is an older, conservative group wary of change. The employees pride themselves on being part of their local hospital but have recently become disturbed at the changes occurring in their health system.

The introduction of managed care into the local marketplace has caused the hospital administration much worry that change must occur to service in the immediate future. Some of the key factors causing concern are as follows:

1. The county in which Clara Maass is located has 14 other hospitals, making the county over-bedded by 200 percent.
2. The competitive environment is enabling managed care companies to force hospitals to take rates below their costs.
3. The hospital's average length of stay and average cost per discharge are significantly higher than those of other hospitals in the area.
4. Many of the physicians are close to retirement and see little reason to change their ways of practicing medicine at this stage of the game.
5. Employee morale is low as a result of cost-cutting, two recent layoffs, and no raises for two years.

Implementation of a CQI program by administration is an attempt to help bring about some of the needed changes in the organization. The hospital CQI program has been approved by the board of trustees and has been in place for almost two years.

Implementation of the CQI program was accomplished through required CQI training for managers, all employees, and as many physicians as possible. Initially, quality action teams (QATs) were chartered to examine clinical and operational issues. The patient services department selected the CareMap format for addressing physician and multidisciplinary issues. CareMaps are multidisciplinary tools for establishing protocols, outcomes, and length of stay.

CareMaps were developed using the primary nurse model, placing the nurse as the responsible party for keeping the patient on the map. Operational QATs were chartered by the steering committee to address processes and procedures that were high-volume, problem-prone, costly, or likely to have an adverse effect on the patient. Elements predictive of patient satisfaction were also used to determine if a QAT should be chartered.

To facilitate integration of CQI principles among all employees, managers attend an ongoing workshop. This monthly meeting is designed to provide a nonthreatening forum for managers to examine their department processes and outcomes and the degree of the department's success in meeting the customer's needs. Ideas from the workshop and suggestions from the

CareMap and QATs are approved by the steering committee and implemented by the team.

Case Questions

1. Employees have the feeling that eliminating "wasted work" and improving processes is a fancy way of eliminating more jobs. Identify strategies to overcome this impression.
2. Managers feel this is the management philosophy of the week. Identify and describe effective means to overcome this barrier.
3. Physicians see CareMaps as cookbook medicine imposed upon them by the nursing department. Describe ways to get them to buy into CareMaps.
4. Identify organizational strategies that the hospital should adopt to make the institution more viable in the marketplace.

Short Case D
ER at Queens Hospital Center

Anthony R. Kovner

Currently 83 percent of patients at the Queens Hospital Center emergency room are treated and released. They wait six to eight hours for treatment. The goal is to decrease waiting time and the number of walkouts and to improve care and patient satisfaction.

Current Procedure:
Step 1. Patient seen by triage nurse.
Step 2. Patient sent to registration.
Step 3. Patient waits to be seen by physician.
Step 4. Patient sent for any necessary lab or x-ray.
Step 5. Patient waits for test results to be reviewed by MD.
Step 6. Patient treated, discharged, or admitted.

Case Question

1. What do you suggest to improve the process? To reduce errors by the triage nurse?

Short Case E
Sparks Medical Center and
the Board of Trustees

Anthony R. Kovner

Sam Phillips, chairman of Sparks Medical Center's board of trustees, wondered why hospital board meetings were so different from those at his spice company, Phillips' Flavors, Inc. The hospital board discussed the reports of various committees, reviewed accreditation and licensing reports, and listened to reports and recommendations about state regulations and reimbursement. At Phillips' Flavors, Inc., the board discussed the future of business, what the competition was doing, and strategies to increase market share and profit margins.

Clara Burns, CEO of Sparks Medical Center, made the following recommendations to Sam Phillips regarding more effective board meetings:

1. Board discussion should focus on the organization's mission.
2. Objectives and strategies should be established.
3. A work plan to plan and measure board performance should be developed.

Sam realized that the problem with addressing these issues was the board structure and organization and the amount of time taken up at meetings by routine committee and management reports. This resulted in a full agenda and little time to deal with issues critical to the future of the Medical Center.

Case Questions

1. What do you recommend that Sam do now?
2. Identify constraints and opportunities that Sam faces in implementing your recommendations.

PART

III

ORGANIZATIONAL DESIGN

To understand how the Professional Bureaucracy functions in its operating core, it is helpful to think of it as a repertoire of standard programs—in effect, the set of skills the professionals stand ready to use—which are applied to predetermined situations, called contingencies, [which are] also standardized.

—Mintzberg

COMMENTARY

Organizations are people and things combined together to achieve an agreed upon goal in a changing and resource-scarce environment. Organizations have socially defined boundaries. They have a structure, process, and outcomes. There are 14 concepts in this definition: (1) people, (2) things, (3) combination, (4) achievement, (5) agreed upon, (6) goal, (7) change, (8) resource scarcity (9) environment or context (10) social definition (11) boundary, (12) structure, (13) process or tasks, and (14) outcomes.

To understand these concepts and how they relate to each other is at the core of organization theory. Every one of these seemingly simple concepts, on close examination, turns out to cover a complex set of ideas.

Organizations are often described at a moment in time (a photograph). They can also be described as changing over time (a movie). It is easier to describe the organization as a photograph, but the leader's task is to guide the organization over time, to envision a future preferred state and get the organization from its present condition to that future.

"I am a nurse working in the intensive care unit of Memorial Hospital." If you have been in an ICU in a hospital, this simple statement describes an organization, its boundaries, and goals, the work being done there, and the technology in use, and a point in time.

In this example, the nurse knows the boundary of the organization. There are also legal definitions of an incorporated organization, which are often but not always similar. Resource scarcity can also be used to understand boundaries. "We do what we can do best and let others do what they do best" is one way of understanding the "make or buy" managerial decisions which define the organization's boundary. Our hospital needs computers and a food service, but we buy the former and contract out the latter because others can make and do these things better than we can. This is the underlying logic behind the Required Reading for this section. Focus on what you are best at and leave everything else to others.

For each of these basic concepts there are ways to subdivide them. People include workers, professionals, managers, and trustees. Things include long-term assets and short-term supplies. Combination includes dividing people and equipment into departments and a hierarchy aligned to the process of work and goals. Resource scarcity implies that achieving the goals of improved health must be constrained by the people and things available. The organization's environment can de described legally (laws governing behavior), economically (competition or monopoly), socially (how people define our work) and historically (our hospital is located where it is because that's where the donor gave us the land a hundred years ago). Goal achievement can be estimated by measuring outcomes (patient census, mortality rates, vaccinations given). For-profit, not-for-profit, and government ownership of healthcare organizations relate to legal definitions and different goals: For example, long-run shareholder value maximization may be the goal of a for-profit organization. Organizations create different internal cultures. A faith-based organization may have a different vision and values than a for-profit even though both may achieve these divergent goals through the provision of high-quality care.

Organizations must transform individual goals (my paycheck, my job satisfaction, my desire to help) into a unified overall good or mission. Everyone who is a member of the organization is there because it fulfills their personal goals. Keeping the balance of all these personal incentives favorable over time and through changing circumstances in a way that achieves the organizational goals is central to the role of management. It is this combining of people and things, setting the boundaries, maintaining the balance of incentives with limited resources, and getting the work done that is the manager's task in organizational design.

There are many different ways to organize work, and some ways work better than others. Strictly causal relationships between technology and organizational design, or between environment and design, have not yet been proven. Mintzberg (1979; 1983) has suggested five basic types of organizational design or structure: simple, machine bureaucracy, professional bureaucracy, divisionalized firm, and "adhocracy" (Mintzberg's term for a mutually adjusting structure).

The basic parts of Mintzberg's organizations are the strategic apex or top managers, middle management, the technological structure (such as planners and industrial engineers), support staff (such as personnel and security), and the operating core (or workers). Each of the five types of organization has a different configuration of these five parts. For example, the simple organization (e.g., a doctor's office) has managers, support staff, and an operating core but little or no technological structure or middle management.

The key means of coordination varies according to the type of organization. In a simple organization, direct supervision is the key means of coordination. In a machine bureaucracy, such as a large outpatient department for the poor, work standardization is the key means of coordination. In a professional bureaucracy, such as a community hospital, standardization of professional skills is a key means of coordinating the work. In a divisionalized firm, such as a multihospital corporation, the key means of coordination is the standardization of outputs, such as profits or market share. Finally, in an adhocracy work is coordinated as the clinicians adjust on the spot to working with one another.

Work is sometimes organized according to the available physical facilities and may be influenced by an organization's history and the initial design of its founders. For example, most doctors still are not employees of hospitals because most physician care traditionally was provided in the homes of the patients.

According to Mintzberg (1979; 1983), work in the operating core can be organized in one of three ways: by process or occupation (e.g., all nurses report to the director of nursing, all physicians to their department chiefs); by purpose or division, cutting across occupational specialties (e.g., all nurses and physicians report to the local clinical leadership, which may be surgery, women's health, or emergency services); or, by both process and purpose, in a matrix organization. Under this matrix method of organization, all nurses report to the clinical leadership of the division for some activities and to the director of nursing for others. Matrix organization solves certain coordination problems by process and by purpose but adds another layer to management, thereby increasing coordination costs. Managers must decide when to use which form of organization and whether the benefits, if any, outweigh the costs.

Today, hospitals are being seen as just part of larger systems of care. Some systems are organized to provide a "continuum of care" from primary care, secondary care in community hospitals, tertiary care, home care, and long-term care all in a single market area. Such integrated delivery systems (IDSs) bring increased managerial challenges in planning organization and performance measurement. Young and Barrett (1997) summarize some of these issues in Table III.1.

Some hospital-centered systems—such as the Hospital Corporation of America, the Voluntary Hospitals of America, or the Veterans Administration —cross healthcare markets. Health maintenance organizations (HMOs) combine the insurance function and provision of care under capitation, which is a reversal of the economic incentives of fee-for-service. Once, one could describe Kaiser-Permanente and say "That is what HMOs are or expect to be." No longer. Organizational variation is unending. One trend is the growth of point-of-service (POS) plans, which give enrollees a choice of care and payment levels. If the core physicians and hospitals are used, patients do not make copayments; if the larger preferred provider list is used, there are copayments. The patient can go out of the network and pay even larger copayments. It is more difficult to control quality and costs in such POS plans, which allow patients more choice of providers than they have in HMOs.

Declining hospital occupancy rates resulting from shorter lengths of stay (largely driven by prospective payment) and fewer admissions (driven by ambulatory surgery and the economics of capitation) combined with the high

TABLE III.1

Managerial
Checklist for an
Integrated
Delivery
System's Senior
Management
Concerning
Cross-
Functional
Process

Planning Processes
Strategy Formulation

- Does the IDS have a clear clinical-integration strategy or are there multiple strategies? If the former, do managers and clinicians at all levels understand the strategy, or is the strategy poorly articulated, or not well understood?
- Is there a formal process of strategy formulation, involving perhaps a board committee, planning staff, and so on, or does strategy evolve more informally?
- Is there a need to convince hospitals to adopt a more peripheral role in the IDS, rather than their traditional central role? If so, how is this being addressed?

Program Adaptation

- Do programs reinforce the IDS's strategy? Are there programs that do not fit it well?
- How does the IDS adapt its programs to provide a better fit with its strategy? For example, if the strategy is to be fully integrated, are programs developed along the full clinical spectrum?
- How are physician requests for capital and programs addressed? Do accepted requests move the IDS toward greater clinical integration?

Budget Formulation

- What kinds of responsibility centers are in place? What kinds of "cost drivers" are being used to build the budget?
- Are there transfer prices? If so, are responsibility center managers allowed to purchase from outside the system if they think a transfer price is too high?
- Do clinical professionals understand the role of each delivery site and its importance for overall care? For example, does a surgeon performing a hip replacement operation understand how the home health agency works, and are the costs of home healthcare part of the budget formulation process?
- Do programs receive the funding and support they need to carry out activities to reinforce the strategy? If there is cross-subsidization among programs and responsibility centers, how are the subsidies determined?

Organizational Processes
Authority and Influence

- How are authority and influence dispersed throughout the IDS? Traditionally, specialists have had more authority than primary care physicians, and the goal was increased admissions. Has this relationship changed?
- Does the authority and influence process reflect the fundamental management and structural changes noted above under the strategy formulation process? How much financial autonomy do program managers have? Is this autonomy reflected in the budget formulation process?
- What informal and formal mechanisms exist for physicians to influence decision making in the IDS?

Client Management

- Where are patients treated most effectively? Is care delivered at the best site, whether it be ambulatory or inpatient, and is it delivered by the most appropriate person?
- How are nurse practitioners and triage functions used?
- Do patients receive preventive care, or (at the other extreme) do they continue using the emergency room inappropriately?

TABLE III.1
(*continued*)

Conflict Resolution

- What *types* of conflict resolution mechanisms are used? These can include paper flows (e.g., interoffice memos), ad hoc task forces, permanent committees, and retreats.
- What *modes* of conflict resolution are used? These can range from "forcing" by a superior to "direct confrontation" among the various parties, perhaps with a mediator present.
- How does the conflict resolution process deal with disputes between, say, physicians and nurses or physicians and social workers, about the most appropriate setting(s) for a patient's care?

Motivation

- Are clinical professionals rewarded for managing a patient's care in such a way that they are motivated to provide treatment at the most appropriate setting in the system?
- As employees are given more discretionary authority for making decisions, is their compensation consistent with these changes?
- Is the incentive compensation system part of the budget formulation process? Where, if at all, is there a lack of goal incongruence?
- How deep into the organization do the risk-sharing and incentive-compensation systems extend? Do they cover nurses and social workers, for example?

Cultural Maintenance

- How does senior management explain and encourage clinical integration?
- How is the IDS using recruitment, hiring, and severance activities to maintain its culture?
- Do training, communication, and support activities validate the importance of clinical integration? How do these activities instill and maintain such values in the organization?

Measurement and Reporting Processes

Financial Measurement and Reporting

- Has the IDS developed a financial measurement and reporting process that measures fixed and variable costs at different levels in the system and reports them to managers?
- How well do the reports help managers to assess their financial performance against budget?
- Do managers have adequate information to make cost-effective decisions? Does the financial measurement and reporting process reflect the effect of capitation?

Program Measurement and Reporting

- Does the program measurement and reporting process include outcomes? If so, how do these efforts relate to the goals of the programs as defined in the strategy formulation and program adaptation processes?
- Are short-term and long-term program objectives consistent? How do program reports help managers to assess their clinical performance (e.g., outcomes and quality-of-care measures)?
- Does the program measurement and reporting process, together with the financial measurement and reporting process, help managers to assess the effectiveness and cost-effectiveness of their programs?

SOURCE: Young, D., and D. Barrett. 1997. "Managing Clinical Integration in Integrated Delivery Systems: A Framework for Action." *Hospital & Health Services Administration* 42 (2): 255–79.

fixed costs of hospitals have fueled the competitive frenzy of the last decade. This heat of competition has led to many new organizational forms, and these changes are far from over. This competition has compelled closer attention to the wishes of the public and a growing emphasis on market understanding and patient satisfaction.

Twenty years ago, a large city may have had 40 independent hospitals. Now these hospitals have either closed or merged into a few large competing networks. These systems are diversifying through vertical integration. At the same time, industry is going in the opposite direction. The conglomerates with many businesses and product lines are dropping the ones that are not doing as well and sticking to "core competencies." Will healthcare follow this lead? Will these large integrated systems be dissolved back into their component parts? In the Required Reading, Herzlinger argues this case using industrial examples to support her predictions.

One key task of today's senior health executives is to try to figure out what organization design will best fit tomorrow's environment and how their organizations can get there ahead of others. This is indeed leading in uncertain times with great rewards for the visionary who understands the environment well enough to predict correctly. If Herzlinger has it right, what are the consequences for today's healthcare organizations?

From Cost Control to Disease Management to Self-Care

The economic logic of capitation for providers is to do less and control costs. This has been done as HMOs have reduced expensive hospital admissions and testing. Providers are paid less and pre-approval for elective procedures has been put in place. The result is a provider, public, and political backlash about "care denied."

A cost-cutting approach can be done with little change in the way care is organized. The next step, then, is to "reengineer" care—or "disease management" as it has come to be called—and is based on answering a question: What is the best care for a defined population and how do we organize to achieve it? For example, how do we keep asthmatics out of the hospital? How do we reduce the loss from work caused by back pain? This calls for transforming the organization of care to improve it and achieving measured outcomes. The Northern New England cardiovascular surgery collaborative as described by O'Connor (see Supplementary Readings) is one such example.

The third stage driven by the economic logic of capitation is self-care. Asthma, diabetes, hypertension, and stress can be largely self-managed. Here the role of community coaches meeting in the church basement with groups of diabetics who are trying to lose weight and exercise may be the future of healthcare focused on wellness in the community.

Performance Requirements

The four performance requirements are discussed below in terms of their importance for organizational design.

Goal Attainment

The appropriateness of a given combination of resources, tasks, incentives, and information systems in a health services organization is defined by its effect on the degree of goal attainment. Hospitals must try to meet many goals, and these goals differ greatly among different types of hospitals. Appropriateness in an army hospital may be defined very differently than in an investor-owned hospital.

At this level, the two overriding measures of goal attainment are efficiency, in terms of costs per unit of output, and quality of care, which is the benefit to the patient from the care received.

System Maintenance

At an implicit level, most of the readings for this section are concerned with developing organizational characteristics that are generally stable, self-adjusting, and permanent. It is perhaps natural to overemphasize change and to forget that the largest part of a manager's work is simply maintaining the organization and opposing the forces of entropy. Employees who leave must be replaced by new employees, who must be trained. Equipment and facilities must be maintained, repaired, and replaced. This information is considered obvious and, therefore, is seldom made explicit in the literature.

Adaptive Capability

As goals, technology, size, personnel, and services change, structure also may need to change. Some structures are easier to change than others. For example, a centralized, hierarchically controlled organization may be changed easily by top management. If change is expected to come from professionals in the organization (as in a research laboratory), then decentralization and professional autonomy may be more appropriate characteristics in the organizational structure. Some changes are easier to implement than others. For example, it may be easy for a hospital to add a new piece of medical equipment but difficult to start a group practice.

A highly formalized organization, with a well-developed structure, task definition, and coordination, may be very efficient under stable conditions. If this organization has been, but no longer is particularly successful, its long-established patterns may be difficult to change.

Values Integration

Clinician values such as independence, special expertise, and commitment to altruistic goals must be brought into organizations where managers set limits on behavior, supervise performance, and maintain economic viability. The attempt to integrate roles and values raises the need for clarification of clinician and managerial interests. To what extent are clinicians economic entrepreneurs or technical experts? Is there a sufficient degree of similarity of interest between clinicians and organizations?

Reference

Mintzberg, H. 1983. *Structure in Fives*. Engelwood Cliffs, NJ: Prentice Hall.
———. 1979. *The Structuring of Organizations*. Engelwood Cliffs, NJ: Prentice Hall.

THE READINGS

H erzlinger proposes a radical transformation of healthcare: Do what you do best, focus all your energy on that, and let someone else do the other things. For business, this would be to focus on the part of a company with the highest long-term rate of return on its invested capital.

This proposal may make the most sense for elective procedures (such as heart surgery) or for specific types of patients with a single condition, such as renal dialysis center patients. Other types of patients, particularly the frail elderly, have multiple health problems. Community general hospitals may serve such patients well where a general internist provides basic care and makes referrals for many other needs as represented by the other specialists associated with the hospital.

Other proposals have been made for improvement. One is the use of practice guidelines for all patients, also called evidence-based medicine. Some examples are beginning to emerge of healthcare systems achieving nearly 100 percent of care under such guidelines.

Another proposal is to create horizontally integrated systems of care for types of patients, setting standards of uniformly high-quality care across all providers. This could take the form of a well-known heart surgery center franchising its services across many states to meet the needs of the workforce of large employers.

These several ideas are not necessarily in conflict, but could be combined together effectively.

Market-Driven, Focused Healthcare: The Role of Managers

Regina Herzlinger
From *Frontiers of Health Services Management* 16 (3), Spring 2000.

Summary

Focused factories will play a positive role in the future U.S. healthcare system. As demonstrated in the revitalized organizations in other parts of our economy, focused factories can provide better, more affordable products. A clear agenda and attention to the customer enable focused firms to develop world-class managerial systems for achieving their goals. These systems codify and integrate many separate functional activities to achieve consistent, high-quality, moderate cost results in each of many separate locations. In healthcare, focused factories can offer care for chronic diseases, frequently performed procedures, and primary and diagnostic care. Such organizations will be able to present clear outcome data, charge lower prices, and enhance customer satisfaction simultaneously.

Remember how the U.S. economy supposedly died, buried by savvier global competitors? Well, it has come roaring back (IMD 1996; Investor's Business Daily 1996). The two primary causes of its revitalization hold important lessons for the healthcare system:

1. Successful firms focused, *focused*, focused on their core competences, shedding distracting side businesses and internal production capabilities that could be better performed by outside providers. For example, Eastman Kodak came back to profit and innovation after it discovered its true inner child—surprise, the photography business—and sold its distracting pharmaceutical and diagnostic businesses (Chakravarty 1997). General Motors too has shed the internal production facilities, such as its parts factories (Bradsher 1998), that hiked its overall costs per vehicle by $598 over the costs of its less-integrated rivals who could buy from efficient, focused, external producers (Blumenstein 1996).
2. Successful firms paid attention to the customer. When J.D. Power surveys revealed continuing customer dissatisfaction with the quality of Chrysler vehicles, its chairman decided to incorporate the J.D. Power criteria into the company's internal quality measures (Woodruff 1994). Small wonder that Chrysler then became among the most profitable automobile firms in the world ("Remaking Ford" 1999).

Organizations with these characteristics are frequently called "focused factories," a name coined in an initially inconspicuous 1974 article in the Harvard Business Review that argued that complex and overly ambitious factories were at the heart of the country's productivity crisis. In this view, later widely adopted by U.S. industry, "simplicity and repetition breed competence" (Skinner 1974). A clear agenda and attention to the customer enable focused firms to develop world-class managerial systems for achieving their goals. These systems codify and integrate many separate functional activities to achieve consistent, high-quality, moderate cost results in each of many separate locations.

As an example, consider the system developed by McDonald's to provide fresh, hot, crisp french fries in more than 11,000 U.S. restaurants, at a low price per sack. They include the following (Upton 1992; Sasser 1980; Smith 1992):

- Nearly as many purchasing specifications for raw potatoes as for a cruise missile;
- Internally developed technological innovations that cleverly automated the frying process and produced a specially designed scoop to speed bagging;
- A 750-page, carefully researched operating manual that details the width of a french fry (9/32 of an inch); the ideal time for frying (two minutes and fifty seconds), shaking (after twenty seconds of cooking), and draining (up to seven minutes); and the process for salting, bagging, and discarding fries;
- Thoughtful training, evaluation, and promotion procedures (many supervisors got their start behind the counter);
- Careful analysis of a mountain of quality, cost, and customer-satisfaction data, including reports by "mystery shoppers" and 332 service "consultants"; and
- The use of the information to continually refine these systems.

Of course, the subject of interest is McDonald's managerial system, not its french fries. If you think McDonald's systems are unworthy of contemplation by healthcare providers, consider the data that underscore the pernicious effect of the absence of such systems in healthcare: approximately 12 percent of hospital patients experience adverse drug events, of which 43 percent were judged as serious or worse and 42 percent as preventable (Bates et al. 1995), and only 45 percent of the hospital patients considered "ideal candidates" for beta-blockers received them at discharge (Ellerbeck et al. 1995). Although dedicated, competent healthcare providers are frequently blamed for such errors—including highly publicized mistakes like the death of a journalist from vast overdosages of cancer drugs (Altman 1995)—the primary fault lies not with them but with the absence of integrated managerial systems that ensure consistent quality and costs (Leape 1995).

Some of the current trends in healthcare are likely to exacerbate this problem. The valiant architects of everything-for-everybody, vertically integrated healthcare systems—by 1996, 44 percent of hospitals (Bellandi and Jaklevic 1999) and more than 48 percent of physicians (Kletke 1998) who were employed were involved in integrated health systems—unfortunately may well find, as the consulting firm McKinsey notes, that "vertical integration [as] a . . . strategy lever . . . is notoriously difficult to set, easy to get wrong, and . . . very costly to fix" (Stuckey and White 1990).

If developing systems for french fries so completely occupies the creativity and energy of the multibillion-dollar McDonald's, imagine the time and effort required to build equivalent systems in healthcare organizations composed of units with vastly different competencies and cultures that provide thousands of services.

The early-stage Humana exemplified these difficulties with its failed attempts to integrate salaried primary care physicians and HMOs with its existing chain of hospitals. Humana's able management simply could not resolve the conflicting motives of the insurance and care-providing units (insurers want to minimize medical care while hospitals want to maximize it); the low productivity of its salaried physicians; and the faltering morale of some of the hospital managers, whose declining occupancy rates had motivated the integration. Paying attention to the customer is difficult too when so many different customers have so many different needs and values (Schiller 1993). Small wonder that a 1998 survey revealed that 57 percent of hospitals are losing money on their owned physician practices (Neil 1998).

Potential Effect of Focused Factories in Healthcare

Increasing focus will ease such problems. Healthcare focused factories that offer care for chronic diseases such as diabetes, cancer, and asthma; frequently performed procedures such as open-heart surgeries; and primary and diagnostic care can simultaneously moderate costs and increase quality. For example, a New York Times article praised the focused factory operated by the eminent cardiac surgeon, Denton Cooley. The 60,000 open-heart operations performed by Cooley surely led to high-quality care (Myerson 1994); in healthcare, ample evidence shows that practice makes perfect (Arndt, Bradbury, and Golec 1995; Grumback et al. 1995; and Kimmel, Berlin, and Laskey 1995). For one, practice creates smoothly functioning teams. As an administrator in a hospital that achieved consistently superior performance in a cardiac procedure noted, "an open-heart patient is cared for by so many people from so many disciplines that building a team is critical." Many of the team members in that hospital had worked together for at least ten years (Gardner 1992). Practice also reduces costs by minimizing errors. For this reason, Cooley charged $27,040 for a bypass in 1994, while the national average hospital price was $43,070 (Myerson 1994). Last, focus simplifies the process of paying attention to the customer, monitoring quality, and measuring costs.

To contemplate how a focused factory might operate, consider the mythical Diabetes Management Center (DMC), a provider-owned and operated organization:

> Its providers include all the specialists needed to treat diabetes and its complications, including endocrinologists, nephrologists, cardiologists, ophthalmologists, dermatologists, surgeons, and many community-based healthcare providers such

as primary care physicians, nurses, therapists, and nutritionists. The DMC owns and operates or has strategic relations with hospitals, kidney dialysis centers that house support groups, healthcare professionals, behavioral and physical therapists, and home healthcare providers. It operates a computer-based Diabetes Helpmate program that routinely tracks enrollee's health status. The system alerts each enrollee's personal "team coordinator" when they are due for certain tests or other measures and tracks whether they have been performed. The DMC newsletter and videos inform enrollees of the latest developments in diabetic care.

The DMC lowers costs and improves quality by continually monitoring its enrollees' health status and providing supportive, convenient assistance for the self-care that is so critical for appropriate management of the disease. The sources of primary care, information, and support could be as near as the neighborhood pharmacy of a DMC-affiliated chain, staffed with trained pharmacists and information kiosks, and a care center, located in the local shopping mall and staffed with a team of healthcare professionals who are focused on diabetes. Neighborhood facilities like these are not nearly as expensive as hospitals. To calibrate their costs, consider that the ubiquitous McDonald's restaurants average a few million in revenues per site (McDonald's Corp. 1996). Indeed, one hospital operates a shopping mall information center at an annual cost of $200,000 ("Hospitals Expand Via Mall Centers" 1996).

The DMC is so confident of the efficacy of its approach that it offers capitated care, with some portion of its payments based on the savings it creates for diabetic care. In the past, a similar real-life provider claimed reduction in costs from $9,500 to $7,500 a year and in absenteeism rates of 10 percent (Southwick 1996).

As in this example, the largest effect of focused factories on both quality and cost will likely emerge when they are applied to chronic diseases. Chronic conditions affect 45 percent of Americans and account for three-fourths of U.S. healthcare expenditures. They limit economic activity, as well; for example, people with chronic conditions accounted for 80 percent of all 1987 hospital days (Hoffman, Price, and Sung 1996). There are many indications of inappropriate care for people with chronic diseases. A study of elderly diabetics found that fewer than 55 percent received the three diagnostic measures generally identified as necessary for optimal care of diabetes (Weiner et al. 1995; "Not All Beneficiaries.." 1997) and an analysis of a large employer's experience with asthma victims concluded that their use of hospitals and emergency rooms could have been substantially reduced with better management of the disease (Boston Consulting Group 1993, 56, 59). Seventy-two percent of physicians agreed that asthma was treated only symptomatically and not to manage the underlying immune abnormality (Southwick 1995).

Although it is tempting to blame doctors and hospitals for such errors, it is more likely that the absence of organized systems for treating chronic diseases is the culprit. A chronic disease–focused factory can alleviate many of these problems. Consider Salick Health Care, a California-based provider of cancer care founded by Dr. Bernard Salick. Salick Health Care's disease focus enables it to achieve better outcomes with breast cancer patients than more general-purpose providers. Salick data show three to four times higher use of appropriate postoperative therapy than National Cancer Institute data indicate nationwide; fewer hospital admissions for chemotherapy compared to local providers; more frequent "good-to-excellent" ratings and fewer complaints than national statistics; and charges at least $20,000 lower than most other providers for blood cell bone marrow auto transplants. Apparently these results—higher patient satisfaction and lower costs—are achieved with outcomes similar to those of other transplant centers (Gale 1997).

Salick's focused-factory approach helps to explain these results. Salick's system includes inpatient, outpatient, and physician providers. Outpatient centers are typically open 24 hours a day, are architecturally designed for the needs of cancer patients, and house a multiskilled team, ranging from oncologists to psychiatrists, social workers, and pain managers. The company believes that the 24-hour availability of services is key to reducing hospital admissions (Gale 1997). The integrated system for cancer care likely explains the higher customer satisfaction rates too. The company is horizontally integrated, with 11 centers across the United States. This size enables the firm to maintain large databases. Its uniform data system contains information on 17 million member-months in 11 states, classified into 23 cost and disease categories. The firm's relatively narrow focus enables it to use this massive database to derive cost data to serve as the basis for capitated contracts (O'Connell 1994, 10). The company's size and focus also enable it to devote substantial resources to the development of clinical practice guidelines (Gale 1997).

As a result of its focus, this organization can present clear outcome data, charge lower prices, and enhance customer satisfaction simultaneously. Although such results could, in theory, be replicated in general-purpose healthcare settings, many hospitals would find it difficult to do so. Hospital administrators may well encounter political problems in singling out a service for focused-factory status. Then, too, most hospitals would struggle to match the level of resources that a focused factory can shower on the development of its system. For these reasons, Salick's management believes that only a small number of existing cancer centers could provide comparable services (O'Connell 1994).

Focused Healthcare Factories: Too Many? Too Few?

Will the United States be overrun with healthcare-focused factories? Surprisingly, a handful of healthcare-focused factories could prove adequate for the needs of a substantial fraction of the sector.

Like many other businesses, healthcare follows Pareto's Law—colloquially known as the "80–20 rule" because its originator, Vilfredo Pareto, derived a curve suggesting that roughly 80 percent of all events can be attributed to 20 percent of their causes. For example, 85 percent of all beer is quaffed by 15 percent of drinkers (Heskett, Sasser, and Hart 1990). Although the precise data needed to validate the theory in healthcare are not readily available, many indications of its applicability exist. Medical care spending is concentrated among small portions of the population: 10 percent of the population account for 75 percent of medical expenditures and 25 percent for 90 percent of expenditures ("The Concentration of Health Expenditures" 1994). Hospital services consumed 37 percent of 1993 national health expenditures, but only about 9 percent of the civilian, non-institutionalized population was hospitalized that year (DHHS 1995). Similar concentrations are seen in diagnoses, procedures, and incidence of chronic diseases. Two diagnostic categories, cardiovascular and injury and long-term effects, accounted for 26 percent of 1987 medical expenditures and ten categories accounted for 75 percent of costs ("Medical-Care Spending" 1994). Similarly, one large employer has found that 33 percent of asthma patients accounted for 73 percent of its cost for treating the disease (Boston Consulting Group 1993, 59, 61). Thus, focused factories concentrated on a handful of diseases and procedures could have considerable effect on the costs and outcomes of the U.S. healthcare system.

Do we have enough resources to support this small number? Consider the case of diabetes. The exact layout of a focused diabetes care system is exceedingly difficult to predict—after all, economics is such an inexact science that economists' original forecasts of 1990 Medicare's costs of $9 billion fell shy of its actual costs by some $58 billion ("Incalculably Inaccurate" 1994). Here is one reasonable scenario: The average state in which roughly $2 billion were spent on diabetes in 1992 (NIH 1995) could sustain 200 neighborhood centers, at $2 million each, and up to 14 specialized diabetes hospitals of 200 to 299 beds, at the average 1992 expenses of $64 million, for that sum—or fewer hospitals and a large number of dialysis centers (DHHS 1995).

The Challenges

Managed care insurers that contract with focused factories will enjoy three advantages:

1. The capitated payment removes the open-ended risk of treating costly patients from the HMO;
2. Enrollees who are very satisfied with focused services are less likely to raise the objections to denial of care that the HMOs might otherwise encounter; and
3. The capitated payment reduces the hefty administrative and marketing expenses of the HMO—averaging 10 percent and running as high as 18 percent (Lothson 1996; McKinsey & Co. 1995).

In contrast, everything-for-everybody healthcare systems that encounter difficulties in measuring their costs for treating diabetics cannot realistically bid for such capitated contracts. And, even if they were to learn their costs, they would likely find it difficult to duplicate the focused provider's managerial system. Focused healthcare factories provide social benefits too: Unlike other providers who are paid for service delivery, their capitated payment provides substantial incentives for preventive and self-care measures for their chronically ill enrollees.

The effect of focused factories raises two important public policy concerns. First, the academic medical centers (AMCs) will find it increasingly difficult to subsidize their important research and education through patient care when they try to compete with efficient focused factories. The American public reveres medical research and technology so much that it is likely to support increasing governmental spending for these activities, but the leaders of AMCs must advance their case with clear, credible measures of the extent of the subsidization of research by patient care activities (NSB 1991; Krakower, Williams, and Jones 1999). The presence of focused factories will also require academic medical centers to focus on their distinctive competences in patient care, which likely lie in high-technology care (Bailey et al. 1999).

Second, at the present time managed care insurers have substantial incentives to avoid sick people. After all, 1 percent of the population accounted for 30 percent of 1987 healthcare expenses ("The Concentration of Health Expenditures" 1994). Limiting such discrimination requires both close governmental scrutiny and research to develop robust criteria for gauging severity of illness. In their absence, the practice of discrimination against the elderly and sick may continue unchecked in focused factories.

The Role of Physicians and Managers

Focused factories hold considerable promise for physicians. The early-stage focused factories I cite—Dr. Cooley's center and Salick Health Care—are physician-led. As the physician who led an effort that reduced hospital stays for acute congestive heart failure by 50 percent noted: "There's a big push to get people out of the hospital sooner. . . . But only physicians know how to take care of patients" (Prager 1996). The statement reminds me of a participant in one of the Harvard Business School's executive programs who explained his remarkable success in the faddy, competitive shoe industry by noting that he had "smelled many feet" as a shoe salesman. Like other successful executives, his experience enabled him to meet his customers' needs.

The advent of focused factories will restore to physicians some of the financial and professional autonomy they feel they have lost to managed care. In my class on "Managing in the New Health Care Sector," I asked how many of my 87 students were the sons and daughters of physicians. A forest of hands shot up—not including the five MDs enrolled in the class. When asked why he had chosen to attend a business school, one said that his mother urged him not to become a doctor because physicians are no longer free to practice medicine. That is not to say that focused factories will lack practice guidelines. As the American Medical News pointed out, "the concentration of 'intellectual capital' is bound to pay off with better outcomes for the patients [and] the tough task for developing clinical standards can be simplified because [they] can draw more readily on a large patient population" (Tokarski 1996). However, such guidelines will be developed by physicians in physician-led focused factories.

Despite a report by California professor James Robinson that early-stage capitated physician groups had already demonstrated their cost-reducing effects (Robinson and Casalino 1995), they are faltering today. The California Medical Association warned that up to 90 percent of the state's physician groups face "imminent bankruptcy" ("Medical Association Says" 1998). Why? Hill Physicians Medical Group is a notable exception because it is led by strong managers as well as strong physicians. As its CEO notes, "(the) core issues . . . are organizational and structural . . ." (Jaklevic 1999).

I choose to use the term "healthcare focused factories," despite its dehumanizing implications, to emphasize that these are not virtual organizations, loosely coupled by electronic media, but rather like factories in which teams of people with disparate skills continually work together to achieve a common aim. These institutions will play a positive role in the future U.S. healthcare system. Like the revitalized organizations in other parts of our economy, they will produce better, more affordable care. Indeed, they can even help to remedy the cruel injustice suffered by millions of poor uninsured by increasing the affordability of the health services.

As in other markets, government must ensure the integrity of these providers, the accuracy of their data and advertisements, the solvency of their finances, the nondiscrimination of their admission policies, and the competitiveness of their market structure. However, the key to this new healthcare system lies not with government, but with the market—the organic confluence of innovative suppliers, both for-profit and nonprofit, and the alert American public.

Acknowledgment

The author is very grateful to Dr. S. Robert Levine of New York for his comments on the Diabetes Management Center.

References

Altman, L. K. 1995. "Big Doses of Chemotherapy Drug Killed Patient, Hurt Second." *The New York Times* March 24: a18.

Arndt, M. R., C. Bradbury, and J. H. Golec. 1995. "Surgeon Volume and Hospital Resource Utilization." *Inquiry* 32 (4): 407.

Bailey, J. E., D. L. Van Brunt, D. M. Mirvis, S. McDaniel, C. R. Spears, C. F. Chang, and D. R. Schaberg. 1999. "Academic Managed Care Organizations and Adverse Selection under Medicaid Managed-Care in Tennessee." *Journal of the American Medical Association* 282 (11): 1067–72.

Bates, D. W., I. J. Cullen, N. Laird, L. A. Petersen, S. D. Small, D. Servi, G. Laffel, B. J. Sweitzer, F. F. Shea, and R. Hallisey. 1995. "Incidence of Adverse Drug Events and Potential Adverse Drug Effects." *Journal of the American Medical Association* 27 (1): 29.

Bellandi, D., and M. C. Jaklevic. 1999. "Still Alone After All These Years." *Modern Healthcare* 29 (14): 44–50.

Blumenstein, R. 1996. "GM's Per-Vehicle Costs Exceed Rivals Due to In-House Parts Work." *Wall Street Journal* June 25: 2.

Boston Consulting Group. 1993. *JDHC Disease Management Strategies*, 56, 59, 61. New York: Boston Consulting Group.

Bradsher, K. 1998. "GM Plans to Spin Off Parts Division." *The New York Times* August 4: d1.

Chakravarty, S. N. 1997. "How an Outsider's Vision Saved Kodak." *Forbes* January 13: 45–47.

"The Concentration of Health Expenditures: An Update." 1994. Intramural Research Highlights-Agency for Health Care Policy and Research (June): 2.

Department of Health and Human Services. 1995. *Health United States, 1994.* Washington, DC: Government Printing Office.

Ellerbeck, E. F., S. F. Jencks, M. J. Radford, T. F. Kresowik, A. S. Craig, J. A. Gold, H. M. Krumholz, and R. A. Vogel. 1995. "Quality of Care for Medicare Patients with Acute Myocardial Infarction." *Journal of the American Medical Association* 273 (19): 1509–14.

Gale, R. P. 1997. Salick Health Care, Inc. Personal Communication.

Gardner, E. 1992. "Study Amends Lore About CABG Volume, Cost." *Modern Healthcare* November 30: 48.

Grumback, K., G. M. Andersen, H. S. Loft, L. L. Roas, and R. Brook. 1995. "Regionalization of Cardiac Surgery in the United States and Canada." *Journal of the American Medical Association* 274 (16): 1282.

Heskett, J. L., W. E. Sasser, and C. W. L. Hart. 1990. *Service Breakthroughs*, 16. New York: Free Press.

Hoffman, C., D. Price, and H. Sung. 1996. "Persons With Chronic Conditions." *Journal of the American Medical Association* 276 (18): 1473.

"Hospitals Expand Via Mall Centers." 1996. *Modern Healthcare* June 3: 50.

"Incalculably Inaccurate." 1994. *Economist* (August 20): 22.

International Institute for Management Development. 1996. World *Competitiveness Yearbook* Lausanne, Switzerland: IMD.

Investors Business Daily. "Capitalism's 'Miracle Period' After WWII." 1996. *Investor's Business Daily* November 27: a17.

Jaklevic, M. C. 1999. "An IPA Success Story." *Modern Healthcare* September 13: 68.

Kimmel, S. E., J. A. Berlin, and W. K. Laskey. 1995. "The Relationship Between Coronary Angioplasty Procedure Volume and Major Complications." *Journal of the American Medical Association* 274 (14): 1137.

Kletke, P. R. 1998. "Trends in Physicians' Practice Arrangements." In *Socioeconomic Characteristics of Medical Practice 1997/98.* Chicago: American Medical Association.

Krakower, J. Y., D. J. Williams, and R. F. Jones. 1999. "Review of U.S. Medical School Finances, 1997–1998." *Journal of the American Medical Association* 282 (9): 847–54.

Leape, L. L. 1995. "Systems Analysis of Adverse Drug Events." *Journal of the American Medical Association* 274 (1): 35.

Lothson, D. J. 1996. *HMO Industry*, 28. New York: PaineWebber.

McDonald's Corp. 1996. *Performance at a Glance.* Oak Brook, IL: McDonald's Corp.

McKinsey & Co. 1995. *1995 Health Care Annual*, 259, 273. New York: McKinsey & Co.

"Medical Association Says HMOs Increasingly Facing Failure." 1998 *Medical Industry Today* Sept. 7: 12–13.

"Medical-Care Spending—United States." 1994. *Morbidity and Mortality Weekly Report* 43 (32): 583.

Myerson, A. R. 1994 "It's a Business, No, It's a Religion." *The New York Times* February 13: d1, d6

National Institutes of Health, Office of the Director. 1995. *Disease-Specific Estimates of Direct and Indirect Costs of Illness and NIH Support.* (unpublished data, November).

NSB. 1991. *Science and Engineering Indicators—1991*, 449, 463. Washington, DC: Government Printing Office.

Neil, R. 1998. "Physicians Deal with Another Blow." *Medical Industry Today* Feb. 16: 23–25.

"Not All Beneficiaries with Diabetes Receive Key Services, GAO Report Finds." 1997. *BNA Health Care Daily* April 14: 23–25.

O'Connell, M. C. 1994. *Salick Health Inc.*, 8–10. New York: Louis Nicoud & Associates.

Prager, L. O. 1996. "Doctor-Driven Utilization Controls." *American Medical News* 39 (40): 10.

"Remaking Ford." 1999. *Business Week* October 11: 136.

Robinson, J. C., and L. P. Casalino. 1995. "The Growth of Medical Groups Paid Through Capitation in California." *New England Journal of Medicine* 333 (25): 1684–87.

Sasser, W. E. 1980. *McDonald's Corporation*, 6. Boston: Harvard Business School Publishing Division.

Schiller, Z. 1993. "Humana Wheels Itself to Surgery." *Business Week* January 25: 58.

Skinner, W. 1974. "The Focused Factory." *Harvard Business Review* (May/June): 113–22.

Smith, L. L. 1992. *McDonald's Corporation*, 8, 16. Los Angeles: Seidler Amdec Securities.

Southwick, K. 1995. "Strategies for Managing Asthma." *Managed Healthcare* (June): dsm8.

Southwick, K. 1996. "A Roadmap for Diabetes Control." *Managed Healthcare* (April): s2.

Stuckey, J., and D. White. 1990. "Vertical Integration (and Disintegration) Strategy." *McKinsey Staff Paper* 51 (November): 1.

Tokarski, C. 1996. "Entreé into World of Managed Care." *American Medical News* 39 (17): 1, 25.

Upton, D. 1992. *McDonald's Corporation, 1992*, 17. Boston: Harvard Business School Publishing Division.

Weiner, J. P., S. T. Parente, D. W. Garnick, J. Fowles, A. G. Lanthers, R. H. Palmer. 1995. "Variations in Office-Based Quality: A Claims-Based Profile of Care Provided to Medicare Patients with Diabetes." *Journal of the American Medical Association* 273 (19): 1506.

Woodruff, D. 1994. "Bug Control at Chrysler." *Business Week* August 22: 26.

Discussion Questions

You are asked to become the CEO of a 200-bed community hospital, one of three in your part of the city, that is trying to be all things to all people. The board has asked you to focus on "what we do best."

1. What are you going to do? Prepare your presentation for the next board meeting.
2. How would you take your organization from its present condition to this future state.

Required Supplementary Readings

Clement, J. P. "Vertical Integration and Diversification of Acute Care Hospitals; Conceptual Definitions." *Hospital and Health Services Administration* Spring 1988, 33 (1): 99–110.

Gillies, R. R., S. M. Shortell, D. A. Anderson, J. B. Mitchell, and K. L. Morgan. "Conceptualizing and Measuring Integration: Findings from the

Health System Integration Study." *Hospital and Health Services Administration* 1993, 38 (4): 467–489.

O'Connor, G. T., S. K. Plum, E. M. Olmstead, J. R. Morton, C. T. Maloney, W. C. Nugent, F. Hernandez, Jr., R. Clough, B. J. Leavitt, L. H. Coffin, C. A. Marrin, D. Wennberg, J. D. Birkmeyer, D. C. Charlesworth, D. J. Malenka, H. B. Quinton, and J. F. Kaspar. "A Regional Intervention to Improve the Hospital Mortality Associated with Coronary Artery Bypass Graft Surgery." *Journal of the American Medical Association* 1996, 275 (11): 841–46.

Questions for the Required Supplementary Readings

1. Integration, diversification, information, and effectiveness and their interrelationships are described by Clement and Gillies. How do you see these concepts relating to each other in healthcare?
2. O'Connor and associates describe a remarkable cooperation effort to improve heart surgery care. What made this a successful effort? Why are such efforts unusual?

Recommended Supplementary Readings

Arndt, M., and B. Bigelow. "The Adoption of Corporate Restructuring by Hospitals." *Hospital & Health Services Administration* 1995, 40 (3): 332–47.

Arndt, M., and B. Bigelow. "Reengineering: Déjà Vu All Over Again." *Health Care Management Review* 1998, 23 (3): 58–66.

Ashmos, D., D. Duchon, F. Hauge, and R. McDaniel. "Internal Complexity and Environmental Sensitivity in Hospitals." *Hospital & Health Services Administration* 1996, 41 (4): 535–55.

Burns, L. R., and D. P. Thorpe. "Trends and Models in Physician-Hospital Organization." *Health Care Management Review* 1993, 18 (4): 7–20.

Burns, L. R., and M. V. Pauly. "Integrated Delivery Networks: A Detour on the Road to Integrated Health Care." *Health Affairs* 2002, 21 (4): 128–140.

Charns, M. P., and L. J. Smith. *Collaborative Management in Health Care.* San Francisco: Jossey-Bass, 1993.

Conrad, D. A. "Coordinating Patient Care Services in Regional Health Systems: The Challenge of Clinical Integration." *Hospital & Health Services Administration* 1993, 38 (4): 491–508.

Conrad, D. A., and W. L. Dowling. "Vertical Integration in Health Services:

Theory and Managerial Implication." *Health Care Management Review* 1990, 15 (4): 9–22.

Cussell, C. K., J. M. Ludden, and G. M. Moon. "Perceptions of Barriers to High-Quality Palliative Care in Hospitals." *Health Affairs* 2000, 19 (5): 166–172.

Eastaugh, S. R. "Hospital Nursing Technical Efficiency: Nurse Extenders and Enhanced Productivity." *Hospital & Health Services Administration* 1990, 35 (4): 561–73.

Glouberman, S., and H. Mintzberg. "Managing the Care of Health and the Cure of Disease—Part I: Differentiation." *Health Care Management Review* 2001, 26 (1): 56–69, 87–89.

———. "Managing the Care of Health and the Cure of Disease—Part II: Integration." *Health Care Management Review* 2001, 26 (1): 70–84, 87–89.

Goldsmith, J. "How Will the Internet Change Our Health System?" *Health Affairs* 2000, 19 (1): 148–156.

Griffith, J. R. "Managing the Transition to Integrated Health Care Organizations." *Frontiers of Health Services Management* 1996, 12 (4): 4–50.

Griffith, J. R., and K. White. *The Well-Managed Healthcare Organization*, 5th edition. Chicago: Health Administration Press, 2002.

Heinbuch, S. E. "Achieving Effective Service-Contracting Results: The Process Is the Key to Success." *International Journal of Health Care Quality Assurance* 1996, 9 (3): 32–41.

Herzlinger, R. E. "The Managerial Revolution in the U.S. Health Care Sector: Lessons from the U.S. Economy." *Health Care Management Review* 1998, 23 (3): 19–29.

Kilo, C. M. "Improving Care Through Collaboration." *Pediatrics* 1999, 103 (1): 384–92.

Kimberly, J. R., and E. Minvielle. "Quality as an Organizational Problem." In *Advances in Health Care Organizational Theory*, edited by S. S. Mick and M. E. Wyttenbach, 205–232. San Francisco: Jossey-Bass, 2003.

Lathrop, J. P. *Restructuring Health Care: The Patient-Focused Paradigm*. San Francisco: Jossey Bass, 1993.

Lawrence, D. *From Chaos to Care*. Cambridge, MA: Perseus, 2002.

Leatt, P., S. M. Shortell, and J. R. Kimberly. "Organization Design." In

Health Care Management, 4th edition, edited by S. M. Shortell and A. D. Kaluzny, 274–306. Albany, NY: Delmar, 1994.

McKay, N. "Rural Hospitals: Organizational Alignments for Managed Care Contracting." *Journal of Healthcare Management* 1998, 43 (2): 169–81.

Misra, D., and B. Guyer. "Benefits and Limitations of Prenatal Care: From Counting Visits to Measuring Content." *Journal of the American Medical Association* 1988, 279 (230): 1661–1662.

Munson, F. C. "What Kind of Unit Management?" In *SUM: An Organizational Approach to Improved Patient Care*, edited by R. Jellinek, F. Munson, and R. L. Smith, 31–56. Battle Creek, MI: W.K. Kellogg Foundation, 1971.

Robinson, J. C., and L. P. Casalino. "Vertical Integration and Organizational Networks in Health Care." *Health Affairs* 1996, 15 (1): 7–22.

Rosenberg, C. *The Care of Strangers*. New York: Basic Books, 1987.

Rundall, T. G. "The Integration of Public Health and Medicine." *Frontiers of Health Services Management* 1994, 10 (4): 3–24.

Rundall, T. G., S. M. Shortell, M. C. Wang, L. Casalino, T. Bodenheimer, R. R. Gillies, J. A. Schmittdiel, N. Oswald, and J. C. Robinson. "As Good As It Gets? Chronic Care Management with Nine Leading U.S. Physician Organizations." *BMJ* 2002, 325 (26): 958–961.

Schweikart, S. B., and V. Smith-Daniels. "Reengineering the Works of Caregivers: Role Definition, Team Structures and Organizational Redesign." *Hospital & Health Services Administration* 1996, 41 (1): 19–36.

Shortell, S. M. "The Future of Hospital-Physician Relationships." *Frontiers of Health Services Management* 1990, 7 (1): 3–32.

Shortell, S. M., R. R. Gillies, D. A. Anderson, K. M. Erickson, and J. B. Mitchell. *Remaking Health Care in America*. San Francisco: Jossey- Bass, 1996.

Shortell, S. M., R. R. Gillies, and K. J. Devers. "Reinventing the American Hospital." *The Milbank Quarterly* 1995, 73 (2): 131–60.

Smith, H. L. "Two Lines of Authority Are One Too Many." *Modern Hospitals* 1955, 84 (3): 59–64.

Tjosvold, D., and R. C. MacPherson. "Joint Hospital Management by Physicians and Nursing Administrators." *Health Care Management Review* 1996, 21 (3): 43–54.

Wachter, R. M., and L. Goldman. "The Emerging Role of Hospitalists in the American Health Care System." *New England Journal of Medicine* 1996, 335 (7): 514–17.

Woolhandler, S., T. Campbell, D. U. Himmelstein. "Costs of Health Care Administration in the United States and Canada Hospitals." *New England Journal of Medicine* 2003, 349 (8): 760–775.

Young, D., and D. Barrett. "Managing Clinical Integration in Integrated Delivery Systems: A Framework for Action." *Hospital & Health Services Administration* 1997, 42 (2): 255–79.

THE CASES

In healthcare, discussion about organizational design occurs at four levels. The first is at the patient care level under capitation and managed care. New questions are being asked: How do we organize the best care for asthma or hypertension or back pain? Answering this question requires a definition of "best," data on the population served, a team of staff members working to achieve these goals, and management support. How does our organization answer these questions? What is excellent diabetes care? How would we know we are achieving it?

At the next level of aggregation are the issues of the design of the hospital, nursing home, and other care organizations. How do we put the component departments together? Restructuring, reengineering, and downsizing are the jargon terms of the moment. The Wise Medical Center case raises some of these issues.

Across the country, hospitals, clinics, and insurers are grouping themselves together as systems of care. In an urban area where 30 separate hospitals once stood, there may now be four competing groups of hospitals. These may be nonprofit organizations, investor-owned, or a mix of both. This new grouping strategy is the third level of organizational design.

One reason for these changes is the recognition that with managed care we will need many fewer hospital beds than we now have. The leaders of a single hospital left out of such a system may well wonder if they will be one of the hospitals that will disappear. One way these mergers are occurring is through the sale of a nonprofit hospital to a for-profit group. The sale price plus the nonprofit hospital's existing endowment is put into a nonprofit foundation. The income from this foundation's endowment is used to achieve the charitable and philanthropic goals of the original nonprofit hospital. The hospital, now part of the for-profit organization, will be run along business lines in a very competitive environment.

In the rush to become one of the three or four biggest groups in the area, the system bases its decisions about organizational design on expediency, comfort level, and speed rather than organizing to provide expeditious, excellent care. The local rush for size is of vital importance in a market oversupplied with hospitals. Any one urban hospital priced too high or of average quality can be ignored by a managed care system. For such a hospital to exist, it will have to accept whatever price the managed care systems choose to offer, which will not be high. If the system is large enough and includes popular, specialized, and prestigious hospitals, then all managed care systems or insurers must deal with them. Such a system will not be a "price taker" but a "price giver." It can charge a full price for its services because the HMO or insurer has no choice.

The fourth level is at the state- or national-policy level. One notable effort to change the context of healthcare delivery was the Clinton administration's unsuccessful national health plan initiative.

The current devolution of decision making related to Medicaid from the federal to the state level will also change the context of care. Some states such as Hawaii and Oregon have provided interesting examples of system reform.

It is the interaction of all four of these levels of organization and system design that makes healthcare delivery a most lively arena. The field is creating unprecedented opportunities for creative leadership and the organization of whole new ways of providing better care at lower cost.

The coordination of many different professional workers with varying skills, views of the world, perceptions of what needs to be done, and licensing statutes lies at the heart of this new design for health services organizations.

Work can be organized in many different ways in large health services organizations: by task or purpose, by facility, or by client group served. Often, several different organizing principles operate in the same organization, sometimes appropriately and sometimes for historical reasons. As Clibbon and Sachs have pointed out, a laboratory is a place, obstetrics is a health condition, outpatients are people, dietary is a service, intensive care is a need, day care is a category of residential status, radiology is a group of techniques, and rehabilitation is a purpose.[1]

The structure of many healthcare organizations was more appropriate for conditions when the organization was founded than it is for today. Organization structure is determined in part by the nature of the work the organization has to do, its physical facilities, the history of the organization, and the culture of the society and of like institutions.

As academic health centers respond to competitive pressures, their organizational structures may have to be adapted for optimum organizational survival and growth. Sam Spellman has devised an ambitious reorganization plan for Wise Medical Center. What would happen if nothing is done and the current organizational structure is retained? What are the costs and benefits of Spellman's proposal? What are the problems and constraints Spellman faces in implementing his proposal? If the new methods for organizing make so much sense, why aren't other academic health centers already implementing them?

Note

1. S. Clibbon and M. L. Sachs, "Health Care Facilities: An Alternative to Bailiwick Planning in Patient Fostering Spaces," *The New Physician* 18 (June 1969): 462–471.

Case 6
A Proposal for the Restructuring of Wise Medical Center

Anthony R. Kovner and Louis Liebhaber

This proposal is written by Sam Spellman, chief operating officer, to stimulate a discussion regarding the future structure of a 700-bed hospital in a large Midwestern city.

Wise Medical Center (WMC) faces the enormous challenge of delivering healthcare services in an external environment whose only hallmarks are chaos and change. Issues of an unprecedented nature confront us and will continue to do so at an increasingly rapid pace with increasingly higher stakes.

Some examples of these issues include:

- epidemics of AIDS, tuberculosis, drug abuse, and mental illness;
- overnight shifts in surgical techniques, such as laparoscopy, that will continue to burgeon;
- significant shifts from inpatient to ambulatory surgery;
- provider shifts such as a major pending penetration of managed care into the urban market;
- tremendous momentum for a significant change in the financing of healthcare;
- regulatory and marketplace controls to support the new financing options;
- greater consumer involvement in treatment decisions;
- biotechnological treatments for diseases, resulting in a variety of dislocations: medical versus surgical treatment of an increasing number of diseases; earlier detection of some diseases; extraordinarily expensive treatment, etc.;
- unprecedented competition among various sectors—hospitals, for-profit niche companies, outpatient options, and physicians;
- state drive for capitation of Medicaid in two years; and
- increasingly expensive—possibly rationed—technology.

In the face of these challenges, and those as yet uncontemplated, the question is: Will the existing organizational structure of an acute care teaching hospital provide enough agility, adaptability, and swiftness to maintain or surpass its current position in the marketplace (financially sound, clinically respected, etc.)?

Lessons from other sectors of the economy would provide us with a resounding word of caution against complacency toward the shape of our organization. Multiple lessons can be learned from what is happening in the world around us. We should examine that world and at least discuss and think through ways for us to adapt to it so that we can remain successful into the future. Below I have set out some thoughts whose origins come from many places, including thoughts and discussion that have already begun to surface at WMC. I pose the following questions as a jumping-off point for discussion and development, not as a complete prescription for the future.

- What are the organizational key concepts to WMC's future given the premise of unprecedented continual change?
- How can an organization such as WMC anticipate change, adjust course, refocus resources and staff, and achieve equilibrium until the next change that must be anticipated and addressed?

I would argue that one response to these questions is to redesign our organization into a manageable number of smaller, more autonomous business entities. These smaller entities (described in detail below) would be organized around the major current businesses of WMC. They would have a degree of autonomy that would facilitate decision making, respond to the environment, and, most important, foster a far greater sense of commitment and purpose to each entity. Such autonomy—with clear accountability—would foster a passionate focus while at the same time adding synergy to the whole. The organization that would evolve would be flatter, more responsive and accountable, much more agile, and cost-effective.

WMC would be divided into at least the following businesses, all linked to the whole through a set of accountabilities and organizational structure and support. There must clearly be a balance, however, recognizing that the success of the whole is more dependent on the success of the individual pieces than in the current structure.

The businesses would be:

- *The Surgical Hospital* (to include all surgical services including the ORs, endoscopy, ambulatory, surgery, etc.)
- *The Private Attending Medical Hospital* (an expansion with the added involvement of the private attendings in the management and definition of the unit)

- *The General Medical Hospital* (the medicine and nonsurgical teaching service)
- *The Maternal and Child Health Hospital* (pediatrics and obstetrics)
- *Ambulatory Care Business* (to include clinics, managed care, and faculty practice)
- *Psychiatric and Substance Abuse Hospital*
- *Rehabilitation Institute*
- *Alternative Site Corporation* (dialysis, home care, and other)
- *Clinical Support Entities* (radiology, lab, cardiology, etc.)
- *Corporate Services*—with potentially several subcompanies (to include food services, housekeeping, security, training, human resources, information systems, etc.)

All of the entities above were given titles that are intended to identify not only the activities and functions that are included, but also to distinguish them as major lines of business; hence, the word "division" is not used, but the word hospital is—to signify a high degree of autonomy and scope.

Each of the major entities would be led by a chief operating officer (COO) or jointly led by a high-level administrative leader and physician. These leaders would be charged with the integrity, bottom-line performance, quality assurance, development, and implementation of a set of strategic and long-range objectives, and each would be accountable to the central management of WMC.

Each entity would have a specific focus. Some are obviously direct providers of patient care. In that role they are charged with developing and growing their piece of the WMC business. Because the management is clearly focused and is responsible for a relatively manageable-sized entity, where all of the employees and medical staff can actually know each other and where a clear ethic, purpose, and accountability can be established, the likelihood of success in meeting the needs of customers and in anticipating and reacting to the environment should be greatly enhanced.

Following is a detailed description of one of these entities.

The Surgical Hospital

The leadership would focus on the present and future environment for surgery. What are the trends? What are the threats and opportunities? What are the needs of our current and potential customers? How do we organize, refocus, communicate, and operationalize the necessary response? Take any specific example, let's say laparoscopic surgery. The surgical hospital leadership would be expected to understand and anticipate the implications of laparoscopic surgical growth and change; confer with its constituents (the surgeons of various specialties); and develop a business approach to the issue, which might include a plan for acquiring equipment, training skilled technical staff, regearing the operating rooms for the technology, providing a marketing plan to HMOs for length-of-stay reduction, and so on. The changing focus, which might also include redirecting resources on the inpatient side, could be communicated to all of the staff in the surgical hospital so that they could in turn prepare for and contribute to the successful implementation of the change.

The proposed reorganization differs from the current environment in several important ways:

- Management of our major businesses would focus specifically on those businesses. The success of those businesses would also be clearly focused on defined individuals with defined resources.
- The size of the entity would be such that the management can communicate effectively with all of the players: the more rapid the need to change, and the more profound the changes that might occur, the greater the need for meaningful, comprehensive buy-in and communication. That communication is infinitely more likely to succeed in an organization one can touch and feel, and also in an organization with which the players can much more closely identify.
- Each entity would be less captive to the bureaucracy and more focused on its mission and customers.
- Each entity, because of its focus and size, increases the likelihood of harnessing the potential of our quality improvement effort and the potential power of the human imagination and the creativity of our workforce.
- These entities are much more likely to operate with a higher degree of internal accountability and consistency. Innovation can be introduced and can take hold much more successfully.
- The new entities will have fewer layers in their organization structure, resulting in lower cost, greater agility, and more resources focused on the end result.
- As described below, the entities become discerning purchasers of service rather than part of the structure that may limit the positive effects of competition and innovation.

If one looks at some of the more successful and market-sensitive (defined as agile and cutting edge) entities in WMC, they are relatively self-contained units managed by a focused group of people with a well-defined mission: hospice, rehabilitation, dialysis, neighborhood health center, the long-term care division (and even specific inpatient units such as substance abuse, medical and surgical intensive care units, etc.).

Corporate Services

For an example of a functional entity as opposed to a direct business entity, let's take a look at corporate services. Corporate services comprises those nonclinical functions that support the direct delivery of our main services (patient care). Corporate services are functions such as billing, housekeeping, food service, security, management information systems (MIS), marketing, human resources, and so forth. Under the proposed plan, they would function much like subcontractors to provide service to the delivery arm, and be held to a standard of performance that one would expect in the competitive world of subcontracting. If the subcontractor for food service, for example, could not demonstrate that it was providing a market-competitive product at a market-competitive price, then the service entity would have the option to subcontract out that service. Even if we were ultimately constrained from actually doing so, the perceived possibility might drive innovation and improvement on the part of the management and workers of food service.

In this scheme every service, almost without exception, could be viewed as a subcontractor with the potential to be replaced by a competitor. The only service that probably would not be subjected to this provision is MIS—and that is only because of the constant state of development in which we find ourselves. It is not inconceivable that we could hire a service bureau and contract out most of MIS also. Even billing could be subjected to a "show me" scenario.

Clearly subcontracting has pitfalls but they may be seriously counterbalanced by the competitiveness, innovation, cost reduction, and flexibility this approach could engender. Further, if our services were so far superior, we could do as we have in food service, and the food service function could seek to provide services on a for-profit basis to other hospitals or businesses.

The raison d'etre of corporate services (as with the other functional support entity, clinical support) is to provide responsive, cost-efficient support to the main business entities of WMC. Corporate and clinical services would provide the services and expertise that would not necessarily be economically feasible to subdivide in each business entity, and the provision of which would simply encumber or sidetrack the efforts of the management of the business entity with tasks that were a tangential, albeit a necessary, part of their business.

The Flatter Organization

The organization described above becomes flatter than the current organization in several ways.

First, each direct care delivery entity—for example, the private attending medical hospital—is of a manageable size (approximately 150 to 225 beds,

400 to 600 employees). All of the direct service providers and subcontractors are accountable to the COO of each entity. Each patient care unit within the entity would have a highly skilled nurse manager and/or head clinician and administrative type (although the latter structure may be less appealing). All of the staff who worked on the unit would be directly accountable to the unit leadership (akin to the Planetree model, although this proposal goes several steps further). The unit managers (whether nurse or some combination) report directly to the COO; with only five to ten units (maximum size), this should be possible.

Second, there would be a natural imperative in this unit-based scenario to innovate and redefine some unit-based jobs to run more smoothly and cohesively—that is, possibly combining patient-focused jobs such as housekeeping, food service, and nurses aide functions.

Third, given the competitive subcontractor model described above, it will be impossible for many services to be market-competitive with the bureaucracy and layering currently in place. These layers are a part of the current fabric and cannot easily be replaced without a different sort of organization to serve.

I am not sure if it is possible to enter into this sort of organizational restructuring on a "pilot" basis, simply because it is so contrary to the current organizational structure. There is far too much potential for undermining, confusion, and waste if two parallel tracks exists.

Sam Spellman convened a meeting of top managers to discuss his proposal for restructuring WMC. These included Paul Bones, chief of medicine; Pam Ewing, vice president for nursing; Tom Starks, director of human services; Tony Rivers, vice president for finance; Lew Oakley, director of planning; and Carl Smith, the WMC CEO. A summary of highlights from their discussion follows.

Tony Rivers: Don't we have enough on our minds without drastically reorganizing patient care services? We should be focusing our energies on organizing for managed care rather than on the internal production of services.

Paul Bones: How are we going to factor in our teaching and research objectives and strategies? We should be paying more attention to teaching and research, since this is what makes us distinctive as a hospital.

Pam Ewing: Where does nursing service figure in all this restructuring? It looks to me as if we would be losing a lot of power with no guarantee that services would be better or cheaper. You're going to put the doctors in charge of the nurses, and I'm not so sure that they ought to be telling us what to do or how we can best work together.

Tom Starks: How are you going to bring the unions into this kind of restructuring?

Lew Oakley: Are you suggesting that we could start contracting out a service like our planning department? Wouldn't there be tremendous costs in developing and evaluating different proposals, plus a lot of uncertainty created among my staff, who are doing the best possible job that they know how to do?

Carl Smith: Sam, I think your scheme is a great idea, and I think the people at Hopkins and elsewhere have carried it out with some pretty impressive results. What worries me is that (1) only a few places nationally have gone into this, and the expenditures in training and planning and executive attention would be very great at a time when we're under a lot of pressure to lower our costs; (2) where are WMC's champions to fight for development and implementation of this imaginative proposal? and (3) do our chiefs really have the skills and experience necessary to run these divisions? We didn't recruit them because they were excellent managers, but rather because of their leadership capabilities to run first-rate teaching programs and stimulate the production of research within their specialty.

Case Questions

1. What are the arguments for and against restructuring?
2. What are the preconditions necessary to allow such restructuring to take place?
3. What are the key obstacles to restructuring?
4. How can these obstacles be overcome?
5. What do you advise Sam Spellman to do? Why?

Case 7
Reorganizing Primary Care
at Blackwell Medical Center

Anthony R. Kovner

Academic Medical Centers

According to Gilmore, Hirschkorn, and Kelly (1999):

We often hear a call for more leadership and strategic planning in academic medicine. The implied paragon typically is a private sector company with an entrepreneurial CEO setting a direction and crafting an innovative strategy to realize the vision.[1]

Academic medical centers (AMCs) differ from private sector companies. Gilmore, Hirschkorn, and Kelly characterize academic medical centers as "loosely coupled" and "church-state"–oriented. A loosely coupled system is a setting where individual units have high autonomy relative to the larger system, often creating a federated character of the institution. In loosely coupled systems, the forces for integration—for worrying about the whole—are often weak compared to forces for specialization.

Organizations that are "church-state"–oriented are those in which one group feels its work is a calling, mission-driven, and another takes up the challenge of providing a productive context for the missionary work. People find it hard to talk directly and openly in church-state organizations, and conversation is constrained either by implicit or explicit church contempt for the managerial role, or by managers who are either unwilling to push back against a poor idea or who are manipulative of the situation out of their own contempt for the "real world" inexperience of the church side.

Dr. Gail Koo, chief of primary care at Blackwell, an AMC, is reviewing her recent reorganization and deciding what else needs to be done. She put down the Gilmore, Hirschkorn, and Kelly article that she was reading and wondered how academic medical centers differed from business organizations.

Blackwell Health System and the Blackwell School of Medicine

These are two separate entities that aim to be strong partners but have separate boards and financial bottom lines. Blackwell Hospital runs the hospital clinics; and the school's faculty practice associates, largely through each academic department, run the faculty practice. What they share operationally are the physicians (who are one and the same), the hospital's medical staff and house staff, and the school's clinician faculty and physicians-in-training.

Two years ago, operating revenues at Blackwell Hospital were $850 million. Operating income (operating revenues less operating expenses) was $40 million. Blackwell then had 1,000 beds, 45,000 discharges, 360,000 outpatient visits, and 75,000 emergency department visits.

The Blackwell School of Medicine's financial results were favorable in this fiscal year with the School's net worth increasing 10 percent to $480 million. Total revenues were $570 million, the investment portfolio grew to $375 million, and research programs grew to $115 million. Revenues from patient care, primarily from the School's faculty practice plan, were $190 million. Currently, the School of Medicine has 430 medical students, 50 MD/Ph.D. students, and 125 Ph.D. students.

The Medical School and Ambulatory Care

Lew Roy, M.D., deputy dean of the School of Medicine, states that "we are unable to grapple with the future of ambulatory care and how services and needed facilities will be funded." Two years ago, hospital-based ambulatory care visits made to the Blackwell campus included 240,000 for specialty care, 120,000 for primary care, 80,000 for emergency services, and 60,000 for behavioral health services. The 120,000 primary care visits included the following: internal medicine, 50,000; geriatrics, 10,000; medicine/pediatrics, 3,000; pediatrics 27,000; OB-GYN, 20,000; and AIDS, 8,000. There is a federated model faculty practice at Blackwell, with a relatively small core budget. All budgets are departmental. The practice is specialty and subspecialty focused. Although the faculty practice and the hospital clinics are physically, managerially, and financially separate, the same faculty leaders and physicians are responsible for the delivery of care in each setting.

As in most academic medical centers, hospital-based ambulatory care at Blackwell loses money. Preliminary estimates for last year indicate that hospital-based practices lose $3 million annually, in terms of direct revenue and expenses (contribution margin) and $30 million, counting indirect expenses. This is offset in the case of primary care by its generating an estimated 25 percent of all hospital admissions, along with 15 percent of ambulatory surgery at Blackwell Hospital.

Blackwell Hospital is currently giving consideration to how large a responsibility it can assume for people who can't afford to pay for their ambulatory care or who are underinsured. This may result in seeing certain kinds of patients only within the hospital's primary care catchment area, however determined. The Medical Center has to determine whether or not to integrate faculty practices and hospital clinics. Such integration has to be considered within the realities of finances and space, social commitment, regulatory and accreditation requirements, the number of patients required for a responsible medical education program, and the patient base necessary to feed a 1,000-bed hospital. "If we don't do anything," Roy summed up "it will be like bleeding from a thousand cuts."

Primary Care in the Department of Medicine

Dr. Sam Winters, vice-chair of the Department of Medicine for Education, describes the department's history of primary care, since he came seven years ago, as having three phases: (1) establishing the culture of quality, (2) programmatic growth to meet educational needs, and (3) recognition as a national and world leader at a scholarly level.

Establishing the Culture of Quality

Dr. Winters arrived at Blackwell seven years ago. He had been recruited by the new chair of medicine, Dr. Marl, as vice-chair and residency director, to build the quality of the residency program in primary care. Before he came, Blackwell was attracting residents from the lower half of the U.S. pool, the residents were demoralized, and the residency was in violation of the accreditation standards. Nationwide, training was shifting from inpatient to ambulatory care, but at Blackwell, the total residency training had occurred in the hospital. Primary care was delivered in a very small, ambulatory clinic, the ground floor of an old and dark apartment building. The seven or eight faculty were unhappy, disgruntled, and delivering a low volume of service. The department had 125 residents seeing 5,500 patients per year. The faculty had little institutional respect and didn't know whether patients were satisfied. Patient no-show rates hit 50 percent. According to Dr. Winters, "We were as close to ground zero as we could go. That was the problem."

The faculty in the clinic setting were marginalized from Blackwell. Most of them were not doing scholarly work and viewed their work simply as a 9-to-5 job. The residents saw the subspecialists in internal medicine as the key faculty. And the ambulatory care space was inadequate to accommodate residents. Before he arrived, Dr. Winters got a commitment from Dr. Ernest Pleasant, the medical center CEO, that an unequivocal goal of Blackwell was to have the top internal residency program and a new facility. The hospital built the department a bright, modern, 27,000-square foot practice building exclusively for ambulatory care practice.

Dr. Winters and Dr. Marl laid down a set of departmental principles as follows, which have guided the development of educational programs in Medicine:

- Residents are assigned only for educational value, not because there is work that needs to be done;
- Everywhere assigned, residents are totally responsible for patients under their care and for a high volume of patients;
- All residents would be trained as competent and confident internists during the residency;
- In all experiences, the program tries to recapitulate the real practice of medicine. Residents must relate to patients, and be available to them. For example, residents have business cars, preprinted prescription pads, and beepers.

Programmatic Growth to Meet Educational Needs

Dr. Winters dramatically upped the job specifications for the faculty and for residents. Residents were to practice regularly in the ambulatory care facility with a fully developed ambulatory curriculum. The faculty was given responsibility for hospital patients, and expected to improve the quality of the practice and productivity. New faculty were hired and almost all of the existing faculty moved on to other positions or took on new responsibilities. The hospital gave the department funds to hire faculty who would increase practice revenues, admit patients to the hospital, and mentor residents. Dr. Gail Koo was recruited to lead the primary care section. All residents were soon practicing in small practices called "firms." Primary care visits increased from 10,000 to 50,000 per year. Faculty grew from 7 to 24. Faculty are now the major core of teachers in the residency program, have high prestige, are involved in major medical center committees, teach in the medical school, and are expected to write scholarly papers. Dr. Koo hired Phil Card as medical director and recruited leadership for the medical firms, giving faculty a sense of ownership for curriculum and firm performance. Faculty are promoted relative to such performance. Primary care faculty gave ten presentations at national meetings last year and have become a major scholarly force.

Dr. Winters said that the Blackwell residency in internal medicine is currently the most competitive in the city, suggesting that "prospective residents actually select the best training program, not the best name." With departmental commitment from the chair, the program is innovative and curriculum-wise. Residents spend 40 percent of their time practicing in the ambulatory care center. The department replaced medical residents with nurse practitioners to cover 40 percent of the inpatient service. Residents were pulled off one of the specialty services because faculty on this service were evaluated as teaching poorly. The prioritizing of teaching was a cultural change for the faculty.

The department has never advertised the primary care practice. But there was an immense need for service in the local community that was not being met, and word-of-mouth was largely responsible for the growth in volume.

Recognition as a National and World Leader at the Scholarly Level

Dr. Koo is currently recruiting additional faculty and giving them protected time to do scholarly work, as they do at Harvard and Hopkins. The department wishes to train future scholars in this area, and Dr. Koo has recently submitted a large grant request to pursue this goal. The program may have outgrown the over 27,000-square foot ambulatory care building. Current challenges involving primary care facing the leadership include the following: better understanding the full revenues and expenses of primary care, both direct and indirect (and the different ways in which this is and can be accounted for); estimating the acceptable cost of a training program at the current level of volume; maximizing collections; and optimizing patient mix. It is important for the primary care practice to reach out to other populations of patients not currently served (e.g., the lower middle-class insured population, union members, and hospital employees). It is important to recruit patients whose private insurance pays for their care, and who have a wider variety of medical problems, given different demographic backgrounds.

The primary care section has developed a doctor house call service— one of the largest of its kind in the United States—to provide care for home-bound persons. Although 40 percent of the patients in this program never used Blackwell Hospital before, they are now heavy utilizers. Residents spend one month making house calls, learning what it means to be a doctor, and keeping a journal on their doctoring experience. According to Dr. Winters, "Private attendings currently don't want most of the clinic patients." The house call service was started by physicians in response to needs articulated by missionary nuns active in the community.

All employees who work in the ambulatory care practice are paid by the hospital. According to Dr. Winters, this has not been a problem. Employees and their supervisors report to the local administrative structure before reporting to anyone external to the building. Dr. Koo has become co-director of the inpatient service, which has helped the primary care program: 25 percent of the department of medicine's residents are now in primary care. Dr. Winters says that he has selectively ignored the economics of all this. "A top-quality program means it's worth investing money into." He adds that "The hospital *does* have a problem with the uninsured, and the program attracts patients from all over the city. The culture of the institutional practices is not to push for payment because of the primacy of the educational mission." The volume of non-pay patients is relatively small. Dr. Winters suggests that priority needs to be given to better billing and collections from Medicaid and Medicare.

According to Dr. Winters, the program does not have to grow beyond the volume required for a first-rate training program. The volume of patients seen in the practice is adequate now, but a different mix might be better for educational purposes. Current challenges involving primary care faculty include continuing to energize the faculty to do the stressful job of managing difficult patients; facilitating faculty to produce sufficient scholarship; "growing" successful mid-level faculty; and helping faculty keep up with change. "Medicine is a moving target," Dr. Winters commented. "We need to develop the people we've recruited here, and to meet the rising expectations of our faculty."

Within Primary Care

Two years ago, Dr. Gail Koo was recruited as the division chief of general medicine (1 of 14 divisions). She also became director of Adult Primary Care and she has a less-defined role in geriatrics, which is a department separate from internal medicine. Her activities fall partly in the medical school and partly in the hospital, where she is co-director of the primary medical care services center, one of the hospital's cost centers. In addition to doing her own research and seeing patients, Dr. Koo has been occupied with six managerial initiatives:

1. *Providing creative leadership for the division.* Dr. Koo has recruited Phil Card as medical director. Dr. Card has focused on continuing to improve the ambulatory care residency program and the clinical practice.
2. *Creating primary care integration.* This is among internal medicine, medicine/pediatrics, and geriatrics, with unified nursing and administrative staff for what formerly functioned as independent programs.
3. *Improving the continuity of primary care.* In past years, faculty saw private patients in a space separate from clinic patients while residents would move from one location to the other, year to year. Patients had difficulty finding their doctors. Continuity required a cultural shift by some doctors who felt "ownership" of the patient was a problem. The faculty practice and the residency practice were integrated. Each of four firms (small groups) now handles their own walk-in and urgent visits rather than these being handled in a central facility. There is improved interdisciplinary cooperation among the four firms, as support staffing is more stable within each firm, and the groundwork has been laid for research through random assignment of new patients to the four firms. Today, all residents will be assigned to a firm. New attendings have been appointed as leaders for each firm and firm leaders have been charged with functioning as in group practice. Dr. Card sees the next step in assuring continuity that of connecting inpatient and outpatient care, with residents seeing their own inpatients, making a courtesy note, and getting information through the Internet on their patient's progress.
4. *Transitioning and reorienting faculty.* Educational programs are being enriched through establishment of an academic half day. At Friday morning conferences, faculty develop and put in place sessions on, for example, evidence-based medicine, women's health, and the economics

of healthcare. Cases are discussed regarding ambulatory care patients seen the previous day. Faculty must be developed and helped in running these sessions.

5. *Building the mission of scholarship.* There are more research funds available than there were five years ago, and the alliance Dr. Koo has been building with the chief of geriatrics should help with this. Dr. Koo has proposals in the pipeline to Health Resources and Service Administration (HRSA) to expand the academic unit and to support fellowships. She is trying to build an infrastructure for research to include hiring a coordinator, considering clinical trials with drug companies, and organizing practice in a way conducive to research. Monies for support staff are written into grant proposals. The division is recruiting more faculty, but this is a slow process, and additional faculty slots are not available. There is also a problem in recruiting faculty to the city. Although they made offers to three to four prospective faculty in July, only one was recruited because of the costs of moving to this city. Dr. Koo observed that "We're limited to recruiting people who already live here or who have compelling ties here so that we can get them."

6. *Removing the stigma of the clinic from private practice.* Dr. Card wants to broaden patient mix beyond Medicaid patients. He has been talking with unions and other groups as the division may lose patients to Medicaid managed care plans. He would prefer a case mix that is 50 percent, rather than 90 percent, Medicaid. New attendings are being recruited that may attract patients with commercial insurance or Medicare.

According to Dr. Koo, the primary care activity has been critical to the success of the internal medicine residency program and in helping to recruit faculty and, therefore, NIH dollars, and the indirect medical education (DME and IME) dollars associated with the training of residents.

Dr. Koo stated that "We outgrew the space from the day we moved in. Visits have increased 15 percent each year. Visits were projected as flat this year, but they will increase by 10 percent. Hours of operation are 9:00 to 7:00, Monday through Thursday; 9:00 to 4:00 on Fridays; and 9:00 to 12:00 on Saturdays. The space is underutilized at some times, such as evenings, because patients don't want to come at those times and because scheduling is dependent on the availability of residents. During the peak hours of 10:00 to 4:00, Mondays through Thursdays, the space is fully utilized. For the faculty practice, attendings can rarely get more than one or two rooms. For efficient practice, they should have three to four examining rooms. There has never been sufficient office space. Doctors and support people are doubled up, and they need to be in this building to be in communication with patients, records and residents."

The Visiting Doctors Program

Dr. Bill Groat is director of the visiting doctors program within primary care. With the consent of Dr. Winters, he and his colleague, Dr. Tony Mills, were given time to work with a community-based nursing agency to launch a pilot program to meet community needs. The visiting doctors program is now in its fourth year, serves the whole city, and has 450 enrolled patients. Staff includes four physicians and four nurse practitioners and an administrative assistant, nurse coordinator, and a senior medical office assistant.

Dr. Groat had to justify the economics of the program to hospital administration. He wrote a business plan. He collected information on every patient and found that revenues (from billings, admissions, ancillary use, and referrals to Blackwell Home Care) far exceeded costs. As a visiting doctor, Dr. Groat can only see 4 patients in a morning rather than 12, as in ambulatory care practice. Payers pay between $80 and $200 for an initial home visit and $60 to $140 for revisits. Most patients are frail and remain within the Blackwell system. The visiting doctors program frees up time and space in the ambulatory care site, as these patients can be seen at home rather than in an examination room. Although there is a problem with staff burnout, as in hospice programs, it is addressed through close relationships between staff and dedicated time for reflection.

Dr. Groat has done a vast amount of work to establish the database, to minimize paperwork and establish a clinical and research base. The program has a broad base of referrals from house staff, inpatient social workers, faculty and voluntary staff physicians, community-based agencies, and family members. Any staff can enter data. Before accepting patients from private physicians, the private physicians have to agree or the family has to tell them of the transfer. The visiting doctors program gets patient referrals now from private physicians who are unable to visit these patients in their homes.

Dr. Groat is considering the following options regarding the future of the program: (1) to stay in the city and continue to grow, (2) to expand into the suburbs, (3) to privatize the service, or (4) to contract with HMOs, as the service can reduce hospital admissions and length of stay. Dr. Groat would like to add to the program infrastructure by hiring a social worker, a Spanish translator/escort and a database manager and statistician. This must be justified financially. He is careful not to rely on foundation funding because this means a lack of hospital support, and typically foundation funding dries up.

Dr. Groat stated that he has received tremendous support within the department of internal medicine. Dr. Winters saw immediately that the program was an important addition to clinical services and that it would make money for the hospital. He made certain that Dr. Groat and Dr. Mills obtained the information to make the economic case, freed up their time, and gave them advice as to the information needed to justify funding.

The Hospital Perspective

Mr. Joel Wrist, vice president of patient services, has worked at Blackwell for 17 years and views primary care as a very successful story. The changes made were substantial and essential for the residency program in internal medicine. The question was what the scale of the practice program should be. A real, finite goal was agreed upon, and leadership in the hospital and in the medical school designed a new building for primary ambulatory care and fast-tracked construction in record time of under two years. The excellent leadership in internal medicine helped the residency program improve greatly during the last seven years.

Mr. Wrist realizes that the primary care building is at capacity. As an educational program, further expansion is not needed, which has been acknowledged by all leaders. Dr. Marl is open to more primary care centers to feed the hospital and serve the community, but this is not required as part of an academic teaching program. Blackwell is partnering now with community-based, lower-cost centers, which are eligible for certain grants, and are doing a good job. In the suburbs, there is an understanding with private medical staff not to compete with them.

Over the last few years, Blackwell opened ambulatory care practices in several locations outside of its primary catchment area. Most of these centers have not succeeded financially, and many of them have been closed. Blackwell's strategy to attract inpatients has shifted away from purchasing or building new ambulatory care practices and toward better linkages with referring physicians through improved communications from attending staff and better use of technology.

Mr. Wrist commented to administration on some issues of importance related to payment for faculty time not devoted to clinical services and regarding productivity. Historically, the hospital has paid for some faculty time devoted to academic pursuits and for related space and support staff. The academic department (medicine) has no funding for this. And the teaching setting assigns far more attending physician time per visit than commercially viable practices would be able to spend. The hospital does not receive adequate DME funds to help support faculty who teach, and faculty's wish for performance-based incentives requires funding through improved clinical productivity. As the economics of hospital management become increasingly difficult, financial support of academic work comes under closer scrutiny.

Mr. Wrist draws the following lessons from the successful experience in reorganizing primary care in the department of medicine: (1) agreement on sizing makes it easier to implement a new strategic initiative, (2) leadership makes a difference, as does (3) a new facility, and (4) Blackwell should have spent more on the new facility to make it more attractive to paying patients. Mr. Wrist has high hopes for a new senior caring initiative that focuses on outreach to the elderly in the neighboring community to screen, educate, case-manage, and refer to existing primary care centers. These centers, in turn, refer to Blackwell for medical services that they do not provide themselves.

Dr. Koo wonders if Mr. Wrist's ideas are right and what he should do next.

Note

1. T. N. Gilmore, L. Hirschkorn, and M. Kelly, *Challenges of Leading and Planning in Academic Medical Centers* (Philadelphia, PA: Center for Applied Research Inc.) 1999.

Case Questions

1. What is different or distinctive about managing in an academic medical center?
2. What are the reasons for success in managing the reorganization of primary care at Blackwell Medical Center?
3. What are the problems and issues currently facing Dr. Koo as Division Chief of General Medicine?
4. What do you recommend that Dr. Koo do about these problems and issues? What are some of her options?
5. What should be done with the Visiting Doctors Program?

Case 8
The Future of Disease Management at Superior Medical Group

Helen Nunberg

Introduction

Five years ago, Superior Medical Group of Paradise County (SMG) entered into a contract with LifeMasters for a disease management program for congestive heart failure. The program achieved improved outcomes, cost savings, and patient satisfaction. SMG's medical director, Dr. Hugh Welly, would like to make a recommendation to the board of directors regarding future chronic disease management. In particular:

- Should SMG develop its own diabetes management program?
- If SMG lacks the resources and competencies to develop its own program, who should SMG partner with?

Dr. Welly, trained as a pediatrician, joined SMG two years ago, after seven years as medical director of Paradise County's Medi-Cal HMO plan. LifeMasters was his first experience with a commercial disease management program. As he prepared for the board meeting, he reflected on the accomplishments and the disappointments of the past year.

Superior Medical Group: History and Development

Prior to the founding of SMG in 1993, the physicians of Paradise County were primarily organized as employees or partners of Northside Medical Clinic, a multispecialty group practice, and as owners of independent solo or small group practices. In addition, there were a small number of physicians in nonprofit community clinics and public county clinics. Sisters of Mercy Hospital acquired the only other hospital in north Paradise County 12 years ago. A second hospital serves the less affluent South County.

The independent physicians organized themselves as SMG, an independent physician association (IPA) soon after Paradise Medical Clinic entered into its first managed care contact. Seven years ago a multi-hospital system acquired Paradise Medical Clinic and began construction of a second hospital in North County. That same year Paradise Sisters Hospital supported the formation of Coast Medical Associates, a primary care group within SMG.

SMG is a private, investor-owned corporation. SMG's current CEO began as the director of contracting in 1994. He is SMG's second CEO. The board of directors makes management decisions based on recommendations from the CEO, the medical director, and board committees. Board members are physicians selected by a formula to balance North and South counties, specialty and primary care, and cognitive and procedural practices (see Figure 8.1).

Physician membership in SMG has been consistent at approximately 200, with recent 20 percent overall turnover, 30 percent in primary care. A physician may choose to become a shareholder after participating in the network for two years by buying shares for a nominal fee. There are currently 140 shareholders.

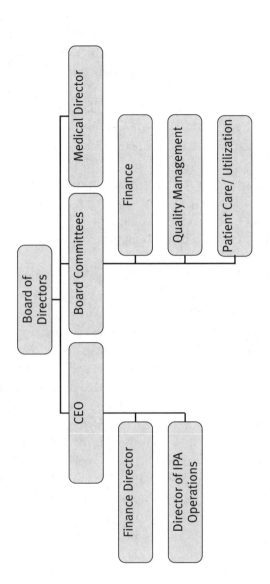

FIGURE 8.1
SMG
Organization
Chart

Patient enrollment, currently 36,000, dropped 12 percent in 2001 because of patients shifting from HMO to PPO plans. SMG is legally able to act on behalf of member physicians only with HMOs, not PPOs. The greatest threat to SMG's continued existence as an organization is the possible "end" of managed care.

In California, 29 physician groups filed for bankruptcy last year; 56 percent of IPAs have problems with solvency. Explanations include unsustainable reimbursement rates, poor management, poor acquisitions, and lack of reinvestment. Fueled by financial stress, SMG has suffered from internal dissension, especially between the primary and specialist physicians. In June of last year, Sisters Hospital's parent hospital system dissolved its relationship with Coast Medical Associates, bringing instability to SMG's largest primary care group. Sisters Hospital had also supported SMG financially four years ago by installing their intranet system, Elysium.

Despite these difficulties, SMG is now solvent and has strengthened its reserves enough to satisfy regulators. SMG's primary income stream is from capitation, a sum equal to the number of patient members multiplied by the contractual rate. The SMG primary care physicians receive capitated payments while specialists are paid fee-for-service. Additional income sources for SMG include grants from pharmaceutical firms for special programs and a contract to provide credentialing services to Coast Medical Associates.

Dr. Welly joined SMG at a time when several specialist groups were threatening to leave unless they received higher reimbursement rates. He identified his role as medical director to be that of "facilitator." He comments, "This person must pay respectful heed to compelling and highly individualized specifics without losing sight of the big picture. The intensified regulatory stringency, escalating consumer activism, and legitimate physician exasperation have made this a delicate balancing act."

Dr. Welly's responsibilities as medical director are primarily in the areas of quality and utilization management. His duties include investigating quality deficiencies; reviewing primary care referrals to specialists; reviewing hospital admissions and length of stay; authorizing high-cost procedures; reporting performance measures to HMOs; and supervising SMG's clinical staff and programs, including disease management. He is SMG's third medical director. He believes that quality management and quality improvement is the essence of what a medical group can do that independent physicians can't do, and believes the continued existence of SMG as an organization depends on its ability to bring something new and valuable to the community.

Dr. Welly communicates continuously with member physicians via the intranet. SMG does not provide significant education or training for its member physicians and does not get involved in the management of physicians' practices. SMG has not implemented quality incentives for the physicians.

Disease Management: Overview

The last decade has seen a wide range of experimentation in healthcare reform intended to contain costs and promote effectiveness. Disease management (DM) is one key tool managed care organizations have attempted to use to control costs and assure quality. The goal of a DM program is to offer a continuum of care that uses guidelines and case management protocols to prevent acute care episodes, achieve improved outcomes, and reduce healthcare costs.

Chronic diseases such as diabetes, coronary heart disease, hypertension, asthma/chronic obstructive pulmonary disease, end-stage renal disease, and HIV/AIDS are the most prevalent and most costly of all health problems. Scientific studies have demonstrated that more intensive management of chronic diseases using evidence-based assessments and interventions leads to prevention or delay of complications. Some studies have shown economic benefits as well.

The distinction between efficacy and effectiveness is critical to DM; treatments with proven efficacy in clinical trials do not always perform as well under conditions typical of clinical practice. Clinical guidelines must be implemented to achieve improved outcomes. Intensive management with evidence-based guidelines requires increased resources. Commercial DM vendors promise high-quality, patient-focused care that is effective and reduces cost. DM is one of the fastest-growing investments in healthcare: "a movement" or a "bandwagon" or a "paradigm shift." Last year DM companies accounted for $600 million in revenue, up from $300 million two years ago and $150 million three years ago.

The Disease Management Purchasing Consortium and Advisory Council's catalogue *DM Vendor Profiles* contains descriptions of 60 independent companies. Health plans and pharmaceutical companies have DM divisions, and physician groups may create their own DM programs. A company or group usually begins with one disease and then expands to multiple disease entities. Vendors primarily contract with at-risk health plans and self-insured employers.

The nonprofit Disease Management Association of America, founded two years ago, defines DM as a system of coordinated healthcare interventions and communications for populations with conditions in which patient self-care efforts are significant. Disease management:

- Supports the physician/patient relationship and plan of care,
- Emphasizes prevention of exacerbations and complications utilizing evidence-based guidelines and patient empowerment strategies, and
- Evaluates clinical, humanistic, and economic outcomes on an ongoing basis with the goal of improving overall health.

Disease management components include:

- Population identification processes
- Evidence-based practice guidelines
- Collaborative practice models to include physician and support-service providers
- Patient self-management education (may include primary prevention, behavior modification programs, and compliance surveillance)
- Process and outcomes measurement, evaluation, and management
- Routine reporting feedback loop (may include communication with patient, physician, health plan, and ancillary providers) and practice profiling

A typical DM program requires clinical protocols, a sophisticated information system, a nurse call center, outcomes reporting methodology, claims analysis capabilities, and patient education materials.

American Healthways identifies three key components that must be present and operational to ensure a program's success:

- Clinical expertise, tools, and interventions
- Data and information management systems
- Experienced personnel (management, clinical, financial, and technical)

To implement a program, these three components come together to identify patients and physicians; stratify patients; collect and track data; scan records to determine when a test, exam, or other type of intervention is due; measure and report outcomes; and effectively communicate with patients and physicians.

Physicians' Views of Disease Management Programs

One physician's response to an *American Medical News* interview with Aetna's CEO: "Personally, I can't think of a bigger waste of money than these programs. I receive these assessments from many managed care companies. I have found they provide no further information to me than what I already know after I have spoken with and examined my patient. I am sure that this costs the managed care companies big bucks. This is a waste of healthcare dollars."

A survey of California primary care physicians published in the *Journal of General Internal Medicine* found over half the physicians surveyed were not hostile to DM programs. The crucial element of a favorable program was that it decrease physician workload without decreasing income.

Physicians voice a number of concerns about DM programs. Whether outsourced to a corporate vendor or performed within a commercial health plan, the profit motive may be in conflict with meeting medical needs. The programs could be made to appear cost effective by favorable selection, or dropping certain populations or diseases because of business considerations. Funds dedicated to DM programs could be taken from primary care physicians. The DM approach could lead to fragmentation of care if patients with multiple chronic diseases were treated in separate disease-specific programs. Primary care physicians who reduce their participation in the care of patients with chronic illness might lose clinical skills, and the physician-patient relationship would be undermined. There is a lack of well-designed peer-reviewed studies to support the claims of the DM vendors that their programs improve outcomes and reduce costs.

DM programs could be perceived as a desirable strategy for assisting busy primary care physicians to care for patients who require considerable attention and time. In-house DM programs that assist physicians in doing a better job at Lovelace Clinic, Kaiser-Permanente, University of Pennsylvania, Harvard Vanguard Medical, and the Henry Ford Health System have been well received by the physicians.

Dr. Welly is not optimistic about SMG developing its own DM programs. "Physicians lack the organizational expertise to make DM programs work. They also don't trust each other with things like this. It's very odd—they'd rather deal with an outsider, and rather still simply get paid more and let things stay as they are."

Physician organizations say compensation for DM is a tricky area that needs to be addressed. The 2,000 physician multispecialty Brown and Toland Medical Group scaled back its DM programs because insurers failed to compensate the group. The group's DM programs reduced overall costs by shifting care from the hospital to the physician's office. "Neither health plans nor employers rewarded us financially for these programs. As we managed these populations effectively and efficiently and hospital costs went down, there was more pressure to reduce the payments coming in to us."

Superior Medical Group's Experience with Disease Management

Congestive Heart Failure (CHF)

SMG entered a contract with LifeMasters four years ago to provide a DM program for patients with Stage 3 and 4 heart failure. The program opened three years ago as a clinical trial; they enrolled 68 patients, mean age 73, monitored by 31 physicians. The first phase was an 18-month period in which SMG's baseline experience was documented. The second phase was an 18-month period in which enrolled patients received frequent telephone check-ins with an experienced nurse, who then initiated alerts to physicians when certain complaints or measurements indicated early signs of deterioration. The calculated savings after fees ($700 per patient per year) was approximately $480,000 due to prevented hospitalizations. Unfortunately, because of the financial structure of the hospital risk pools, the savings did not translate into additional income for SMG. Although the program saved almost half a million dollars, other costs pushed expenses over the global budget.

SMG physicians resisted the program because it incurred new costs in lean times. They resented outside commercial "skimmers," third-party intrusion into the doctor-patient relationship, and the implication that existing care was deficient. Physician acceptance was facilitated by the experimental study design, existence of credible previous studies showing improved outcomes in CHF with DM programs, and the time LifeMasters staff spent in visits and presentations. "Physician involvement from the outset was a critical component of the success, and response to physician criticisms greatly strengthened the program." However, criticism from some physicians continued regarding cost ("Give me the money instead"), and "false alerts" that caused increased patient contacts and staff overhead, resulting in reluctance to refer newly identified patients and cynicism regarding SMG's administrative efforts in the quality improvement arena. Dr. Welly noted "Physicians have a hard time understanding the global aspects of these systems. If they get no check, they become angry and consider the system a failure."

Dr. Welly joined SMG as the study period was ending. It was his first exposure to a commercial DM program and he was impressed with the results. There was, however, a serious structural flaw—lack of financial rewards at the level of the physicians' offices. The physicians were required to look at the alerts that came in from LifeMasters nurses, and respond to them, with no reimbursement for their time. He recognizes the resources LifeMasters brought that SMG lacked—the experienced personnel and the physical space in this rural area and the information systems. Nonetheless, he doesn't believe SMG would enter into the same partnership now; LifeMasters would have to take financial risk and financially reward the physicians for their cooperation.

Osteoporosis

With the support of a pharmaceutical grant and the technical assistance of a member rheumatologist, SMG developed a program to rationalize osteoporosis screening. SMG mailed osteoporosis patient education materials to all female enrollees above a certain age. Physicians were required to fill out a questionnaire to establish patient risk in order to refer a patient for a bone density study. The patient score on the questionnaire determined which, if any, study would be performed. The cost was $70,000; women at risk received appropriate osteoporosis screening, and inappropriate studies were reduced.

Diabetes

The current age-standardized prevalence of diabetes in the United States is 8 percent, a rising prevalence associated with increases in obesity and sedentary lifestyle. Diabetes is the leading cause of new cases of blindness in adults 20 to 74 years old. Approximately 500,000 hospitalizations per year list diabetes as the primary diagnosis. Cardiovascular disease, kidney failure, amputations, and ketoacidosis are complications that frequently require hospitalization. In 1997, more than 33,000 new cases of end-stage renal disease were attributed to diabetes. Long-term complications of diabetes can be prevented through glucose, lipid, and blood pressure regulation, and early detection and treatment of eye, foot and kidney abnormalities. Improved patient education and self-management, and the provision of adequate and timely screening services and medical care can prevent complications.

Last month SMG launched a patient education promotion project supported by a grant from Aventis, a producer of insulin. Using claims data, physician offices were prompted to refer their diabetic patients to the diabetes education program at Sisters Hospital. With grant funds, SMG financially rewarded cooperating physicians and their staffs.

Dr. Welly is on the steering committee of the California Cooperative Healthcare Reporting Initiative's (CCHRI) Diabetes Continuous Quality Improvement project, a statewide collaborative to improve diabetes management. CCHRI is a program of the Pacific Business Group on Health, a large purchaser that negotiates rates with 12 HMOs for 21 companies. The mission of CCHRI is to measure performance and cooperate in quality improvement programs at the level of the physician group. SMG will be one of five medical groups participating in a pilot data-sharing project seeking to improve electronic data exchange between health plans and provider groups to routinely track services to diabetic patients.

CCHRI has developed basic guidelines for diabetes care (Table 8.1), endorsed by all the major health plans. Dr. Welly's efforts to have the guidelines incorporated into practice are primarily a "consciousness elevation" approach, with frequent communications on the subject. He believes that close to 50 percent of SMG's diabetic patients receive care that fulfills most of the guidelines.

TABLE 8.1

Components
of Diabetes
Disease
Management

Periodic Physical and Emotional Assessment

- Blood pressure and weight each visit, adjust medications to control blood pressure
- Foot exam—visual exam every visit, pulses and neurological exam annually
- Dilated eye exam annually by ophthalmologist
- Depression screen annually—treat with counseling, medication and/or referral
- Dental exam twice annually

Self-Management Training

- Assess patient knowledge of diabetes, medications, self-monitoring, and complications
- Home blood-sugar testing by patient, clinician reviews results
- Counsel on weight loss and nutrition, assess progress toward goals, and identify problem areas
- Smoking cessation—screen, advise, and assist
- Physical activity—assess and prescribe activity based on patient's needs/condition

Laboratory Exams

- Hemoglobin A1C (marker for diabetic control) quarterly if not meeting goals, 1 to 2 times per year if stable, treat with diet and medication.
- Microalbuminuria (marker for early kidney disease) annually
- Blood lipids—treat aggressively with diet and medication; measure quarterly if not meeting goals, annually if stable

An endocrinologist and internist from Coast Medical Associates worked with SMG's intranet provider, Axolotl, to develop a computer-based decision support diabetes program that would have provided clinical reminders in patient charts. However, because Axolotle is restructuring to focus on web-based upgrades, the SMG program has been delayed. The web-based program is expected to be expensive.

SMG collects data on the monitoring of diabetes patients, both to comply with the Health Employers Data and Information Set (HEDIS) and for its own quality management. SMG has provided written feedback reports to physicians regarding their performance in diabetes care, but this is difficult using claims data only.

SMG Support for DM

Dr. Welly's involvement with DM is still a fairly lonely crusade. "The physicians don't know what is going on in the larger field." Dr. Welly believes it is politically impossible to take money out of patient care revenue to invest in a DM program, whatever the return on investment or guaranteed savings. SMG currently shares financial risk for hospitalizations with HMOs. A budget is negotiated with each HMO based on historical utilization rates and blended with regional utilization rates. The difference in hospital costs above or below budget is evenly divided between SMG and the HMO.

HMOs are insisting medical groups implement disease management. HMOs have an "extremely condescending attitude to physician groups because it takes physicians so long to get anything done," so HMOs contract with commercial vendors or have their own DM divisions. Some DM companies are willing to share financial risk with health plans.

Commercial Diabetes DM Programs

McKesson CareEnhance, Pfizer Health Solutions InformaCare, Merck & Co., Inc., Health Management Services, American Healthways, Health Management Corporation Healthy Returns, Cor Solutions, and Matria are a few diabetes DM vendors. The programs are variations on a basic design of population assessment and data analysis, predictive modeling to stratify patients into high and low risk, targeted interventions, physician communications, and tracking utilization data.

Diabetes Healthways uses an engagement model, aggressively contacting patients. The company projects a $1.5 million annual diabetes care savings for an average 100,000-member commercial HMO. A retrospective analysis of 7,000 patients in their NetCare program found a $50 per member per month savings in diabetes treatment costs over 12 months and an 18 percent drop in hospital admissions.

Matria refers to the scientific literature to support claims of clinical effectiveness and economic benefit. The Diabetes Control and Complications Trial concluded that intensive management focused on reducing Hemoglobin A1C levels in patients with Type 1 diabetes prevented or delayed the onset of complications and significantly reduced the impact of these complications. The United Kingdom Prospective Diabetes Study reached similar conclusions for patients with Type 2 diabetes. "A 1997 study concluded that reducing Hemoglobin A1C from 9 percent to 7 percent reduced average diabetes-related medical costs by $1,200 per patient." However, this study by Gilmer did not compare pre- and post-DM program medical costs; it was a retrospective analysis that found charges for medical care from 1993–1995 were closely related to patients' Hemoglobin A1C levels in 1992.

As Dr. Welly reflected on his recommendation to the board, he wondered whether it was his role to get physician buy-in on DM programs, or whether he should limit his efforts to what was necessary for compliance with HMO contracts. He wanted to be realistic about how much he could expect to accomplish given the low level of integration of the independent physician offices. He wasn't sure whether a DM program would increase SMG revenue, savings, or costs. How would SMG pay for the increased coordination and intensity of services to patients with chronic illness? Dr. Welly had been successful with small pharmaceutical grants and hoped to realize larger grants, knowing the large resources of pharmaceutical companies and the incentive they have to fund programs which would increase the sales of their products. He didn't think this presented a conflict of interest, or an ethical dilemma, but wasn't sure he should push for a DM program not knowing with certainty that the funding would be available.

Case Questions

1. Would a diabetes DM program increase SMG revenue, savings, or costs?
2. What is it about the organizational structure and culture of an IPA that facilities or blocks quality improvement (QI)?
3. Should Dr. Welly recommend to the SMG Board of Directors that they contract for a diabetes DM program? Should he recommend that they develop their own, with or without a partner?
   - If yes, how could Dr. Welly increase support from SMG physicians and management for DM programs?
   - If no, what should Dr. Welly recommend to the Board to improve SMG's diabetes management?
4. Is the diabetes DM program a strategic decision?

PROFESSIONAL INTEGRATION

. . . in the United States, the physician is
not so much part of the hospital as the
hospital is part (and only one part) of the
physician's practice.

—Freidson

COMMENTARY

The integration of clinician and organizational goals is one of the key challenges facing managers in healthcare organizations today. Increasingly, managers are being asked to link clinician objectives to organizational objectives. This assumes that clinicians are willing to consider being so linked, when changing clinician behavior may require prior changes in organizational performance for which managers are primarily accountable. These issues play out differently in various types of organizations such as hospitals, nursing homes, group practices, visiting nurse services, and HMOs.

Most of the physicians who work in hospitals are independent contractors who are not employed by the hospital. In nursing homes, there are fewer physicians who visit patients, and the patients frequently do not return to their homes and to the physician's private practice. In the group practice, the physicians own the organization and are the top managers; non-physician managers work for them. Visiting nurse services are typically run by professional nurses, and very few physicians play any major role in such organizations. HMOs are typically run by professional managers, some of whom may be physicians; however, it is crystal clear that organizational rather than clinician concerns are paramount.

The issue can be framed into more standard labor relations terms, where managers in organizations have to negotiate contracts of work with unions representing workers. Hundreds of thousands of health workers are unionized; among them, very few physicians. What makes physicians different from the other health professionals is that no one bargaining agent in the hospital represents most of them; physicians differ among themselves in their relationships to healthcare organizations they do not control. For example, in the hospital, radiologists, anesthesiologists, and pathologists are commonly employed. Surgeons may be dependent upon the hospital as a primary work place, while dermatologists and psychiatrists, for example, do not include the hospital as an important part of their practice.

There are over 200 different healthcare occupations, including highly trained professionals such as optometrists, dentists, podiatrists, pharmacists, and physical therapists. For reasons of space, we will concentrate here on relations between hospitals and physicians, with some mention of nurses.

Physicians and Hospitals

A study of the key drivers of physician loyalty carried out by the Health Care Advisory Board concluded that clinical quality, efficiency, and convenient access were at the center of the physician agenda, with most hospitals not meeting (admittedly high) physician standards as to operational efficiency and staff competency (Health Care Advisory Board 1999).

Some divergence between hospital and physician objectives is functional. Physicians are concerned with the best possible care for their patients. Managers are concerned with the best possible care for all patients and potential patients. This divergence is functional to the extent that claims for resources to attain both objectives can be effectively represented and adjudicated in the hospital decision-making processes. If there is no divergence, the result may be a lack of sufficient hospital or physician response on behalf of their different constituencies. If the divergence is too great, the result may be sub-optimization, as physician objectives are achieved at the expense of hospital objectives or vice versa.

Our views on physicians and hospitals, echoing those of Griffith and White (2002), are that the business of the healthcare organization is healthcare. This means that physicians and managers must be allies. Buyers/customers want high-quality care at the lowest possible price. They will increase the market share of any hospital that they believe provides it. Managers must develop relationships with physicians so that the market gets the healthcare it wants. Managers cannot run for any period of time a hospital where the mission is at odds with the physicians who operate the core technology.

Again, following Griffith and White, physicians can expect from hospitals the following: a reasonable income and lifestyle, professional recognition, and participation in decision making (2002). Of course, everyone wants this where we work; life teaches that many of us, some would say most of us, cannot easily get it. What is a reasonable income anyway, relative to whose income? Some physicians, and some professors for that matter, can never get sufficient professional recognition. Some physicians do not want to participate in hospital decision making; others want to participate too much, given their limited skills and experience and given conflicts of interest. Bottom line, an important part of the manager's job is managing the expectations of physicians so that they will get a clearer, realistic view of these issues. The goal is for all parties to see and hopefully move toward more of a win-win situation (not that win-win is always possible either). When there is conflict, Griffith and White (2002) suggest that market share maximization is the mutual benefit criterion—that is, not paying physicians enough leads to low quality and loss of market, while paying them too much leads to market share erosion as customers seek lower cost, acceptable-quality alternatives.

Senior managers are few, and physicians are numerous. Can managers achieve hospital objectives when they conflict with the priorities of physicians? Some opportunities for managers result from the following characteristics of hospitals.

- *Key interest groups in the organization have different objectives.* For example, intensivists may oppose while family physicians and the governing board may favor increased hospital emphasis on chronic and ambulatory care.
- *Physicians often compete among themselves for scarce organizational resources.* For example, radiologists could urge purchase of new radiologic equipment while internists prefer investments in physician order entry systems.
- *There may be goal divergence among physicians in the same clinical area.* Full-time surgeons are probably more interested in research than surgeons in private practice.

Physicians and hospitals can be viewed as partners joining their skills and resources with a mutual interest in adapting effectively to a rapidly changing competitive environment. In certain joint ventures, both may provide capital and commitment. These ventures may be carried out by new corporate entities that are for-profit and jointly-owned. "Intrapreneurs" are entrepreneurs within an existing organization who are encouraged to create and develop new programs and services. Encouraging affiliated physicians to develop new programs is one form of this intrapreneurship. Describing these activities with new words like joint ventures and intrapreneurs reflects the greater attention now being paid to them.

Physicians respond differently to the changing environment for hospitals. Some will wish to respond in the direction of change, others to resist changes that seem to be fads or ill-advised responses. Physicians differ in their responses to newer clinical programs such as hospices, urgent care centers, pain management, and alternative medicine programs, as well as in their responses to newer management initiatives such as paperless records, performance budgeting, and patient-focused care. Physicians favor, are indifferent to, or oppose some or all of these programs and initiatives, some of which are more suited to or affordable for some organizations than others. Managers must test the external and internal environments of their organizations and adapt to inevitable change. Managers must differentiate between the inevitable and the uncertain and choose programs and directions after the pioneers have worked out the bugs, but before the latecomers have jumped on the bandwagon. No mean feat, but this is what effective managers, after all, are paid well to do.

Physicians, Nurses, and Managers

The power of physicians and nurses has changed over time. Before the Flexner reforms that started in 1910, a few months of education would qualify one to become a physician, and there were lots of hungry physicians. A wealthy patient could and did pay for a full-time physician or private-duty nurse. Although many medical schools were closed during the Flexner reforms, there was a long delay in reducing the number of practitioners. Many physicians struggled during the Depression of the 1930s, while hospital managers took big pay cuts to hold their jobs (Neuhauser 1995). The growth of health insurance after World War II in 1945 led to a so-called golden era of medicine as cost-based reimbursement of Medicare and Blue Cross supported the growth of hospitals and nursing education largely moved out of the hospital and into the college and university.

From 1950 to 1970, the power of physicians was great. The most likely reason a hospital administrator would lose his job was because the medical staff wanted to get rid of him. Physicians, if displeased with a hospital, could easily shift their admissions to another nearby facility. Hospitals added new equipment and services to attract medical specialists. Reaction to increasing costs included prospective payment (DRGs), capitation (HMOs), and price competition among managed care plans.

Once nursing and teaching were among the few professions available to women. The opening up of other professions such as medicine, law, and accounting has forced nursing to compete to attract students, including encouraging men to become nurses. The shortage of professional nurses affects hospitals where half of all nurses work on salary.

The acute shortage of professional nurses in hospitals is giving nurses greater power. California has regulated the hours required in hospitals for nursing staff per patient, and nurses are increasingly organized in unions or professional associations that bargain more aggressively over the conditions of work. Aiken (2001) has written extensively of complaints from nurses about working conditions, which are often primarily not about pay but rather about inadequate staffing and the unwillingness of management to listen to nurse suggestions for improving patient care or to staff nursing services so that nurses can provide a high quality of care.

References

Aiken, L. 2001. "Evidence-Based Management: Key to Hospital Workforce Stability." *Journal of Health Administration Education* Special Issue: 117–124.

Griffith, J. R. and K. White. 2002. *The Well Managed Healthcare Organization,* 5th edition. Chicago: Health Administration Press.

Health Care Advisory Board. 1999. *The Physician Perspective: Key Drivers of Physician Loyalty.* Washington, DC: Health Care Advisory Board.

Neuhauser, D. 1995. *Coming of Age,* revised edition. Chicago: Health Administration Press, p. 76.

THE READINGS

The required readings for Part IV are a series on the future of healthcare professions. The authors urge conversion of our healthcare system to one that is more patient-centered and where clinician and organizational goals are better integrated to achieve that purpose. Making changes in the training, culture, and behavior of healthcare clinicians will not, however, be easy. Yet, this is the type of healthcare system envisioned by the Committee on Quality of Health Care of the Institute of Medicine (2001) in their widely circulated report *Crossing the Quality Chasm*. The committee has recommended the following six redesign imperatives, all of which are affected by the relationships among doctors, nurses, and managers.

1. Redesigned care processes
2. Effective use of information technologies
3. Knowledge and skills management
4. Development of effective teams
5. Coordination of care across patient conditions, services, and settings over time
6. Use of performance and outcome measurement for continuous quality improvement and accountability

What is required is a focus by healthcare organizations on patient trajectories through episodes of illness rather than on procedures of care and professional prerogatives and convenience.

Reference

Committee on Quality, Institute of Medicine. 2001. *Crossing the Quality Chasm: A New Health System for the 21st Century*. Washington DC: National Academy Press.

The Drivers of Change

Mary E. Stefl, Ph.D.
From *Frontiers of Health Services Management* 18 (2), Winter 2001

Imagine a healthcare system that is truly patient centered. Sick patients would not wait days for an appointment with their primary care physician and then hours in the front office. Referrals to a specialist would be scheduled promptly, at a convenient location, and at a convenient time.

In this system, providers would respect patients' wishes and understand cultural differences in healthcare practices. Care protocols would be designed in collaboration with the patient and, when desired, the patient's family. Providers would readily share information about the patient's condition and discuss treatment alternatives, and full disclosure would be made about the costs involved.

In this system, both clinical care and healthcare management would be evidence-based, so that the most appropriate care would be provided in the most efficient, effective, and safe manner. Patient outcomes, and not cost or organizational structure, would be the guiding force behind care design. Errors would be documented and studied so that processes could be improved, and any harm caused to the patient would be readily disclosed.

In this system, physicians, nurses, healthcare executives, and a host of other healthcare practitioners would work together in teams because they all believe it is in the best interest of the patient. Their efforts to improve the health of the patient would rely on highly sophisticated and integrated information systems that have been designed to ensure confidentiality.

This is the type of healthcare system envisioned by the Institute of Medicine's (IOM) Committee on Quality of Health Care in America (IOM 1999; IOM 2001). At its core is the patient, but it relies on finely tuned care processes or systems and integrated information technology to deliver patient care. Achieving this vision will require fundamental changes in the healthcare system operating today, changes that were thoroughly explored in a recent issue of *Frontiers* (Detmer 2001).

But a new healthcare system also means important changes for healthcare professionals who will need to learn new skills and new values, and educational and training programs will need to respond appropriately. Making these changes in the training, culture, and behavior of healthcare professionals will not be easy. Some direction can be found in the series of ten rules for twenty-first century healthcare that were enumerated in the IOM's Quality Chasm (IOM 2001) report. These rules were formulated as a guide to achieving patient-centered care, and they have obvious implications for health professionals.

New Rules for Health Professionals

1. *Care should be based on continuous healing relationships.* Patients need care on a 24-hour-a-day, 7-day-a-week basis, but the current system is largely limited to workday office visits. To provide this continuous care, new modes of communication will be necessary, and the Internet provides great potential. While face-to-face visits will continue to be

important, much follow-up care can be accomplished in other ways. Electronic and other modes of communication could make care more continuous and enable clinicians to have more office visit time to devote to each in-person encounter.

2. *Care should be customized based on patient needs and values.* Variability in treatment will be based only on individual patient needs and values. Clinicians will use information technology to determine the various courses of action for a given condition, discuss these treatments and the associated probabilities of success, and then select the course of action that fits best with the patient's wishes and needs. Clinicians will learn to harvest the information infrastructure for treatment alternatives rather than attempt to memorize an unwieldy amount of information. They will also need strong communication skills, including the art of listening to the patient.

3. *The patient will be the source of control.* At the present time, professionals maintain control over the time, place, and type of care provided. Under the new rule, patients will share in the decision-making process with care providers (to the extent patients wish to be involved). This implies that professionals will freely share information with the patient. Closely related to the second point above, this rule also assumes clinicians will possess good communication skills.

4. *Knowledge will be shared and information will flow freely.* According to the Quality Chasm report, transfer of personal and scientific information is the foundation of the patient-clinician relationship. Patients should have unrestricted access to their medical records, and they should be able to find out which providers have accessed and annotated them. To prevent confusion or fear on the part of the patient, providers will need to find ways to educate patients.

5. *Decision making will be evidence-based.* Clinical care should be based on the best and most recent available information. With an appropriate information infrastructure, care protocols can be constantly updated to include the newest knowledge and to account for patient variability. At the same time, the design and management of care processes should be based on systematic study.

6. *Safety will be a system priority.* The healthcare system and healthcare providers should not tolerate preventable errors. Rather than blaming individuals for mistakes, errors should be systematically studied so that processes can be designed to prevent future events. Healthcare professionals should learn from other industries that make systematic improvements based on the study of errors. The culture of hiding mistakes should give way to one in which errors are openly reported and shared with the patient.

7. *The system should be transparent.* The Quality Chasm report states quite simply: "Have no secrets." Healthcare professionals and organizations should be accountable to the public. The results of their care should be freely available so that patients can make informed choices. The culture that routinely withholds information will have to be replaced.

8. *Needs should be anticipated.* The system should not wait for problems to occur, but anticipate needs based on patient history, local circumstances, and knowledge of the patient's disease. Healthcare providers will be responsible for linking patients with community resources and providing systems (e.g., e-mail or telephone reminders) that assist patients in managing chronic conditions. Besides improving patient care, the anticipation of needs can save costs as some disease management programs have demonstrated (Tieman 2001).

9. *Waste should be continually decreased.* A culture of continuous improvement should be built into each component of the healthcare system. All healthcare providers should have training in improvement techniques. Healthcare executives have a special responsibility for ensuring that these techniques are put to good use.

10. *Clinicians need to cooperate.* If care is to be patient centered, it will involve the services and skills of a variety of healthcare providers who cooperate and communicate with one another. At certain times, these professionals will need to work together as teams to provide the most comprehensive patient care. When care involves special resources, management professionals may join the care team. The current culture of autonomy will need to give way to one of cooperation, and education for healthcare professionals will need to incorporate team-building techniques.

Applied to healthcare professionals, these ten rules can drive changes that will vastly improve patient care. They will require changes in our existing educational curricula and in the culture of the settings in which care is practiced.

Technological Advancement

The work of the IOM can and should drive changes in healthcare delivery in the near future. However, both current practitioners and educators need to be aware that breakthroughs in technology, especially in genomics, robotics, and nanotechnology, have the potential to significantly alter the practice of medicine and healthcare delivery. A new delivery system and culture of care cannot ignore these inevitable trends.

For example, genetic therapies are already being practiced, albeit on an experimental basis. And while the role of genetics in health and illness has been understood for some time, the recent completion of the mapping of the human genome suggests that developments in medical genomics will accelerate.

Genetic screening will become more sophisticated and reliable, and techniques will follow for repairing pieces of DNA that cause disease or dysfunctional mutations. As a result, much of healthcare delivery may shift from middle and old age to youth (Myers, Paulk, and Dudlak 2001) and more care will be delivered in ambulatory settings. Geneticists will likely become an integral part of the healthcare team, and the role of pediatricians will be greatly enhanced. Advances in pharmacogenetics, where drug therapies are devised for an individual based on his or her genetic code, will make treatments far more effective.

Robots and robotic devices have already entered healthcare delivery. Robotic drug dispensing systems may redefine the role of clinical pharmacists (Barcia 1999) and service robots can deliver medications to patient rooms 24 hours a day without error (Robbins 2001). Robotic surgery shows great potential (e.g., Noonan 2001). The FDA is now sponsoring seven clinical trials of surgical procedures ranging from bypass operations to prostate surgery. All contact with the patient is made through robotic devices. Dexterity and precision is enhanced; all of the unnecessary movement made even by the steadiest of surgeons is eliminated. The outcome is a nearly bloodless, minimally invasive procedure with reduced postoperative pain and recovery time. In most current cases, the surgeon manipulates the robotic controls in the same room as the patient. Once the technology becomes more refined, physical proximity will no longer be required.

Nanotechnology is robotics on a molecular scale, for it involves building machines on the atomic level, one atom at a time (Kurzweil 1999). Interest in the potential of nanotechnology has blossomed in recent years, as scientists and engineers learn more about the basic building blocks of life and fabricated materials (National Nanotechnology Initiative 2001). Futurists envision microscopic machines introduced into the bloodstream with a mission to fix diseased cells, destroy arterial plaque, or eliminate pathogens. These nanoscopic machines could, without triggering an immune reaction, repair damaged organs or deliver therapeutics at the cellular level.

Medical treatment through nanotechnology would eliminate the need for most surgery and recovery time. Treatment would be highly specific to the individual patient's biochemistry, and consequently efficient and effective. Most treatment could be performed in an outpatient setting or in the patient's home.

Crossing the Quality Chasm (IOM 2001) is an immediate action call to healthcare professionals, both practitioners and educators alike, to create a delivery system focused on patients. Doing so will require considerable effort and enormous changes in existing behaviors and attitudes. But the change process must also consider the opportunities and challenges that advances in genomics, robotics, nanotechnology, and other emerging new technologies will create for medical practice and healthcare delivery in the future.

The articles that follow examine the potential effect of these trends on three of the most visible and important healthcare professions: medicine, nursing, and healthcare administration.

References

Barcia, S. M. 1999. "Man vs. Machine." *Health Management Technology* 20 (9): 24–25.

Detmer, D. E. 2001. "A New Health System and Its Quality Agenda." *Frontiers of Health Services Management* 18 (1): 3–30.

Institute of Medicine. 2001. *Crossing the Quality Chasm: A New Health System for the 21st Century.* Washington, DC: National Academy Press.

———. 1999. *To Err Is Human: Building a Safer Health Care System*, edited by Lt. T. Kohn, J. M. Corrigan, and M. S. Donaldson. Washington, DC: National Academy Press.

Kurzweil, R. 1999. *The Age of Spiritual Machines.* New York: Viking Penguin.

Myers, C., N. Paulk, and C. Dudlak. 2001. "Genomics: Implications for Health Systems." *Frontiers of Health Services Management* 17 (3): 3–16.

National Nanotechnology Initiative. 2001. http://www.nano.gov.

Noonan, D. 2001. "The Ultimate Remote Control." *Newsweek* (June 25): 70–74; 76.

Robbins, J. V. 2001. "Nuts, Bolts and Brains." *Hospitals & Health Networks* 75 (2): 48–50.

Tieman, J. 2001. "Coming of Age." *Modern Healthcare* 31 (28): 26–27; 38.

Substance, Form, and Knowing the Difference

David C. Leach, M.D., and David P. Stevens, M.D.
From *Frontiers of Health Services Management* 18 (2), Winter 2001

Substance is enduring; form is ephemeral; failure to distinguish between the two is ruinous. Success follows those adept at preserving the substance of the past by clothing it in the forms of the future. Preserve substance; modify form; know the difference.
—Dee Hock, *The Birth of the Chaordic Age*

Trekkies among the readers of this journal will be familiar with the various iterations of physicians in "Star Trek," the classic science fiction series. The starship Enterprise was on a mission—to explore the universe—"to boldly go where no man has gone before." In the first iteration, circa 1966, the physician in the series was Dr. Leonard "Bones" McCoy, a crusty Georgia general practitioner who did not trust technology, was a fierce advocate for his patients, and who was, in short, an ideal physician as viewed by the public at the time. The second iteration, "Star Trek: The Next Generation," premiered in 1987, and presented Dr. Beverly Crusher, a woman, fluent in technology and gifted with interpersonal skills, again reflecting the ideal as viewed by the public of the time. By 1995 the physician was gone. She was replaced by a hologram, infinitely accessible, absolutely current in both information and skill, and able to wing the interpersonal. If prescient, this may not bode well for physicians. In any event it may be best to begin by accepting the possibility that none of us will be indispensable.

While it is difficult to predict the future, it is not too far-fetched to imagine a world in which reliable information is available to patients who seek routine preventive measures, personalized advice for common medical problems, and connection with other patients facing similar issues—all in the absence of a face-to-face meeting with a physician. It is more likely that, if physicians are needed, it will be when the human condition runs its course and the "mirage of health" (Dubois 1971) is replaced by the reality of illness and the person becomes a patient.

The future will engage our will as well as our intellect. We will be expected not only to discern the truth, but also to make judgments about the degrees of goodness of various options. The raw utilitarian approach of science requires further illumination in the particular case; it needs to be integrated with the art of medicine. A drug that works, but bankrupts the patient and family, cures the disease and damages the patient. End-of-life heroics may attack the patient as well as the disease, offering neither comfort nor cure. If we are to add value, we have to offer ourselves as well as our technology.

Even then, however, it seems likely that technology will do the heavy lifting needed to establish an accurate diagnosis and to clarify the best treatment. Our value will come from the fact that we share with the patient human vulnerability; that fact may prove comforting. This fundamental contribution will be enhanced if we apply intelligence and thoughtful reflection to experiences with similar patients, so that we can answer questions relevant to the situation—answers based on true stories and human interpretations of reality that may supplement the cold facts that surround but don't comfort the patient. We might be needed for other reasons, but this human element seems bedrock; all else will be built on this.

It may be time to review our most potent arsenal—not our technological arsenal, but our values, our time-tested truths, our best behaviors as physicians. It may be time to identify the substance of medicine, to be clear about what we will carry into a complex emerging future. Clarity about substance and form will allow us to preserve our best and be malleable about the rest.

Relationship

A case may be made that the durable substance of medicine is relationship, that is, humans relating to other humans. Relationship deals with vulnerability, values, and dignity. All else is modifiable form.

Substance involves competence, but also compassion. Competence and compassion are inseparable. Either without the other cannot suffice. Competence without compassion is not really competence, and compassion without competence is not compassion. The nexus of competence and compassion comes back to relationship; only a clear and open understanding of one person by another can illuminate the best path.

The current healthcare system sabotages relationship. Relationships with patients, with society, with professional colleagues, and with self all have been compromised. Make no mistake, some heroes and heroines in the system find a way to keep relationships with patients alive, but the system makes it very hard to find the time needed to listen, to develop trust, and to really connect patient and doctor. Heroes and heroines exist, but the villain is time.

We have lost control of time; it now dictates who we are. How we spend our time defines us. We spend it on form rather than substance. Care of the system has compromised care of the patient. If we are to improve healthcare we must pay more attention to time; we must use it to strengthen relationships between physicians and patients, physicians and colleagues, and physicians and society. The system has undervalued its greatest asset—it has preserved form and sold substance short. Technology has enhanced our capacities to recognize disease but lack of time and skill have inhibited our abilities to recognize the patient. Ken Ludmerer (1999) has developed this thesis extensively in his book, *Time to Heal*.

Common purpose is important; it binds the community together. When it is lacking, tyranny and command and control behavior take its place (Hock 1999). Common purpose will be hard to establish. As we enter the twenty-first century, the surviving systems will have clarified purpose so that all components of the system are aligned. Three words will suffice—improve patient care.

Simple Rules for the Twenty-First Century Healthcare System

The Institute of Medicine (2001) has offered ten simple rules for the twenty-first century healthcare system. Each supports deepening of human relationships and thereby reinforces the substance of medicine. The rules are organizing principles for an emerging complex world. Each requires that we distribute our time differently. They invite experiments and local interpretation, and offer hope that best practices will emerge.

But some problems exist. The rules expose the absence of a healthcare system.

Parts of the system frequently work at odds with one another, and these fragments are too fragile to support the rules.

For example, consider the rule: Care is based on continuous healing relationships. The fragment "physician" cannot attempt to implement the rule without engaging the rest of the system. Assumptions about encounter-based modes of healthcare are deeply entrenched in all parts of the system. What changes would have to be made in the insurance industry, medical group practice mores, hospital and outpatient facilities, home support systems, information systems, and communication systems to support this rule? What is the likelihood of a physician implementing this rule without realignment of all the other parts? Without these changes it remains just a good idea. Is it possible to have a common purpose sufficient to redesign all of these elements of the system? Are we skilled enough and committed enough to make the fundamental design changes that are needed for patients to benefit from this rule?

Consider another example: the patient as the source of control. This rule is designed to empower the patient with information, time, and access to expertise. Paradoxically, this will strengthen relationship, but it may increase conflict between the doctor and the patient. Inevitably some patients will choose options that may be in conflict with the best science. They may have control but their interest may not be best served by that control. A deep and trusting relationship is needed to make this work. The insurance industry may have trouble with this rule, and if we are to develop a true system, they have to be at the table. Yet patient control coupled with unlimited expectations will ultimately challenge whatever system is bankrolling care. What happens to trust when the best advice is not "covered?" This rule, as with the others, requires all parties serving all of the truth, not just selected pieces. Otherwise the fragments will be pitted against each other. Parker J. Palmer quotes Abba Felix that "to teach is to create a space in which obedience to truth is practiced" (Palmer 1993). This educational mantra could be modified to: to practice medicine (and, of necessity, to create a system) is to create a space in which obedience to truth is practiced. If the system is designed to support this rule we can achieve a true system; otherwise we will just increase conflict.

As one reflects on each of the proposed rules it becomes apparent that the entire system would need to be redesigned to derive the full benefit of them. This is a tremendous opportunity. Can common purpose bind us together?

Organizational Models

What type of organizational model could be robust enough to embrace these new rules and new technologies and allow us to adapt intelligently to an unknown future? Dee Hock (2000) has an interesting answer. He writes, "organizations [are] increasingly unable to achieve the purpose for which they were created, yet [they] continue to expand as they devour scarce resources, demean the human spirit, and destroy the environment . . . We have unhealthy healthcare systems." He suggests an alternative to hierarchical command and control mechanistic organizational models. He has created the term the "chaordic organization." As the founding CEO of Visa he created a prototype organizational model that encourages simultaneous cooperation and competition, unleashes intelligent adaptation to local environments, yet insists on common purpose and supports the free flow of information, knowing that information is needed to ensure that all parties do adapt intelligently. What would a chaordic healthcare organization look like? His paper, "Gone Chaordic" (Hock 2000) describes the principles necessary for such an organization as well as a tantalizing, radical vision.

Educating Physicians for the New World

Teaching medical students and residents provides a test of our own understanding of substance and form. In recent decades teaching models have been designed to accommodate an exponential increase in biomedical knowledge and technology. Techniques have focused more on content and less on person. Many teachers and learners have attempted to compensate but are thwarted by "the system." Time is compressed; hospital stays are short. Residents need to be efficient. Listening deeply to the patient is not always an option. Education has been utilitarian rather than Aristotelian, a "this works and this doesn't" approach, rather than an attempt at full development of a good citizen, a citizen capable of making and recognizing right judgments, judgments that harmonize goodness and truth. This is tricky business and will call upon our deepest traditions, traditions made more, not less, relevant by the press of technology.

What does this mean for education? Context—the organizational model—is important. Teaching high-quality medicine in a dysfunctional system is becoming, by its very definition, impossible. Education, like patient care, is rooted in relationship. There are things in teaching hospitals that support and things that inhibit relationship. Teaching substance requires closeness between teacher and student. A computer can teach form. A computer can be a role model for holograms but not for humans.

Essentials for teaching include memory, hope, and reality: memory of our previous experiences and own attempts at learning; hope for both the student and the teacher; and the reality of a patient accompanied by shared discovery of that reality with a student. In professional education the memories, hopes, and realities are not just personal. They are the memories of the profession, the hopes of the profession, and the realities the profession has encountered over millennia.

Time and space for reflection are essential, but we need to be practical. Both patient care and medical education are best when pragmatic. How should our students spend their time if we are to arm them with substance, teach them to discern and be malleable to form, and have them contribute to the larger system so that the purpose of improving patient care is achieved? Corollary rules for learning in the twenty-first century health system might include the following:

- Spend the bulk of time practicing relationships with self, colleagues, society, and most of all with patients.
- Understand and respect human beings; become effective champions of the human spirit.
- Center relationships around discernment—knowing how to know.
- Learn to use one's hands, to develop procedural skills, to become effective.
- Constantly analyze experiences and use those experiences as a major source of knowledge.
- Learn improvement skills by making changes and testing to see if improvement has occurred.
- Understand duty, competence, and what it means to put the patient's interest first.
- Work with others to improve the system.

Accreditation

Finally, and this is not totally science fiction, imagine that you have been charged with accrediting an institution as worthy of supporting the training of physicians who will function in the twenty-first century. Imagine that you agree with the premise that the substance of medicine is more important than form, and that the true substance of medicine is human relationships. What would you look for?

Unfortunately, you find an immediate problem. You are charged with accrediting an institution only to find on careful inspection and reflection that institutions don't exist. They are mental constructs. The only things real in an institution are the people and the relationships they have with each other. Yes, there are bricks and mortar, but people make an institution what it is. So what are you accrediting? Fundamentally it comes down to relationships between humans.

But you conclude that you need to measure something. After all, that is what accreditors do. So you decide you want to focus on things that facilitate and things that inhibit human relationships.

Think of things that inhibit human relationships: a lot of them have to do with how we spend time. Lack of time, interruptions, distractions during conversations—these inhibit in all settings and seem especially prevalent in hospitals. Osler said, "Medicine is a jealous mistress" (Osler 1932). In the modern hospital, form is an avaricious thief stealing what is due to substance.

As a cross check you also may want to measure things that the students have learned: what can they now do that they could not do before? What might you measure? Maybe you should measure how students and faculty spend their time. You can ask patients and students if their doctor/teacher spent enough time with them, whether they listen, nurture true relationship, and communicate openly. You can ask the students for a portfolio of their experiences; their stories about their patients can be revealing. Each student and resident should have his or her procedural skills observed directly and clearly demonstrated to be done well. You can test their knowledge.

Ultimately then, we are back to the classics. What is different is that this time we have to take it seriously. Otherwise the holograms may await.

References

Hock, D. 2000. "Gone Chaordic." *Health Forum Journal* (Mar/Apr): 20–25, 68–70.
———. 1999. *Birth of the Chaordic Age*. San Francisco: Berrett-Koehler Publishers, Inc.
Dubois, R. 1971. *The Mirage of Health*. New York: Perennial Press.
Institute of Medicine. 2001. *Crossing the Quality Chasm: A New Health System for the 21st Century*. Washington, DC: National Academy Press.
Ludmerer, K. 1999. *Time to Heal*. New York: Oxford University Press.
Osler, W. 1932. "The Student Life." *Aequanimitas*. Philadelphia: Blakiston.
Palmer, P. J. 1993. *To Know as We Are Known*. San Francisco: Harper.

The Challenge for Nursing

Linda R. Cronenwett, RN., Ph.D.
From *Frontiers of Health Services Management* 18 (2), Winter 2001

Whether the topic is evidence-based care, patient safety, continuous quality improvement, or the drivers of future change described earlier in this issue by Dr. Stefl, our ability to "cross the chasm" from the present healthcare system to a preferred future is limited if our prevailing strategy is to do more of the same with fewer resources. But when and how will the learning occur to stimulate a different response?

In the education of healthcare professionals, the primary focus is the transmission of disciplinary knowledge. In healthcare practice, we function in disciplinary teams, knowing and caring little about the work of other professionals who provide services to patients (except, of course, when their work impedes our own efficiency or quality of work life). As a result, healthcare professionals are ill-equipped to provide leadership for the new health system and quality agenda described by Detmer (2001) and the Institute of Medicine (IOM) *Quality Chasm* (2001) report.

During the 7th Annual Summer Symposium, "Building Knowledge for the Leadership of Improvement of Health Care," at Dartmouth led by Paul Batalden (July 2000), participants challenged each other to consider how health professions education might need to change to better prepare healthcare professionals for the future. Participants began by sharing stories of heroes in nursing, medicine, and healthcare administration during two periods: 1850 to 1950 and 1950 to 2000. We worked first in single discipline groups to answer the questions:

- What values were important to the professionals in your discipline during this time period?
- What behaviors were needed to perform the daily work with the values stated above?
- What key aspects of professional preparation were needed to achieve the work, values, and behaviors?

Members of each discipline discussed the characteristics of heroes in each time period and how they related, if at all, to the values, behaviors, and methods of professional preparation of the period. We then formed multidisciplinary groups, presented our summaries to each other, and looked for themes across professions. During other parts of the symposium, we learned about the projected effects of genomics, robotics, and nanotechnology on the future of the health professions and spent time imagining what would be required of the health professional hero of the future.

The results of the group exercises were enlightening. The characteristics of heroes across disciplines were more alike than different. Furthermore, the characteristics of heroes of the past, present, and future were similar as well. Abilities possessed by heroes across disciplines and time periods included:

- Ability to identify the human elements of need and keep that vision central to any enterprise

- Ability to use information for learning, as an individual and within systems
- Ability to function as a member or leader of an effective team
- Ability to create and be part of a learning community
- Ability to sustain a commitment to service, always demonstrating a moral and ethical compass
- Ability to listen, communicate, and manage conflict

These abilities often made the difference between people referred to as heroes, and other professionals who may have had an equal or greater mastery of traditional disciplinary knowledge. If the above behaviors have been associated with professional heroes in the past and present, and we need heroes in healthcare today, then the question is: What ought we to be doing within our professions to induce learning about these behaviors?

The nurses at the symposium (to whom I am indebted for the development of the basic ideas but who are not accountable for the examples elaborated below), wrestled with the question: What would it take in nursing to better educate health professional heroes for the future? The following ideas emerged.

Increase the Availability of Clinical Role Models

Learners are most likely to develop the values and behaviors they see demonstrated in the context of clinical practice. A significant percentage of nursing faculty members do not practice. Others have limited exposure to students during faculty practice time. As a result, nurses in practice are the primary or sole role models for the values and behaviors that we want future healthcare professionals to learn.

In the current environment, the instability of nurses' schedules makes even a consistent preceptor a treasure. Furthermore, faculty members rarely select, prepare, or nourish the preceptors who serve as primary role models for students. If faculty members do not serve as role models for the behaviors we wish students to adopt in clinical practice, and if we do not nourish preceptors who are strong role models, then how do we ensure that students learn the behaviors and values needed for the future?

Academic nursing leaders could use a variety of strategies to enhance the quality of role models for students in clinical practice, such as:

- Establish intentional partnerships between faculty members and clinical leaders to develop plans for identifying and nurturing good preceptors
- Increase the presence of practice experts on nursing faculty through adjunct or regular appointments; institute methods of rewarding their contributions; fully legitimize them as teachers

- Decrease barriers and increase incentives for faculty practice
- Increase the number of school of nursing practice/service initiatives in which students might learn
- Develop multiple strategies for integrating faculty into the work of patient care in each of the traditional research, teaching, and service missions

The above strategies will work best if students see nurses and other healthcare professionals working in systems that are testing innovations that respond to the challenge of the ten rules as proposed in the IOM (2001) report. Because most settings and professionals are only beginning to grapple with the changes required to transform healthcare systems, other teaching strategies for the next generation of health professionals are needed.

Increase Opportunities for Learning Outside of Disciplinary Silos

Current health professional students graduate knowing little about each others' knowledge bases and even less about the daily work challenges of each others' professional lives. Furthermore, by the time they graduate, health professionals have been exposed to numerous examples of ineffective, even hostile, interprofessional communications. As Detmer (2001) noted, "Teamwork means that each player knows who comprises their team, what the roles and responsibilities of each team member are, and how their performance can both help and hinder those with whom they work." Dramatic changes in health professions education are required if new professionals are to better learn how to work in interprofessional teams. If nursing leaders were to contribute to solving this problem, we might:

- Require nursing students to shadow other professionals and share observations about the roles, knowledge base, and work challenges of multiple disciplines
- Include objectives for student learning about effective teams/crews and the importance of good communication for patient safety
- Set goals for a minimum number of interdisciplinary learning experiences during the course of undergraduate and graduate education; if courses are impossible, use classes, modules, or observational learning exercises
- Use technology to promote simulated or virtual collaborations where barriers to simultaneous team learning exist
- Partner with administrators of clinical agencies to develop learning opportunities for students that would provide opportunities for interprofessional team learning

- Require that all faculty members be involved in some interdisciplinary enterprise, such as participating actively or taking leadership in interdisciplinary research and practice organizations, presenting papers at interdisciplinary meetings, publishing in interdisciplinary journals, and teaching in interdisciplinary courses

The last point may be one of the most important. If faculty members are not involved in interprofessional work, students lose the opportunity to learn from some of their most important role models. Furthermore, nursing faculty members are unlikely to understand students from other disciplines if they are not actively involved in interdisciplinary work, thereby limiting their effectiveness as teachers of interdisciplinary groups of students.

At a minimum, nurses need to eliminate rhetoric that denigrates physicians, administrators, or other colleagues. We need faculty members and preceptors who challenge nurses when hostile remarks about colleagues are made. A commitment to continuous improvement in interprofessional collaboration should be a core goal that permeates every facet of nursing education and practice.

Exemplify Commitment to Continuous Learning and Improvement

Whether healthcare professionals are using new technologies, new knowledge, or new concepts of patient-centered care, it will be incumbent on heroes of the future to be committed to continuous learning and improvement. Without this commitment, the inertia embedded in complex systems will continue to prevent or minimize the effect of potential innovations.

In spite of the current emphasis on continuous improvement in healthcare settings, it remains the norm for nursing students to move through their clinical learning experiences without observing interdisciplinary teams working on improvements to care. Students are unlikely to observe improvement work in universities either. To enhance the education of nursing students, faculty leaders and accrediting bodies could require that all nursing programs include content about the concepts and methods of continuous improvement. Students could be assigned to observe or participate in improvement projects as part of their learning activities, in either academic or clinical healthcare settings.

For faculty members to teach about continuous improvement, they must understand the concepts and methods of improvement work themselves. Faculty who pay attention to what students, future employers, and communities want from nurses modify curricula and measure the effect of their changes in continuous cycles of learning from the information they gather. Students who observe these values and behaviors in action are better prepared for continuous improvement work in the healthcare settings in which they practice.

Finally, student learning could be improved through exposure to current nursing heroes who are making contributions to the improvement of healthcare. The work of continuous improvement in the practice setting is frequently interdisciplinary work where nurses are not the identified leaders; however, nurses often are the people who identify the opportunity for improvement and do the work necessary to make the improvement project succeed. Faculty members and healthcare administrators can create opportunities for nurses who were formal or informal leaders of healthcare improvements to be featured speakers for professional and student audiences. By honoring nurses who play key roles in improvement projects, administrators and faculty members create an incentive for the behavior in others.

Focus on the Big Issues of Human Need

Much of nursing care takes place at the intersection of technology, patients, and families. In fact, one common view of nursing depicts the nurse as the person with the responsibility to ensure that technology is working and works for patients: "educating patients about new devices, getting patients to accept and comply with their use, and alleviating patients' fears about them" (Sandelowski 2000).

Emerging technologies always present opportunities for changing—and sometimes improving—healthcare, but people need to know that future healthcare professionals will stay focused on the needs of human beings. The IOM's Quality Chasm (2001) report emphasizes this point with proposed rules for care based on continuous healing relationships, care customized to patient needs and values, and the mandate to keep the patient as the source of control.

When nurse clinicians focus on the needs and preferences of patients, they understand and embrace the need to work with other professionals, because no one professional or profession can meet the needs of patients alone. When nursing scientists understand the magnitude of patient or community problems, they pull together interdisciplinary teams to conduct the research necessary to find solutions to those problems. When nursing faculty members understand the magnitude of the systems problems in healthcare, they move away from a sole focus on disciplinary knowledge to include learning about systems of care. The focus on the central issue of human need makes the difference.

In spite of nursing's history of focusing on the whole human being, nurses sometimes refrain from tackling the big issues of human need. A major reason is nursing's position with respect to the other dominant players in healthcare—medicine and healthcare administration. Neither profession embraces nursing as a full partner. After several experiences where a team's accomplishments are attributed to physician or administrative leaders, nurses sometimes retreat to work on problems of lesser scope that do not require interdisciplinary work. When this happens, nurses sometimes resort to blaming them (physicians and administrators) for problems we've quit trying to solve.

If nurses retreat, we give away our place at tables where nurses' voices in generating solutions to the big problems in healthcare are required. Given the interdependence of nurses, physicians, and healthcare administrators when the patient is the focus of concern, nursing leaders need to continue to expose students to functioning, effective interdisciplinary teams who are working on the big problems of human need, and the professional lives of nursing faculty members need to demonstrate the priority placed on this work.

Patient advocacy organizations are often places where patients, nurses, physicians, and other healthcare leaders join forces to promote legislative or policy initiatives that create the kinds of change needed by patients and communities. The behaviors of health professional heroes are often on display in these organizations and, if observed, could motivate the next generation of professionals. Nursing students could be assigned to service-learning experiences in patient advocacy organizations where nurses are participating in policy-making efforts to improve care. At a minimum, leaders in patient advocacy organizations should be as visible and accessible to students as are the leaders of the associations where the profession is the focus of concern.

Final Thoughts

The agenda for change is staggering in scope. With the current pressures on the healthcare workforce, most would agree that conditions to support transformational work are suboptimal. But the ideas proposed above are possible—today, now. Nursing has leaders who are capable of initiating changes in our educational and clinical systems that would prompt necessary shifts in thinking and better prepare nurses for partnering with physicians and healthcare administrators in the days and years ahead.

In addition, faculty from nursing, medicine, and healthcare administration can change, right now, how we teach about errors. If we do, the next generation of professionals would expect to learn from, rather than be punished for, mistakes. The same professional leaders can immediately embrace the necessity for safe, respectful interprofessional communication and commit to providing students in all disciplines the mentoring needed for strong and productive interdisciplinary collaboration.

The 7th Annual Summer Symposium participants envisioned healthcare that would be changed forever by robotics, nanotechnology, and genomics, but we envisioned health professional heroes of the future who closely resembled heroes of the past. The ideas developed in response to the question "What could nursing do?" were not dissimilar from the ideas proposed by physicians and healthcare administrators. All of us have work to do to prepare the health professional of the future for the heroic actions patients, families, and communities will need in the twenty-first century.

Acknowledgments

The author would like to acknowledge the influence of the other nursing participants in the 7th Annual Summer Symposium at Dartmouth, including: Jane Barnsteiner, Patty Gerrity, Marjorie Godfrey, Iain Graham, Creigh Moffatt, Linda Norman, Richard Redman, Jean Sorrells-Jones, Marcia Starbecker, and Marita Titler.

References

Detmer, D. E. 2001. "A New Health System and Its Quality Agenda." *Frontiers in Health Services Management* 18 (1): 3–30.

Institute of Medicine. 2001. *Crossing the Quality Chasm: A New Health System for the 21st Century*. Washington, DC: National Academy Press.

Sandelowski, M. 2000. *Devices and Desires: Gender, Technology, and American Nursing*. Chapel Hill, NC: UNC Press.

Healthcare Managers in the Complex World of Healthcare

G. Ross Baker, Ph.D.
Excerpted from *Frontiers of Health Services Management* 18 (2), Winter 2001

Simple Rules

The idea that a set of simple rules and a shared vision for healthcare will transform working relationships and engender more effective outcomes for patients and caregivers is a compelling one. The genesis of this idea stems from complex adaptive systems theory and fundamental work done in biology and physics. The application of complex adaptive systems thinking to human systems and organizations is a rapidly evolving field (see, for example, Axelrod and Cohen 1999; Stacey 1996; Stacey 2001; Pierce 2000; McKenna 1999; Anderson and McDaniel 2000; Zimmerman, Lindberg, and Plsek 1998; Brown and Eisenhardt 1998). Consistent with this approach, the IOM report authors note that creating a common purpose or shared goals and identifying a few simple rules to guide behaviors for those in the healthcare system will create a context for "a healthcare system capable of dramatic changes in quality." What is less clear, however, is how to create that agreement on the shared vision and how to develop a political, economic, and social environment where such simple rules can be freely adopted and used.

For guidance, we might refer to the two examples used in the IOM report to illustrate this point. However, these examples seem instead to indicate how far the current healthcare situation is from other experiences where a shared vision and simple rules have created successful change. The first example is the development of the Internet, whose designers focused on creating shared computer communication protocols and conventions to ensure effective data exchanges, not on dictating the number and locations of computer servers and other hardware necessary to transfer data. A few simple rules enabled computer users around the world to easily access the Internet. As a result, its growth was rapid and unhindered by unnecessary regulation and requirements. Users could link into the system from a variety of computer platforms. The ease and minimal costs of participating in the Internet attracted users; the growth in users created even greater interest and increasing use of this technology.

The second example focuses on the credit card company Visa, whose members (the banks issuing its credit cards) have agreed on a few key elements: the use of the logo and visual layout of the card and a common clearinghouse that permits Visa cards to be used worldwide. Visa now has yearly sales over $1 trillion, but, as Dee Hock, the former CEO of Visa notes, few know much about its structure and organization, "the better an organization is, the less obvious it is. . . . It's the results, not the structure or the management that should be apparent" (Waldrop 1996).

One might question whether either of these examples provides a good analogy for healthcare organizations. The Internet built its success on a new technology that developed first as a military, then a largely academic, network. Its initial appeal was based on simplicity, low cost, and easy access. Rapid growth has transformed the Internet, and while its commercial potential is immense, many organizations have stumbled trying to employ Internet strategies to sell goods and services and interact with customers. Clearly the technology is still developing, and the social organization needed to reap the benefits still lags.

The Visa card developed as a new strategy for an old problem: providing a means to exchange currency for goods and services. The vision of a highly decentralized and highly collaborative organization that linked competing banks emerged as a solution to a fundamental tension between the member financial organizations. The banks issuing Visa cards competed between each other for business. But this competition led to indiscriminate distribution of credit cards and high levels of fraud, resulting in major losses. Cooperation was necessary to ensure that banks established minimal rules for designing and issuing cards and creating a common clearinghouse to enable merchants to accept any Visa card.

These examples suggest that simple rules may emerge where new technologies provide opportunities in environments with limited regulation. In both cases the innovations transformed previous means of interaction and altered social relationships among users. The Internet was supported by a largely informal organization of users, while the credit card business emerged as only one line in a wide array of services offered by financial institutions. Innovation was possible because in neither case were established organizations betting their futures on its success.

What situations and opportunities exist to create a common vision and simple rules to improve healthcare? How many large integrated delivery systems are capable of the decentralization of decision making necessary to allow simple rules to influence behaviors? Most of these delivery systems have spent the last five to ten years pursing integration strategies; assembling clinics, hospitals, and physician practices; and trying to create common identities among them. The increased complexity and size of these organizations has meant that many senior leaders have focused considerable effort grappling with the economic, legal, and organizational problems of creating these new organizations. Shortell and colleagues (2000) note that the purpose of many of these mergers was to improve the coordination of care for patients across the continuum. Yet many delivery systems have stalled while trying to integrate their various parts and to create common human resources, information management, and planning activities (Shortell et al. 2000). The huge costs associated with mergers along with increasing competition on the price of care has also meant that many delivery systems have had to lay off staff and limit services to maintain viability. As a result, these organizations have increased, not diminished, their controls on local operating units, trying to standardize procedures and eliminate duplication in facilities and staff.

Skunkworks and Microsystems

Paradoxically, the difficulties faced by integrated delivery systems in the current environment may hold the keys to improving healthcare. It would be unrealistic to expect these organizations to commit entirely to a strategy built on the vision of the IOM and the simple rules, if only because the risks of such a strategy are unknown. At the same time, however, these organizations do have substantial resources and skilled managers and clinicians who could experiment with new approaches in selected areas. Healthcare delivery systems might identify divisions or units, including primary care clinics and specialty units, to operate as "skunkworks," that is, as experimental units focused on developing new skills and trying new approaches, free from the constraints of operating under current organizational policies. Clinicians and managers in these units would set aims and then experiment with new ways to improve care, create better patient experiences, and reduce costs. Lessons learned from these experiences could be shared across the larger systems, creating new energy and new possibilities for broader innovation.

Given the evident need for change, such local experimentation with new models of care might seem like too slow an approach. Some organizations that have already been successful with piloting new models of care might commit to a more intensive change strategy that builds upon previous efforts to improve care. For most organizations, however, a more measured approach will balance the risks of abandoning current strategies with an opportunity to invest in different approaches. Freeing some parts of healthcare organizations to experiment with new models and ideas could create considerable momentum for improvement across the system.

Greater experimentation with new approaches will also help identify breakthrough changes. Much of the change occurring today in healthcare does not fundamentally alter current patterns of work and/or empower patients. New investments to develop information technology and buy physician group practices, for example, do not create new systems of care; they preserve the old ones. Other industries that have achieved breakthrough levels of performance have relied on "disruptive innovations": cheaper, simpler, and more convenient approaches and services that meet needs and alter the status quo among those providing these products and services (Christensen, Bohmer, and Kenagy 2000). In healthcare many dominant organizations, including teaching hospitals and large delivery systems, are committed to providing increasingly specialized services and more sophisticated technology. However, much of the illness burden is created by chronic diseases that could be better managed by generalists, or by patients themselves with appropriate training and supporting technology. Such care can be more effective and less expensive (Wagner, Austin, and Van Korff 1996), but such breakthroughs in cost and quality will only emerge if we start investing in alternative approaches.

The innovations needed will emerge from redesigning care at the front lines, not reorganizing large systems. Paul Batalden, Eugene Nelson, Julie Mohr, and others (Batalden et al. 1997; Nelson et al. 1998; Mohr 2000) have argued that healthcare quality and costs could be improved by focusing on changes in "microsystems" of care. Microsystems consist of "caregivers and support staff who work together daily to treat illnesses and injuries and to promote the health and well-being of a defined patient population" (Nelson et al. 1998). These teams of clinicians and support staff care for "panels" of patients, using information on these patients and their care to improve outcomes and reduce costs.

This focus on microsystems contrasts with some of the dominant themes over the last decade in clinical practice improvement and organizational change. Clinicians have been advised to identify "best practices" and "evidence-based healthcare" to improve the choice of specific therapies and procedures for patients. This approach emphasizes individual change, helping practitioners in a specific profession to identify and adopt the most appropriate practice for a specific illness or condition (e.g., "evidence-based medicine" or "evidence-based nursing"). At a macro level, as we have already suggested, managers have focused on creating large integrated delivery systems, designing these structures from the top down (i.e., based on the coordination and communication needs of the organization and its staff) rather than from the bottom up (based on the needs of patients and communities). By contrast, a focus on microsystems recognizes the important middle ground that links individual practice to larger organizational systems. Practitioners in microsystems still need to identify the "best practices," and larger delivery systems still need to integrate services across the continuum of care. However, these efforts will be more effective if linked to improvements in coordinating the work of all the caregivers in the microsystem who share responsibilities for patients, improving this care by using information about each individual patient's prior experiences and evidence of the outcomes of all similar patients who have been treated in the microsystem.

Creating Change

Developing effective microsystems will require intensive work with clinical teams to redesign patient care processes, collect and use information from patients, and share knowledge of effective practices (IOM 2001). Many healthcare organizations struggle with these challenging tasks. For example, many healthcare organizations have invested resources in redesigning patient care processes to reduce costs and improve outcomes. But research suggests that organizational barriers and traditional patterns of professional relationships have limited the effect of these efforts (Savitz and Kaluzny 2000; Shortell et al. 2000). Considerable evidence indicates that clinical process redesign can improve patient results (Classen et al. 1992), but studies of the use of these techniques across organizations show little or no affect on process improvement on clinical outcomes (Shortell, Bennett, and Byck 1998; Goldberg et al. 1998).

Similarly, while some organizations such as Group Health Cooperative of Puget Sound have been able to implement collaborative learning models to develop better care for diabetic patients (Wagner et al. 2001; Wagner 2000), many organizations have labored to transfer learning from one clinic to another. In part, this difficulty stems from the need for learning to occur at a group and organizational level, not just among individuals. The experience of northern New England academic medical centers illustrates that improvement in cardiac bypass surgery comes not just from improvements in surgical technique, but also from collaborative efforts by physicians, nurses, and others to change the organization of care, the layout of operating rooms, and interaction among OR and recovery room staffs (O'Connor et al. 1996).

Even when the changes needed for improvement are relatively simple and straightforward, they can be difficult to implement. Like other organizations, healthcare suffers from the "not invented here" syndrome that leads staff to resist adopting changes that have been shown to be effective in similar settings. As Pfeffer and Sutton (1999) note in discussing this problem in industry, "the success of most interventions designed to improve organizational performance depends largely on implementing what is known, rather than from adopting new or previously unknown ways of doing things." In healthcare the recent efforts of the Institute for Healthcare Improvement, in its Breakthrough Series on Reducing Adverse Drug Events and Medical Errors, demonstrate that clinical teams who are given a list of improvements for reducing errors and simple methods for testing and implementing these changes can reduce errors in the use of high-risk medications such as insulin, heparin, and warfarin (IHI 1997). Absent such methods and support from senior leaders, however, these changes are less likely to occur.

Healthcare professionals and healthcare teams possess key knowledge that is often poorly used. Brian Quinn and colleagues (1996) argue that healthcare organizations, like other professional firms, need to do a much better job in leveraging the knowledge and skills of these professionals. They identified a number of key practices in the most effective organizations that contribute to success. These include recruiting the best performers, supporting their work with well-designed information technology, overcoming professionals' reluctance to share information, and organizing operations around the work and needs of professionals. Progress in the performance of healthcare microsystems will require continued experimentation with new innovations, a greater tolerance for making and learning from mistakes, improved knowledge of clinical process improvement skills, and better skills for putting this knowledge about what works into action. Making this happen will require new behaviors and new skills of leaders supporting those working in these microsystems.

References

Anderson, R. A., and R. R. McDaniel, Jr. 2000. "Managing Health Care Organizations: Where Professionalism Meets Complexity Science." *Health Care Management Review* 25 (1): 83–92.

Axelrod, R., and M. D. Cohen. 1999. *Harnessing Complexity: Organizational Implications of a Scientific Frontier.* New York: Free Press.

Batalden, P. B., J. J. Mohr, E. C. Nelson, S. K. Plume, G. R. Baker, J. H. Wasson, P. K. Stoltz, M. E. Splaine, and J. J. Wisniewski. 1997. "Continually Improving the Health and Value of Health Care for A Population of Patients." *Quality Management in Health Care* 5 (3): 41–51.

Brown, S. L., and K. M. Eisenhardt. 1998. *Competing on the Edge: Strategy As Structured Chaos.* Boston: Harvard Business School Press.

Christensen, C. M., R. Bohmer, and J. Kenagy. 2000. "Will Disruptive Innovations Cure Health Care?" *Harvard Business Review* (Sept/Oct): 102–111.

Classen, D. C., R. S. Evans, S. L. Pestotnik, S. D. Horn, R. L. Menlove, and J. P. Burke. 1992. "The Timing of Prophylactic Administration of Antibiotics and the Risk of Surgical Wound Infection." *New England Journal of Medicine* 326 (5): 281–86.

Goldberg, H. I., E. H. Wagner, S. D. Fihn, D. P. Martin, C. R. Horowitz, D. B. Christensen, A. D. Cheadle, P. Diehr, and G. Simon. 1998. "A Randomized Controlled Trial of CQI Teams and Academic Detailing: Can They Alter Compliance With Guidelines?" *Joint Commission Journal on Quality Improvement* 24 (3): 130–42.

Institute for Healthcare Improvement. 1997. *Breakthrough Series Guide to Reducing Adverse Drug Events and Medical Errors.* Boston, MA: IHI.

Institute of Medicine. 2001. *Crossing the Quality Chasm: A New Health System for the 21st Century.* Washington, DC: National Academy Press.

McKenna, S. 1999. "Learning Through Complexity." *Management Learning* 30 (3): 301–320.

Mohr, J. J. 2000. "Forming, Operating and Improving Micro-systems of Health Care." Ph.D. thesis, Dartmouth College.

Nelson, E. C., P. B. Batalden, J. J. Mohr, and S. K. Plume. 1998. "Building a Quality Future." *Frontiers of Health Services Management* 15 (1): 3–32.

O'Connor, G. T., S. K. Plume, E. M. Olmstead, J. R. Morton, C. T. Maloney, W. C. Nugent, F. Hernandez, Jr., R. Clough, B. J. Leavitt, L. H. Coffin, C. A. Marrin, D. Wennberg, J. D. Birkmeyer, D. C. Charlesworth, D. J. Malenka, H. B. Quinton, J. F. Kasper. 1996. "A Regional Intervention to Improve the Hospital Mortality Associated with Coronary Bypass Graft Surgery." *Journal of the American Medical Association* 275 (11): 841–6.

Pfeffer, J., and R. I. Sutton. 1999. "Knowing 'What' To Do Is Not Enough: Turning Knowledge Into Action." *California Management Review* 42 (1): 83–108.

Pierce, J. C. 2000. "The Paradox of Physicians and Administrators in Health Care Organizations." *Health Care Management Review* 25 (1): 7–28.

Quinn, J. B., P. Anderson, and S. Finkelstein. 1996. "Managing Professional Intellect: Making the Most of the Best." *Harvard Business Review* (Mar/Apr): 71–80.

Savitz, L. A., and A. D. Kaluzny. 2000. "Assessing the Implementation of Clinical Process Innovations: A Cross-Case Comparison." *Journal of Healthcare Management* 45 (6): 366–80.

Shortell, S. M., C. L. Bennett, and G. R. Byck. 1998. "Assessing the Impact of Continuous Quality Improvement on Clinical Practice: What It Will Take to Accelerate Progress [see comments]." *Milbank Quarterly* 76 (4): 593–624.

Shortell, S., R. R. Gilles, D. A. Anderson, K. M. Erickson, and J. B. Mitchell. 2000. *Remaking Health Care in America*, Second edition. San Francisco: Jossey-Bass.

Stacey, R. D. 2001. *Complex Responsive Processes in Organizations. Learning and Knowledge Creation.* London: Routledge.

———. 1996. *Complexity and Creativity in Organizations.* San Francisco: Berrett Koehler.

Wagner, E. H. 2000. "The Role of Patient Care Teams in Chronic Disease Management." *BMJ* 320:569–72.

Wagner, E. H., N. Sandhu, K. M. Newton, D. K. McCulloch, S. D. Ramsey, and L. C. Grothaus. 2001. "Effect of Improved Glycemic Control on Health Care Costs and Outcomes." *Journal of the American Medical Association* 285:182–189.

Wagner, E. H., B. T. Austin, and M. Van Korff. 1996. "Organizing Care for Patients with Chronic Illness." *Milbank Quarterly* 74 (4): 511–42.

Waldrop, W. W. 1996. "The Trillion Dollar Vision of Dee Hock." *Fast Company* (8): 75.

Warden, G. L., and J. R. Griffith. 2001. "Ensuring Management Excellence in the Healthcare System." *Journal of Healthcare Management* 46 (4): 228–37.

Zimmerman, B., C. Lindberg, and P. Plsek. 1998. *Edgeware: Insights from Complexity Science for Health Care Leaders.* Irving, TX: VHA, Inc.

Discussion Questions

1. How realistic are the authors in their "new rules for health professionals"?
2. How will providers be persuaded to see that the new rules are in their own interests?
3. What are some of the problems for patients caused by lack of integration of clinician and organizational goals in healthcare?
4. Why does this lack of integration occur?
5. What are some of the opportunities available to managers to better integrate the goals of physicians and nurses with those of the organization?

Required Supplementary Readings

Griffith, J. and K. White. "Organized Physician Services." In *The Well Managed Healthcare Organization,* 5th edition. Chicago: Health Administration Press, 2002, 279–326.

Griffith, J. and K. White. "Nursing Services." In *The Well Managed Healthcare Organization,* 5th edition. Chicago: Health Administration Press, 2002, 371–406.

McNeese-Smith, D. K. "A Nursing Shortage: Building Organizational Commitment Among Nurses." *Journal of Healthcare Management* May–June 2001, 46 (3): 173–187.

Stewart, L. J. and D. Greisler. "Measuring Primary Care Practice Performance Within an Integrated Delivery System. *Journal of Healthcare Management* July–Aug 2002, 47 (4): 250–262.

Discussion Questions for the Required Supplementary Readings

1. How does organizational structure influence physician integration with healthcare organizational goals?
2. What are the causes of nurse dissatisfaction in hospitals, and what can hospital managers do to improve nursing morale?
3. How can organizational mission and goals influence clinician integration?
4. How does clinician payment influence clinical integration with organizational goals?

Recommended Supplementary Readings

Aiken, L. "Evidence-Based Management: Key to Hospital Workforce Stability." *Journal of Health Administration Education*, Special Issue, 2001, 117–124.

Coile, R. C. "Magnet Hospital Use Culture, Not Wages, to Solve the Nursing Shortage." *Journal of Healthcare Management* 2001, 46 (4): 224–247.

Delbecq, A. L., and S. Gill. "Justice as a Prelude to Teamwork in Medical Centers." *Healthcare Management Review* 1985, 10 (1): 45–51

Detmer, D. E. "A New Health System and Its Quality Agenda." *Frontiers of Healthcare Management* 2001, 18 (1): 3–30.

Eisenberg, J. M. *Doctors' Decisions and the Cost of Medical Care.* Chicago: Health Administration Press, 1986.

Freidson, E. *Medical Work in America.* New Haven, CT: Yale University Press, 1989.

Health Care Advisory Board. "The Physician Perspective: Key Drivers of Physician Loyalty." Washington, DC: Health Care Advisory Board, 1999.

Hoff, T. J. "Exploring Dual Commitment Among Physician Executives in Managed Care." *Journal of Healthcare Management* 2001, 46 (2): 91–111.

Hoff, T. J. "The Physician as Worker: What It Means and Why Now?" *Health Care Management Review* 2001, 26 (4): 53–70.

Holm, C. E. "The Future of Physician-Health System Integration." *Journal of Healthcare Management* 2000, 45 (6): 356–368.

Lake, T., K. Devers, L. Brewster, and L. Casolino. "Something Old Something New: Recent Developments in Hospital-Physician Relationships." *Health Services Research* 2003, 38 (1): Part II, 471–488.

Lewis, J. E. "Improving Productivity: The Ongoing Experience of an Academic Department of Medicine." *Academic Medicine* 1996, 71 (4): 317–328.

Parker, V. A., M. Charns, and G. J. Young. "Clinical Service Lines in Integrated Delivery Systems: An Initial Framework and Exploration." *Journal of Healthcare Management* 2001, 46 (4): 261–275.

Robinson, J. C. "Theory and Practice in the Design of Physician Payment Incentives." *The Milbank Quarterly* 2001, 79 (2): 149–178.

Simendinger, E., J. D. Sedberg, and D. Vizzi. "When Your Orthopedic Group Threatens to Walk." *Journal of Healthcare Management* 2001, 46 (6): 359–360.

Zuckerman, H. S., D. W. Hilberman, R. M. Anderson, L. R. Burns, J. A. Alexander, and P. Torrens. "Physicians and Organizations: Strange Bedfellows or a Marriage Made in Heaven." *Frontiers of Healthcare Management* 1998, 14 (3): 3–34.

THE CASES

The two case studies in this section exemplify different approaches to reorganizing hospital operations, which are increasingly physician-led. The "Physician Leadership: MetroHealth System of Cleveland" case describes the overhaul in management/medical staff relations brought about by a new leadership. Of note is the successful effort of this leadership to compete in the Cleveland market as a public hospital. The "Breast Service at Easter Medical Center" case shows why ineffective leadership and lack of integration of physician and hospital goals leads to poor unit performance.

Today, the medical profession yet retains its basic and legally enforced monopoly over the key functions of healthcare, as physicians are the sole authority in diagnosing and carrying out the treatment of health problems. The basis of their decision making has been experience and clinical judgment. Increasingly, this informal unchallengeable mode of decision making is being replaced, however, under physician supervision, by "evidence-based" medicine, and even "evidence-based management." This includes data gathering that is based on population-based reasoning, clinical decision analysis, cost-effectiveness analysis, clinical paths, guidelines or algorithms, process improvement thinking, outcomes analysis, statistical process control, quality of life measurements, and comparative cost analysis.

Physicians can rely on numerous sources of power in dealing with managers, including the protection afforded them by organizations or through negotiated contracts. Physicians may use the authority based on their knowledge to demand resources from the managers such as additional staff, space, and equipment. Physicians are often respected by the public, certainly more than healthcare managers. They may have access to board members and community leaders who are their patients. Their power may stem from the ability to unite and to withdraw their services from organizations whose behavior is unacceptable to them.

Physicians expect recognition, acceptance, and trust from managers, and they expect that their livelihood will not be threatened by managerial initiatives. Physicians are concerned about their status and power compared to other occupational groups, to other physicians within an organization, and to physicians working at competing institutions. They want to determine their own working conditions and to be provided with support services adequate to house, feed, and care for their patients. Physicians do not like to waste time in

221

endless or frequent meetings, and they expect to be consulted if organizational policy changes will affect them.

Many of these seem reasonable expectations. Why, then, do physicians feel that expectations are not met by the organization and its managers? Other physicians may be competing for limited resources of funds, space, and staff; demand may change for one specialty compared to others. The manager may have a different concept of time wasting. To the physician, completing records represents time unreimbursed or ambulatory care not delivered. To the hospital, it is required for necessary cash flow. Sometimes events move too quickly for adequate consultation, or there is a lack of communication among physicians and lay managers.

For example, a manager may ask the chief of staff, a department head, or the medical board for approval of implementation of a risk management program, provision of financial guarantees to recruit family practitioners, or appointment of a new chief of emergency medicine. Medical officials may give informal approval and get back to physicians in each department for further discussion and recommendations for action. In the interim, however, time, money, and skilled personnel may no longer be available. Even after policies are agreed upon, the manager may find that medical leadership has misinterpreted what was agreed to at joint meetings. Following implementation of new policies, physicians may personally object, and subsequently provide care of poor quality. Yet they may fail to understand why managers do not honor what seems to them to be legitimate requests. Further, as physicians are independent contractors, they may have goal conflicts with organizations within which they practice.

Similarly, the manager expects recognition, acceptance, and trust from the physician. Managers expect physicians to be concerned about organizational goals such as cost containment and quality improvement. Managers expect physicians to fulfill specific organizational commitments agreed to in advance, such as punctual attendance at hospital meetings. The manager does not expect to be attacked personally when she and a physician disagree. She expects respect for her organizational role and responsibility for internal coordination of activities and adaptation of the organization to external pressures. The manager expects physicians not to waste the manager's time but to, for example, try to solve a problem first with the involved department head whose lack of timely response to the physician's request may, after all, be reasonable. The manager expects to be consulted if an action by a physician will affect the organization's goal attainment or system maintenance.

Many of these expectations seem reasonable. Why then don't physicians meet them? Physicians may not view the manager as she views herself. Physicians may view the manager as a supporter for their medical work rather than as an organizational coordinator or integrator. They may see the manager as working *for* physicians rather than *with* them to attain organizational goals. Many physicians may fear the manager because of increasing dependence on the organization for their livelihood. Managers, through their influence on budget determination and their control of information, may affect the physician's access to scarce resources.

If physicians can discredit the manager, the manager will have less power over them. Physicians are accustomed to giving orders, not to taking them. If the manager is actively attempting to increase revenues and decrease expenses, physicians can surely find fault. (The manager did not consult sufficiently with them, she did not consult sufficiently in advance, or she has favored certain other departments in budget and staff.) Further, physicians may object to the manager's tone, style, travel schedule, number of assistants, size of office, or amount of salary.

Physicians will often disagree with the manager over policy. For example, physicians at Alpha Hospital may decide that expensive equipment will help in their daily practice, and surgeons at neighboring Beta Hospital are getting more sophisticated equipment. Alpha Hospital's policy of providing services to the chronically ill will therefore not help surgeons stay competitive or increase their incomes. Or physicians may have a conflict of interest with the hospital; extra nursing staffing will reduce the operations surplus or lead to operations deficits.

There is often no effective organizational responsibility system for most physician behavior. Physicians can take "cheap shots" at the manager if they are not effectively accountable to anyone in the organizational structure for incurring costs or ensuring quality and access. Non-paid physician department chiefs and committee chairs are usually more interested in maintaining their physician networks of patient referral than in attaining organizational goals. Physicians work long hours and they consider the competing and conflicting demands on their time more important than certain organizational obligations, even those to which they have agreed in advance.

Finally, physicians may distrust the manager, find the manager incompetent, or dislike the manager personally. This may be because of the manager's actions or inaction, ranging from gaining board approval for a CT scanner to responding inappropriately to low nursing morale. Increasingly physicians are being hired as managers by HCOs, in part because they are more likely to be obeyed than non-physician managers. Many physician managers quickly learn, however, that, to the extent they are paid by the organization and no longer practice, they are increasingly viewed by many physicians as one of "them," rather than as one of "us."

Given the inherent difficulties, what opportunities do managers have to perform effectively and yet maintain decent working relationships with physicians? Is this even possible? Managers can exchange scarce resources of money, staff and space with physicians in return for assistance in goal attainment. Managers can order physicians to implement decisions, calculating that physicians lack the power to resist effectively. Managers can persuade physicians to act in the long-term interest of the organization, the patient, and the consumer. The manager has a limited amount of political "chips" to spend, just as she has a limited amount of organizational funds available. The manager can invest in political power by building good informal relationships with key physicians, or she can spend power in making decisions opposed by key physicians or groups. Timing, tone, body language, and judgment are all important for the manager whose tenure may well vary conversely with activism.

The manager has resources available that the physician lacks. She may have influence with the governing board regarding long-range planning decisions, influence on appointment of physicians to paid and unpaid positions or access to grants and gifts, and influence on rates of physician remuneration. The manager may have special knowledge useful in advising physicians on business and personal problems and to do personal favors for them. The manager has information concerning results of implementing proposed strategic initiatives at other HCOs.

Even as physicians have authority for patient care decisions, the manager has authority for support decisions, based on expertise in, for example, marketing and compliance with government regulation. Often competitive and regulatory requirements can be interpreted by managers to rationalize decisions that will benefit patients and consumers at the expense or inconvenience of physicians. The manager may also accrue a certain authority because of long tenure in a position, having gained the trust of physicians with similar tenure. When a manager has gained such trust, others will back critical decisions or disagree in private or in advance, without personal attacks.

The manager can persuade physicians of the justice or advantage of policy or administrative decisions. Of course, some physicians will not wish to be persuaded. It is not difficult to wake up someone who is sleeping, but it is hard to awaken someone who is pretending to be asleep.

The manager can help physicians obtain the resources they need, which may be in the organization's interest as well. The manager may delay implementation of what physicians oppose until a more favorable future time. Above all, the manager must know what she is doing, be sure of her facts, and be conservative in her forecasts. As in other fields, nothing succeeds like success or fails like failure, and often the failing manager will not be given a second chance.

The two cases "Physician Leadership" and "The Breast Service at Easter Medical Center" approach similar organizational problems of remaining competitive by improving quality, making services more customer focused, and containing costs. Both cases focus on physician leadership to bring along the physicians, sooner rather than later.

Case 9
Physician Leadership: MetroHealth System of Cleveland

Anthony R. Kovner

As of fall 1998, key changes shaping the Cleveland health system included the following: increasing concentration in the hospital market, expansion of high-end medical services, health plans facing stiff price competition and internal administrative difficulties, and employers not pursuing aggressive purchasing strategies.[1] Three local institutions—the Cleveland Clinic, University Hospitals Health System (UH), and the former Blues plan, Medical Mutual of Ohio—retain dominance in the market.

Market Description

The Cleveland Clinic owns 40 percent of the hospital beds in Cuyahoga County (population 2.2 million) and 30 percent in the broader six-county primary metropolitan statistical area (see Figure 9.1), compared with UH's 11 percent. While the two local not-for-profit hospital systems have grown, the two for-profit systems have lost market share over the last two years. Metro-Health, the county's public hospital, continues to be the leading provider of charity care and Medicaid services (see Figure 9.2). Metro retains a close relationship with the Cleveland Clinic, participating as a lead member of the Cleveland Health Network (CHN).

Cleveland has been viewed as a specialty-oriented healthcare market with considerable excess hospital capacity. The expiration of Ohio's certificate-of-need has resulted in new construction and technology investments by hospitals. Clear competition also exists among health plans. Premium levels have been flat or have declined during the past year. Most plans share the same broad provider networks. Purchasers (employers) have not increased their demands for highly managed care insurance products nor turned to direct contracting to get more control over costs and quality.

Medicaid plans are having financial difficulties. The state's payment rates have declined and competition among the plans has increased. The number of Medicaid plans is expected to decline further as the state implements

FIGURE 9.1
Cuyahoga
County
Hospitals

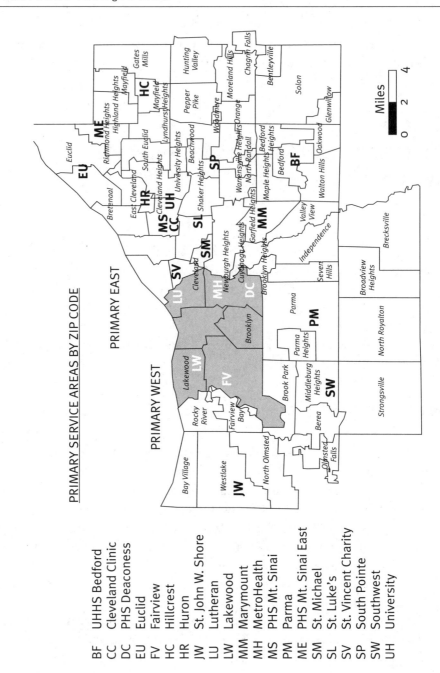

PRIMARY SERVICE AREAS BY ZIP CODE

PRIMARY EAST

PRIMARY WEST

Miles

0 2 4

BF   UHHS Bedford
CC   Cleveland Clinic
DC   PHS Deaconess
EU   Euclid
FV   Fairview
HC   Hillcrest
HR   Huron
JW   St. John W. Shore
LU   Lutheran
LW   Lakewood
MM   Marymount
MH   MetroHealth
MS   PHS Mt. Sinai
PM   Parma
ME   PHS Mt. Sinai East
SM   St. Michael
SL   St. Luke's
SV   St. Vincent Charity
SP   South Pointe
SW   Southwest
UH   University

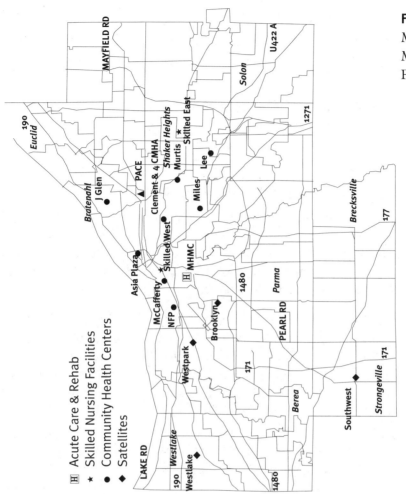

FIGURE 9.2
Map of
MetroHealth
Facilities

enrollment floors in each county, under which only plans that enroll 10 percent or more of the eligible population will be allowed to contract with Medicaid. MetroHealth is Ohio's largest provider of Medicaid services.

Overview of the MetroHealth System

The mission statement of the MetroHealth System is as follows:

> The MetroHealth System commits to leadership in providing healthcare services that continually improve the health of the people in our community. We offer an integrated program of services provided through a system that encompasses a partnership between management and physicians and reflects excellence in patient care supported by superior education and research programs. We are committed to responding to community needs, improving the health status of our region, and controlling healthcare costs.

Metro is licensed to operate 680 beds, of which 524 are staffed and in use. Metro also operates two skilled nursing centers with an additional 490+ beds, a network of 16 ambulatory care centers offering primary care services in various locations, and three substance abuse treatment centers. The medical center's 41-acre campus is located on the near west side of the city of Cleveland, approximately two miles from downtown. All facilities are fully accredited.

Since 1914, Metro has been a major teaching affiliate of Case Western Reserve University and provides 40 to 50 percent of all clinical hours for university medical students. Grant funding for Metro's Center for Research and Education from the National Institutes of Health was more than $10.8 million in 1997, as compared with $3.8 million in 1992.

Cuyahoga County provides financial support for Metro through annual appropriations from a portion of the proceeds of two voted property tax levies for health and human services and, from time to time, its general fund. Metro trustees are appointed jointly by the Board of County Commissioners and the senior judges of the probate and common pleas courts. They serve without compensation for six-year overlapping terms and may be reappointed upon the expiration of their terms. By law, the composition of the trustees must be bipartisan with equal representation from the two major political parties.

Metro houses a Level I (highest level of complexity) trauma center, serving as the regional burn center for northeast Ohio and northwest Pennsylvania. The Neonatal Intensive Care Unit is one of three Level III (highest level of complexity) nurseries in Cleveland. The Center for Rehabilitation is a distinct 143-bed acute rehabilitation center and one of the largest in the country. Metro operates Metro Life Flight, the nation's second busiest aeromedical transport service, with four owned helicopters.

TABLE 9.1
MetroHealth
Medical Center
Utilization
Statistics,
1995–1997

Indicator	1995	1996	1997
Staffed Beds	532	532	524
Occupancy Rate*	65.5	58.6	56.9
Occupancy Rate**	64.8	58.4	57.2
Licensed Beds	728	728	728
Occupancy Rate	47.9	42.9	41.0
Discharges	21,603	19,913	18,036
Patient Days	127,180	113,868	108,863
ALOS (no newborns)	5.9	5.7	6.0
Newborn Bassinets	48	48	48
Number of Births	3,823	3,910	3,719
Newborn Days	10,010	9,755	10,531
ALOS (including newborns)	5.4	5.2	5.5

*Excludes newborns
**Includes newborns
NOTES: Effective May 13, 1996, 29 Rehabilitation beds were changed to Skilled Nursing beds.
1. Staffed Beds, 1995–1997 all exclude Nursery bassinets. However, 1996 and 1997 include 29 Subacute beds.
2. Licensed beds include 48 Nursery bassinets and the 29 Subacute beds. (In 1995 the 29 beds were Rehabilitation.)
3. The discharges and patient days for 1996 and 1997 *exclude* both newborn and subacute activities.

Two-thirds of Metro's 21,536 discharged patients (excluding normal newborns) live in its primary service area, whose population is approximately 500,000. In 1996, Metro accounted for 9.18 percent of the 193,802 county patients (excluding normal newborns) discharged from Ohio hospitals. In the primary service area, which alone accounted for 46.4 percent of all discharges in the county, Metro captured the largest share of the market at 16.7 percent. Metro was a market leader in burns (70.7 percent), rehabilitation (58.3 percent), neonatology (19.2 percent) and obstetrics (18.5 percent). Metro provided more than 500,000 outpatient visits in 1997 (see Table 9.1 for Metro utilization statistics).

Metro's medical staff is organized into 16 major departments, each with a full-time chair. There are more than 350 employed physicians in each of these departments as of 1998, as shown in Table 9.2, and more than 300 residents. Total medical staff includes 238 associate staff, 193 adjunct or affiliate staff, plus 71 bioscientific, emeritus, or honorary staff members. Metro employs 5,562 full- and part-time employees, including the active medical staff. Approximately 2,000 of these employees are union members.

Relationship Between Management and the Medical Staff

Metro's CEO, Terry White, has previous leadership experience at Lutheran Hospital, University Hospital of Cleveland, and University Hospital of

TABLE 9.2
Number of Physicians by Major Medical Departments (as of July 22, 1998)

Department	Active Staff
Anesthesiology	18
Dentistry	7
Dermatology	4
Emergency Medicine	19
Family Practice	27
Medicine	95
Neurology	2
Ob/Gyn	21
Orthopaedics	14
Otolaryngology	2
Pathology	9
Pediatrics	52
P M & R	18
Psychiatry	21
Radiology	24
Surgery	31
Total	364

Cincinnati. He has been the MetroHealth CEO for five years. According to Mr. White, organizations are made up of people, structure, and process. In 1994, the hospital lacked such proper structure and process. Since then, Mr. White has been developing a grand alliance with the medical staff to have one rather than two management groups. He has tried, in his direction of the institution, to create a culture incorporating physician leaders. Going beyond the tokenism of board representation or the installation of a medical director, he has tried to build a physician-driven organization, with medical leadership and accountability.

When Mr. White started at Metro, a high-quality medical staff was in place, functioning under an employment model. This model had 17 different medical departments, with separate practice plans, and no oversight and accountability. Chairs were responsible for more than $100 million dollars of budget, half of which came from practice revenue and half from hospital subsidy. The senior medical officer position was short-tenured and the occupants were neither respected nor empowered. The credentials of chief medical officers were mediocre in research and in business. No one wanted a really strong person to occupy this post. Under the previous CEO, the chairs had direct access to the CEO for most key management decisions.

In 1995, the interim chief of staff retired, and Mr. White hired a national search firm to recruit a successor. The search committee, led by a physician who was not a department chair, was composed of "physicians of the future," rather than being chair-dominated. Dr. Melinda Estes, who was finally selected as chief of staff, had unassailable credentials (including an MBA), a great number of publications, impeccable training as a neuropathologist, and her own research lab; in addition, she was the first woman on the board of governors at the Cleveland Clinic, where she was also associate chief of staff. Dr. Estes was articulate, with good interpersonal skills.

Mr. White wants Metro to be a physician-led organization; therefore, he sees his job as empowering the chief of staff to do this. She is in charge of the medical staff, and the department chairs—who are not allowed to make end runs to the CEO—report to her. In addition, the MetroHealth Management Council (MMC) was created. Before any major recommendation goes to the governing board, it must be agreed to and processed by the MMC. (See Appendix 9.1 for the MMC management protocol.)

What Mr. White has asked of physicians in return is accountability—that they support the institutional mission and be accountable for it. For the first time, the budget for 1999 integrated medical and hospital revenues by service. Results for physicians are measured in terms of productivity rather than revenues—otherwise, practice plans could be successful but slip into providing a lower standard of care for non-paying patients.

Mr. White sees his main CEO functions as helping develop Metro's vision and strategy, managing the board relationship, supporting the organization and fundraising, and building a structure to accomplish the Metro mission. He carries out his duties as CEO through a goals-and-objectives process.

Participation in Managed Care

Metro has approximately 35,000 covered lives in managed care, approximately two-thirds of whom are women and children covered by Ohio's mandatory Medicaid program. More than 12,000 covered managed care lives are not on Medicaid. Metro employees have a fee-for-service insurance program and managed-care contracts with all the major insurance companies. Metro is part of the CHN network for managed-care contracts, which was set up with the Cleveland Clinic. Being part of a network has also enabled economies in purchasing, as Metro is able to access Premier, a multi-hospital organization that negotiates national contracts with suppliers for a broad range of products. Collaboration with other providers has also involved clinical services. For example, Metro was losing $1.7 million annually on renal inpatient services until it formed a joint venture with another provider of renal services. The partnership has resulted in a $400,000 annual surplus that enables Metro resources to capitalize satellite centers, which results in more people served in a more cost-effective way. By gaining control of these costs, Metro's 1998 costs were below those in 1994.

Metro is the largest Medicaid provider in Ohio, both in terms of fee-for-service and managed care. Managed-care revenue makes up less than 20 percent of total Metro revenue. (Metro still has a large fee-for-service Medicaid business because of turnover of beneficiaries who lose eligibility in the Medicaid program and because the disabled are not yet included in the mandatory program.) A number of competitors in this market have either pulled out or gone bankrupt, and only four HMOs in Cuyahoga County cover Medicaid managed-care beneficiaries.

Metro receives full-risk capitation under its Medicaid HMO contracts. HMOs administer payment for services rendered by other providers to Metro Health Services members. This typically accounts for 15 to 20 percent of the premium and is applied against MHS gross capitation. Metro receives the net premium less HMO management fees (which average 15 percent). The state and county have retained vendors to manage enrollment. Metro is losing money on Medicaid managed care because of a variety of factors, including utilization, inadequate premiums, and high HMO administrative costs. Although Metro is losing 10 to 15 percent on every contract, providing services to these beneficiaries is part of Metro's public mission; therefore, it must continue these contracts.

Metro's managed care panel includes 107 primary care practitioners and 366 specialists. Before contracts are negotiated they are reviewed by the MMC. Metro issues quarterly statements and reports on inpatient utilization, showing where they are losing money. Metro views the Medicaid managed care capitation rate set by the state as too low. In addition, the utilization targets that form the actuarial premises for these premiums are not realistic, given the population served. Metro's Utilization Committee now has data on a per-doctor level which may, in the future, be related to physician compensation.

Development of Ambulatory Care Networks

Eight of Metro's satellites are in the city and four are in the suburbs, in addition to ambulatory care provided at the main hospital site. These satellites were developed to expand access and support managed care penetration for all payers. Set up to work like private practice models, the suburban satellites grew 20 percent in 1998. Patients are attracted to their own physicians, who are employed by Metro, and who often have roots in the community. The suburban satellites break even and the urban centers lose money.

Physicians under managed care are under pressure to be more productive. Base salary is now structured so that part is variable based on relative value units delivered. The physician leadership in ambulatory care is integrated within the system leadership structure, sits on all committees, and is involved in future planning. The medical operations unit provides support to the physician leadership in ambulatory satellites. Ambulatory care is a competitive market, with other hospital systems locating new sites to funnel off paying business from the Metro satellites.

Regarding ambulatory care strategy, Dr. Harry Walker, the medical director for the Center for Community Health, put it this way: "It's hard to be successful if you lock yourself into being only a public hospital. We can't lose the mission, but economic realities have to be co-equal. We must be efficient even where we are losing money, so as to use precious resources to the best advantage." Dr. Walker finds physicians more committed now to the defined strategic goals of the organization. "There is a challenge in staying alive in a competitive market, facing up to reality, but physician leaders have been brought in who want the system to work. There is a higher trust level now, more of a shared responsibility; before, there were two separate decision making groups—medical and administrative."

Keeping Financially Healthy

Metro financials are healthy (see Table 9.3 for 1995–1997 comparative data) and have improved since 1995. Comparing 1997 to 1995, occupancy is down 13 percent (to 57 percent), discharges are down 16.5 percent, and inpatient days are down 14.4 percent. However, total outpatient visits are up 12 percent, and gross revenues are up 1.7 percent. This total includes a 21 percent increase in commercial insurance revenues. Net revenues are down 0.25 percent. Total gross revenues were $341 million and charity and bad debt costs were almost $44 million, a 13.6 percent decrease from 1995. Metro received a $17.8 million governmental subsidy in 1997. This subsidy will be $24 million for 1999.

Healthcare is a large part of the Cleveland economy. According to surveys, Metro has a positive image with the public, and residency programs have a good image with those seeking residencies, as reflected in the match results. Although many people in the greater Cleveland area may not know that Metro is a public hospital, MetroHealth lags in awareness by the public and favorableness relative to its primary competitors. The system approach with satellites has improved its image. Metro's primary care community is mainly the working poor, rather than the unemployed. And it is not located in an area with many competing hospitals of comparable clinical stature and capability.

Several of the current top Metro managers came from the Cleveland Clinic. Physicians working at Metro are proud of their mission and excited by taking cases that others don't want. But Metro cannot just rely on government status and subsidies, and physicians understand this—1999 was the first year in which medical and administrative budgets were integrated. Department chiefs became accountable, fiscally, for their whole product line.

TABLE 9.3

MetroHealth Medical Center Comparative Data, 1995–1997

	1995	1997	% Change		
Number of Staffed Beds	532	524	−1.50%		
Number of Births	3,823	3,595	−5.96%		
Occupancy Rate	65.50%	56.92%	−13.10%		
*Discharges**	1995	1995%	1997	1997%	% Change
Medicare	5,372	24.87%	4,330	24.01%	−19.40%
Medicaid	8,753	40.52%	7,177	39.79%	−18.01%
Commercial Insurance	4,672	21.63%	4,560	25.28%	−2.40%
Self-Pay	2,806	12.99%	1,969	10.92%	−29.83%
Other					
Total Discharges	21,603	100.00%	18,036	100.00%	−16.51%
Inpatient Days	1995	1995%	1997	1997%	% Change
Medicare	41,175	32.38%	31,758	29.17%	−22.87%
Medicaid	46,611	36.65%	38,392	35.27%	−17.63%
Commercial Insurance	29.699	23.35%	30,556	28.07%	2.89%
Self-Pay	9,695	7.62%	8,157	7.49%	−15.86%
Other					
Total Inpatient Days	127,180	100.00%	108,863	100.00%	−14.40%
	1995	1997	% Change		
Total Emergency Department	58,176	51,445	−11.57%		
Total Outpatient Department Visits	560,670	628,328	12.07%		
Total Outpatient Visits	1995	1995%	1997	1997%	% Change
Medicare	79,110	14.11%	96,386	15.34%	21.84%
Medicaid	196,235	35.00%	223,371	35.55%	13.83%
Commercial Insurance	141,233	25.19%	177,691	28.28%	25.81%
Self-Pay	144,092	25.70%	130,880	20.83%	−9.17%
Other					
Total Outpatient Visits	560,670	100.00%	628,328	100.00%	12.07%
Gross Revenues (in thousands)	1995	1995%	1997	1997%	% Change
Medicare	$82,651	24.64%	$79,707	23.35%	−3.56%
Medicaid	$118,588	35.35%	$109,519	32.09%	−7.65%
Commercial Insurance	$85,499	25.48%	$103,550	30.34%	21.11%
Self-Pay	$48,750	14.53%	$48,527	14.22%	−0.46%
Other					
Total Gross Revenues	$335,488	100.00%	$341,303	100.00%	1.73%
Net Revenues (in thousands)	1995	1995%	1997	1997%	% Change
Medicare	$74,421	28.07%	$71,786	27.14%	−3.54%
Medicaid	$85,163	32.12%	$72,967	27.59%	−14.32%
Commercial Insurance	$61,504	23.20%	$67,495	25.52%	9.74%
Self-Pay	$2,115	0.80%	$2,570	0.97%	21.51%
Medicaid DSH	$30,905	11.66%	$31,852	12.04%	3.06%
Local Gov. Appropriation	$11,012	4.15%	$17,800	6.73%	61.64%
Total Net Revenues	$265,120	100.00%	$264,470	100.00%	−0.25%
Uncompensated Care Costs (in thousands)	1995	1995% of Costs	1997	1997% of Costs	% Change
Charity Care & Bad Debt Costs	$50,846	16.33%	$43,918	14.68%	−13.63%

*This data does not include subacute discharges or newborn days and discharges.
SOURCE: NAPH Survey for both years. Only reflects the Medical Center activities.

One result of the integration was to change physicians' schedules to enhance productivity. For example, in surgery, schedules were changed from whatever surgeons wanted to what maximizes revenue utilization and level scheduling. Prior to the schedule changes, a surgeon had a clinic schedule every day, that was never filled, and all the patients were directed to show at 1:00 p.m. Now the surgeon is scheduled for one or two afternoons and the schedule is full.

For medical operations support, departments are organized into a small number of clusters. One such cluster is surgery, ENT, orthopaedics, anesthesia, cardiology, and pulmonary. The operations manager is taking scheduling away from medical secretaries into a central scheduling system. Waiting lists are being reduced. Because of better scheduling, for example, the wait for eye exams has been reduced to three to four weeks from six to eight. Physicians stay later, allowing for three additional appointments per physician each afternoon. Metro collects only 30 percent of billings from the surgical cluster patients, and the new operations manager is working on improving pricing and coding with the help of a consultant.

Developing Information Systems

Metro is making a big transition to more modern systems. Previously, individual departments had their own information systems. They are now installing an integrated system (except for inpatient care) that will cost $20 million over the next three years. The Information Systems Committee started out searching for a purely clinical system and instead replaced a number of systems, looking for one vendor to replace the paper records. They chose Epic Systems as the new vendor because its system included scheduling for physicians and ancillaries, professional billing, managed-care referrals and authorizations, and an electronic medical record.

The new system was justified on financial terms to the Metro board, based on labor savings. But the new system will also be more accurate, produce information in a timelier way, help Metro satisfy external data requirements, and provide clinical decision support. An intensive training program will have to be conducted for physicians, who have recently been surveyed. According to Dr. Estes, most physicians have some experience with information systems and are not opposed to implementing the new system.

Measuring Quality, Improving Outcomes, and Increasing Patient Satisfaction

Metro is part of the Cleveland Health Quality Choice outcomes-measurement program, in which hospitals play a more active role in managing length of stay. As a result of government mandate, attending physicians must be personally involved in care, so Metro has transitioned from a resident-based to an attending-driven model.

Metro has a quality department and a case-management department that do concurrent quality and financial reviews of patient stay. Quality and utilization committees collect this data and then share it with the relevant department. If multiple departments are involved, the physician in charge of quality improvement addresses the issue. For example, one such issue was communication of abnormal findings in x-ray. Radiologists didn't call the requesting doctor in all cases. The quality department did a root case analysis of the problems. Now physician-to-physician verbal communication is required to close a radiology file. Metro has an open communication system regarding errors, and the Quality Improvement Committee looks at how to improve the processes. For example, patients receiving anti-coagulation medicine were being dosed too heavily and the process was not being monitored carefully enough. An interdisciplinary initiative was launched and three to four protocols were reduced to two with a single pharmacy-based mixture instead of one mixed by a nurse according to physician order.

The director of the quality department spends 10 percent of his time on this function and there are 12 FTEs in the quality department. Case management has 35 to 40 FTEs. Each year the Quality Improvement Steering Committee reviews the prior year's accomplishment and has a prioritization session for the next year (see Appendix 9.2 for Quality Improvement Steering Committee minutes, 1998 Performance Improvement Selection grid, Performance Improvement Initiatives 1998 and 1999, and Quality Improvement Report Schedule). The top quality improvement priority last year was customer service, specifically, and developing an organizational culture to support customer service. Next year the committee is planning to focus on improving emergency department throughput.

The quality department reviews medical records to meet managed-care requirements and reviews ambulatory care charts quarterly. An ombudsman directs complaints to supervisory staff for response. The most frequent complaint was rudeness by employees, which led to the customer service program.

Physician leadership is directly involved in improving patient satisfaction. For example, the new chief of pediatrics found long waits and dissatisfaction in the clinics, with idle time in the morning and overcrowding in the afternoons. Residents were canceling sessions to take elective courses. Now after residents schedule sessions, they can be canceled only 45 days in advance. The number of schedulers was increased and they were moved to the patient care area. A nurse advice line was installed, which improved service to patients regarding prescription refills. As a result of improved scheduling, more pediatric services are provided by appointment rather than as walk-ins. The chief is now working on extending hours of operation in the evenings and on Saturdays. He says, "I've had administrative support. I have faculty support to do what is good for the patient. We are not compromising education. I lead by example, doing clinics myself, and once a month being on inpatient service. So I know what the problems are."

The Role of Medical Leadership

In addition to being chief of staff, Dr. Melinda Estes is the senior vice president for medical affairs. Dr. Estes has worked in the Cleveland market for 15 years, and has been at Metro for two. (See Figure 9.3 for an organizational chart of the department of medical affairs.) She is supported by four associate chiefs of staff in the following areas: inpatient services, ambulatory care, managed care and utilization, and professional staff affairs. Only four of the chairs who were there when she was hired remain two years later.

In 1997, Dr. Estes found that the quality of physicians was excellent but many had a "victim mentality." Data for effective management was lacking. "We didn't know who we were admitting, how long they were staying, who was taking care of them, and how well we were billing. We had the information somewhere, but not in usable form." Multiple decision-making groups were meeting in parallel fashion, including the multispecialty group practice, the faculty business office, and the physician-hospital organization. The physicians were not taking responsibility for making decisions.

Department chairs, always key leaders at Metro, are now leaders of the institution as well. The new philosophy is (1) departmental business is everyone's business; (2) the office of medical affairs is looking at what departments are doing; (3) the leadership is to deliver bad news without blaming scapegoats; (4) department chairs understand and craft the institutional vision, and must buy into and sell that vision; and (5) department chairs must understand their business—operationally, fiscally, and strategically. Dr. Estes has begun to set clear expectations. For example, when she came, "no one would send anyone they knew" to the department of dentistry. The area was physically dirty, faculty providers rarely, if ever, provided care, the support personnel were rude and unhelpful, little attention was paid to billing, revenue collections were low, it was a 9 to 3 operation, and their phone abandonment rate (callers hanging up when no one answered) was 70 percent. Dr. Estes reviewed performance with the chair and set expectations using MGMA standards for benchmarking, as adapted by standards at the dental school. She set modest expectations, moving from three to five patients per dentist during a four-hour shift. There was no progress over six weeks. She was visited by two young faculty dentists who said they could "clean matters up." She shared their recommendations

FIGURE 9.3

The
MetroHealth
System
Organization
Chart (Medical
Affairs)

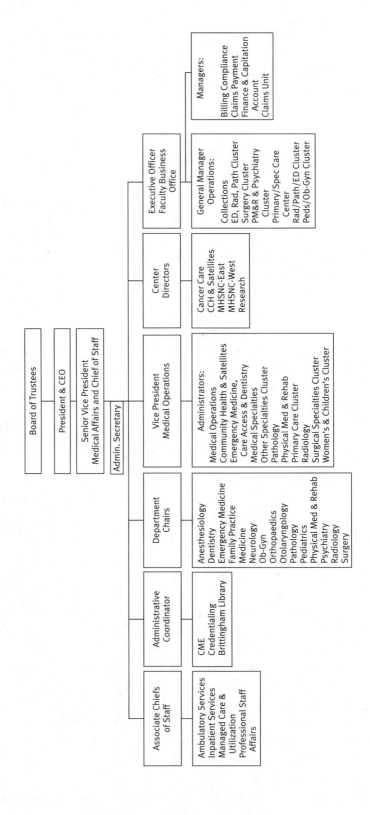

with the chair, who replied that the department was functioning optimally and that Dr. Estes didn't understand dentistry. She asked him to step down as the chair. An interim chair was appointed and dentistry is now one of Metro's most productive, respected, and profitable departments. Metro employees now use it. This was accomplished over 12 to 14 months, with a unionized workforce.

The medical operations group provides support to the departmental chairs. Between 75 and 80 persons work in this group, which serves as the administrative side for the medical groups. Previously these staff had worked in the individual departments. The group has seven cluster departments for administrative purposes, each headed by an administrator. These staff changes were made in a budget-neutral manner.

Dr. Estes chairs the MetroHealth Management Council (MMC). This group makes policy, develops strategy, and has fiscal responsibility. The MMC has seven physicians and three hospital managers (the CEO, the chief financial officer, and the chief nursing officer). The vice president for medical operations provides administrative support and is a nonvoting member. The president of the medical staff is ex officio. (They have never had to take a vote.) Dr. Estes selected a balance of primary care and specialty care physicians to serve on this committee, all acknowledged leaders who could think institutionally. The chiefs of surgery and medicine are on the MMC, as are the chief of radiology, the chair of pediatrics, the chair of ob-gyn, the director of community health, and the director of ambulatory care. There are two women.

Since August 1997, the MMC has had three all-day retreats, the last one addressing educational affiliations: what to get from them, and how to renegotiate affiliation contracts. The CMO sets the agenda for MMC meetings. After each meeting, executive summaries are sent to the department chairs. These summaries are discussed at monthly medical staff meetings and by the medical executive committee. Dr. Estes attends departmental meetings, as invited, at least once a year. She holds quarterly lunches with 12 different physicians whom she usually doesn't otherwise see, and walks around and tours departments by design. She writes 15 to 20 personal notes a week to physicians recognizing service or effort and communicates with physicians by e-mail and by appointment. Dr. Estes believes that to be effective, the physician leader must communicate, communicate, communicate, be a problem solver, and be proactive in leading change.

Notes

1. Center for Studying Health System Change, *Community Report Cleveland, Ohio* (Washington, DC: Center for Studying Health System Change, Fall 1998).

APPENDIX 9.1
MetroHealth
Management
Council
Protocol

Vision

The MetroHealth Management Council (MMC) will play a key leadership role in establishing and maintaining the MetroHealth System (MHS) as a highly competitive, cost-effective and compassionate provider of improved healthcare to the Cuyahoga County and Northern Ohio community. This will be accomplished in a setting that continues to support health education and research.

Mission

The MMC will define and oversee the implementation and evaluation of MHS healthcare initiatives including strategic, financial and operational practices. It will also develop and maintain an effective partnership between healthcare provider and hospital economies.

Objectives

Activities of the MMC will be consistent with the established vision and mission and will focus on:

1. Definition of strategic business opportunities, ventures and partnerships.
2. Identification and prioritization of opportunities that will lead to cost and operational improvements.
   • Set priorities for the allocation of resources.
   • Review and approve budgets.
3. Initiation and oversight of ad-hoc committees established to analyze operational change, develop market opportunities and prepare business plans for recommendation to the MMC.
   • The MMC will define the initial mission, objective and charge for ad-hoc committees. This may be subsequently refined by the Ad-hoc Committees and approved by the Management Council.

Committee Composition

The MMC will be chaired by the Sr. Vice President and Chief of Staff and will be composed of seven physician staff, the President of the Medical Staff, and three Hospital representatives.

As of July 24, 1997, members of the MMC are:

Melinda Estes, MD Chair	Mark Malangoni, MD
Terry White	Chris McHenry, MD
Errol Bellon, MD	Les Nash, MD
Roxia Boykin, RN	Greg Norris, MD
Pat Catalano, MD	Richard Olds, MD
Ann Harsh	Harry Walker, MD

Governance & Process

The Chairperson of the MMC is responsible for setting the agenda for each meeting. Other processes will function as detailed below and as graphically illustrated.

A. *Member Terms*
   a) The Senior Vice President for Medical Affairs will chair the MMC.
   b) The Chief Executive Officer, Chief Financial Officer, Vice President for Patient Care Services and the President of the Medical Staff will be permanent members of the council.
   c) The chairperson annually at the first meeting of the MMC in July will appoint all Council members, excluding those indicated in b) above.

d) Members are expected to attend all council meetings and the attendance of alternates will not be allowed.

B. *Reporting*
   a) The MMC will report through the CEO to the Board of Trustees.

C. *Communication of MMC Meetings and Activities*
An objective of the Council is to communicate their activities to all levels of the organization. The Council will communicate through a single out-going communication that will be in the form of an executive summary. Other forums of communication will include:

- MHS Medical Leadership Council
- MEC
- Department Meetings
- Town Hall Meetings
- Management Meetings

Minutes will be maintained for the use of the Council.

Communication from MHS staff to the MMC should flow through the members of the Council with any MHS staff having the opportunity to communicate to the Council.

D. *Committee Meeting Process*
   a) An Executive Session will be used for sensitive issues as determined by the chairperson.
   a) Reports of Other Committees.

Formation and Process for Standing and Ad Hoc Work Groups and Task Forces

The Chairperson of the MMC is responsible for establishing standing and ad hoc work groups and task forces, assigning a chairperson for the committee and identifying an initial charge and focus for the work groups or task forces. In the case where a member of an ad hoc work group or task force is not a member of the MMC, the MMC Chair will assign a member of the MMC to be the primary interface to the ad hoc work group or task force chair.

Communication through an MMC Council representative is designed to ensure consistent communication and to facilitate requests for information or other resources that may be required by the work groups or task forces. The MMC will set standard of performance for the work groups or task forces and will monitor and adjust implementation strategies as necessary.

A. *Responsibilities of Ad Hoc Work Groups and Task Forces Chairs*
   a) Communicate and refine the work groups or task forces mission and charge with members.
   b) Assure that a meeting schedule is established and meetings are held.
   c) Assure that minutes are recorded.
   d) Work with group to establish list of deliverables and time frames.
   e) Apprise the MMC of critical issues and report to Management Council as requested by the Management Council.

B. *Evaluation of Work Groups and Task Forces Rcommendations:*
The MMC will evaluate all work groups and task forces recommendations. Once these recommendations and plans are accepted by the MMC, the designated representative will be assigned for oversight of implementation.

APPENDIX 9.1

Graphical
Representation
of MMC
Decision Process

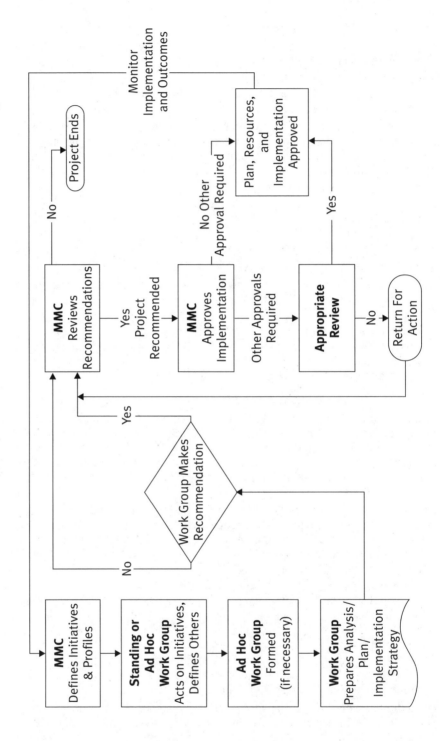

APPENDIX 9.2

MetroHealth
System Quality
Improvement
Steering
Committee
Minutes

MetroHealth System Quality Improvement Steering Committee	1/21/99 1:00 PM–2:30 PM K-101 ← NOTE: Change in Location for 1999 Meetings

Meeting Called by:	Brendan Patterson, MD		

Attendees:	S. Amin	M. Legerski	J. Schlesinger
	B. Averbook, MD	T. Lukens, MD	D. Smith, MD
	R. Boykin	M. Malangoni, MD	J. Tomashefski, MD
	B. Brouhard, MD	R. Olds, MD	W. West
	R. Blinkhorn, MD	A. Petrulis, MD	T. R. White

Please Bring:	*Minutes, Agenda, Attachments*

AGENDA

	TOPIC	PRESENTER	TIME
1.	Approval of minutes - November 19, 1998		2
2.	Tentative Report Schedule - 1999 (Attachment A)	B. Patterson, MD	5
3.	Brainstorming & Multi-voting - PI Priorities for 1999 (See 1998 Priorities - Attachment B)	Group	30
4.	Evaluation of Program - 1998 (Attachment C)	S. Amin	5
5.	ORYX • Indicator Selection • Data 3rd Q 1998 (Attachment D)	R. Boykin S. Amin	5
6.	P & T Report	B. Averbook, MD	5
7.	Ethics Report	D. Smith, MD	5

APPENDIX 9.2
MetroHealth System 1999 Quality Improvement Steering Committee Report Schedule*

Reports/ Discussion Topics	Frequency per Year	1/21/99	3/25/99	5/27/99	7/22/99	9/23/99	11/18/99
Benchmark Data							
• Cleveland Health Quality Choice Reports	x2			X			X
• ORYX Data	x2	X			X		
• Anthem Report Card	x1				X		
Accreditation Committee	PRN						
Customer Service Performance Improvement Team	x2			X			X
Ethics Reports	x2	X			X		
External Request Oversight Activities	PRN						
Infection Control Reports	x2		X			X	
Mortality Summary	x1			X			
P&T Reports	x2	X			X		
Pathology Quality	x2		X			X	
Risk Management Reports	x3		X		X		X
Safety Report	x4		4th	1st		2nd	3rd
Transfusion Review Summary (include as part of Pathology Quality Report in 1999)	x1						
Utilization Management Reports	x2		X			X	
PI Priorities	x1 & PRN	X					
Evaluation of Program	x1	X					
QI Plan Review	x1	X					
Plan for Next Year	x1						X
PI Initiative Updates	PRN						
New Business	PRN						
Total # Scheduled Reports		6	5	4	5	4	5

*NOTE: If emergency discussion/actions required when regular report is not scheduled, add as an agenda item under new business.

APPENDIX 9.2
MetroHealth
System 1998
Performance
Improvement
Selection Grid

Selection Criteria
(factors considered during brainstorming & multi-voting processes)

A. Accomplish mission & goals; actualize vision (Strategic Priorities 1–7)

B. Hospital-wide function not currently being assessed (Strat. Pr. 2,4,7)

C. Current or previous compliance issue (Strategic Priorities (1,4,7)

D. UR, RM, QC, Infection Control issue (Strategic Priorities (1–3)

E. High cost or significant savings potential (Strategic Priorities 3)

F. Benchmarking information available (Strategic Priorities 4,7)

G. Evidence of variations in practice (Strategic Priorities 1,4)

H. External customer expectation/need (Strat. Pr. 1,5)

I. New process or problem-prone activity (Strat. Pr. 2,4,7)

J. Strong internal interest (Strategic Priorities 1–7)

K. High Volume

L. High risk

Total Points

Potential projects identified by MHSQISC members during brainstorming session (February 1998)

MULTI-VOTING RESULTS*
(3 points if selected as highest priority
1 point if 3rd highest priority
0 points if not selected as one of the top 3 choices)

Potential Projects	
Customer Service (Int. & Ext.)	23 points
Error Management/Root Cause	14 points
Specific Disease Management	12 points
Ambulatory Operations	7 points
Presurgical Evaluation	5 points
Abnormal Labs/Communication	3 points
Billing Issues	2 points
Surgical Waiting Area	0 points
Transportation/East Side	0 points
ORYX/SB50/Sentinel Events	
JCAHO	

*Based on responses from 11 individuals

APPENDIX 9.2

MetroHealth
System Quality
Improvement
Steering
Committee
Performance
Improvement
Initiatives,
1998*

Committee Oversight Activities
- Set performance improvement priorities for 1998 (2/98, 4/98)
- Restructured committee membership and reporting relationships (4/98)
- Developed tentative reporting structure for activities in 1999 (11/98)

Customer Service
- Developed an improvement team to address customer service issues (2/98)
- Identified key deliverables (7/98)
- Developed timeline to accomplish identified strategies/tasks (9/98)

Data Review
- Cleveland Health Quality Choice (4/98, 6/98, 11/98)
- Mortality summary data (5/98)
- Transfusion appropriateness data (5/98)
- ORYX indicators (11/98)

Ethics Committee
- Provided several patient care consultations (9/98)
- Participated in ethics-related educational activities (9/98)
- Discussed/made recommendations regarding ethical concerns of "Do-Not-Resuscitate" policies/procedure, informed consent, advance-directives, managed care

Joint Commission
- Notified that the Joint Commission Type I Recommendations were addressed satisfactorily (2/98) & of revised Joint Commission grid score (4/98)
- Had a Mock Joint Commission Survey by a consulting team (7/98)
- Received results of Mock Survey & developed action plan (9/98)

Infection Control Committee
- Summarized reorganization activities of Employee Health program (9/98)
- Reviewed data regarding care of inpatients with pulmonary tuberculosis in 1997 (9/98)

Informed Consent
- Formed a sub-committee to address informed consent issues (5/98)
- Identified methods to document informed consent (7/98)
- Identified educational needs (7/98)
- Classified major vs. minor procedures needing informed consent (11/98)

Managed Care
- Anthem
  - Notified that actions taken in response to 1996 Report Card were accepted (2/98)
  - Collected & submitted required data for 1997 (4/98)
  - Notified of passing 1997 Report Card score (5/98)
  - Collected & submitted required data for 1st half 1998 (11/98)
- Cleveland Health Network
  - Provided results of medical record audits, office site reviews, & long-term care site review (5/98)
- Explored alternative methodologies for conducting required medical record audits & office site reviews (7/98)

Pathology Quality Committee
- Implemented new reporting structure for related committee activities (Tissue Committee, Transfusion Committee, Point of Care Testing Committee & Departmental QI Committee) (9/98)

- Evaluated the performance of INR testing in a proposed Anticoagulation Clinic (9/98)
- Implemented efforts to reduce wastage of fresh frozen plasma & platelets (9/98)
- Implemented a new mechanism to improve turnaround time for specific test results in pediatrics (9/98)

Pharmacy & Therapeutics Committee
- Revised restriction policy for pharmaceutical representatives
- Implemented corrective actions relative to administration of heparin (11/98)

Risk Management
- Coordinated activities to:
  - Reduce frequency and severity of patient falls (4/98, 7/98, 11/98)
  - Reduce elopements from the Emergency Department (4/98)
- Conducted critical incident reviews with corrective actions for:
  - Administration of heparin (4/98, 7/98, 11/98)
  - Antibiotic administration in the Operating Room (5/98)
  - Administration of conscious sedation (7/98)
- Clarified appropriate use of terms "sentinel events" and "critical incidents" (7/98)
- Shared plans for a "Mock Trial" educational session in 1/99 (11/98)

Safety
- Reviewed the annual summary of activities for all Environment of Care components (4/98)
- Summarized capital expenditures to remove physical barriers & improve ADA compliance (5/98, 11/98)
- Noted activities aimed at reducing employee injuries (5/98, 7/98, 11/98) & exposure to latex products (7/98)
- Clarified staff roles regarding the use of restraints in conjunction with patient care (5/98)
- Noted reduction in general liability claims due to efforts by Facilities Engineering to correct hazards on grounds & by Logistics Department to train staff in safe/defensive driving (5/98)
  - Training of staff (5/98)
  - Revision of emergency preparedness & disaster planning (7/98, 11/98)
- Shared activities to integrate Life Flight safety into general safety activities (5/98) and results of inspection of the helipad by the Cleveland Fire Department (11/98)
- Summarized activities taken to improve safety within the physical plant (7/98, 11/98)
- Addressed storage practices in the Quad & the basement of Bell Greve buildings (7/98)
- Noted results of inspection by State of Ohio OSHA that was conducted in response to an employee complaint regarding air quality in the Quad (7/98, 11/98)

Utilization Management
- Provided denial data for delegated utilization management plans (11/98)

---

*As documented in 1999 minutes from MetroHealth System Quality Improvement Steering Committee

Case Questions

1. What are the most important factors at MetroHealth which affect physician-management relations?
2. What are some of the ways in which integration of physicians relative to the goals of a hospital system can be effectively measured?
3. To what extent does the payment system at MetroHealth influence physician performance?
4. In what ways is Dr. Estes a successful physician leader?
5. To what extent is physician commitment to organizational mission and strategy key to MetroHealth's success in the market place?
6. To what extent is physician commitment to organizational mission and strategy key to MetroHealth's relative success in the market place?

Case 10
Organization Design for the Breast Service at Easter Medical Center

Chiara del Monaco and James Paul Volcker

Internal Issues: Background and Unit Organization

Established in early 1992, the breast service seeks to deliver comprehensive care to women with breast disease. The service is a part of the Department of Surgery at Easter Medical Center (EMC), which over the last few years has undergone a wide reorganization focused primarily on information management, operations, employee development, and marketing. The department feels that weaknesses in these areas have stifled its ability to provide quality service and, ultimately, increase market share.

Tangible signs of the reorganization include a restructuring of the Department of Surgery (Figure 10.1). Physicians have been appointed as vice chairmen for information systems/research, operations/quality management, medical education/employee development, and external affairs. These doctors are responsible to the department chairman for overseeing the redesign of their respective areas. A chief financial officer supervises the business office in the department and provides financial guidance to the vice chairmen and division chiefs in their work. In addition, because physician autonomy and decision making are highly regarded as strengths in the department, a series of division chiefs remain as governors of their respective surgical services.

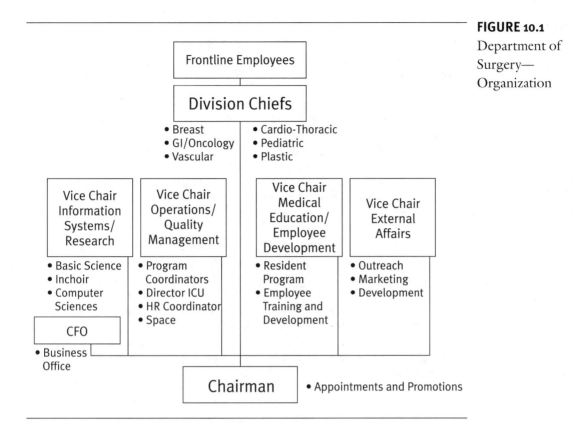

FIGURE 10.1
Department of
Surgery—
Organization

The chiefs provide strategic planning within their specific areas and are given discretion to access input from the vice chairs as necessary.

In addition to modifying its hierarchy, the department has created a vision statement and a new "commitment to partnership" (Figures 10.2 and 10.3, respectively). The latter document in particular, which includes goals for patient care, has been the impetus for a series of front-line employee workshops to bring about self-awareness and a unified approach to servicing customer needs. In general, departmental leadership has encouraged all employees to voice opinions to improve department service.

FIGURE 10.2
Vision

We, the members of the Department of Surgery, are committed to be a continuously improving professional and academic culture dedicated to prolonging and enhancing human life through excellence in clinical practice, teaching, research, and the development of surgical treatment. We will accomplish this by working in close partnership with each other, our patients, and our colleagues throughout the medical center and the larger community.

FIGURE 10.3

A Commitment
to Partnership

We, the members of the Department of Surgery, are committed to providing you, our patients, referring physicians, and colleagues throughout the medical center, with the highest quality service. We will endeavor to do this by holding ourselves to the following standards.

- We will respond to your inquiries and requests promptly, courteously, and thoroughly.
- We will provide you with relevant, comprehensive, and timely information, explanations, and materials.
- We will listen carefully, acknowledge your point of view, and encourage your questions so we may better understand your expectations.
- We will engage you in a collaborative decision-making process to produce the best possible outcome.
- We will work in close partnership with you and use all available resources to solve any problem you might be experiencing.
- We will take the initiative to put you in direct and timely contact with the person who has the knowledge and experience to best serve you.
- We will consistently demonstrate a willingness to meet your needs by going beyond the boundaries of our individual jobs.
- We will treat you with a depth of courtesy that demonstrates dignity, empathy, sensitivity, and utmost respect for the diversity of those we serve.

It is a strength of the Department of Surgery that it has taken the steps to reorganize as it has. With the advent of managed care, the healthcare industry is no longer "business as usual." Competitive pressures have generated the need for providers to focus not only on delivery of services, but also increasingly on how those services are delivered. Issues of efficiency within the industry have meant that outcomes assessment has become essential. The contemporary healthcare provider needs to be able to monitor quality of service and have access to data through which to assess outcomes. These new needs have, in turn, required new types of training for the healthcare professional.

The continuance of the division chiefs' structure, with the separate surgical services, is a potential weakness of the reorganization. In effect, the surgical fiefdoms remain, governed by the service chiefs. Physician autonomy remains a feature of the department; at best, limited mechanisms of accountability exist within the new structure. Mandating that the surgical services comply with the new way of doing things is nearly impossible—yet it is crucial that the chiefs and the service physicians "buy in" to the reorganization. They have to feel that the changes are positive steps in their work, or the hoped-for improvements will not happen.

Within this context of reorganization, the breast service has tended to maintain the status quo. Nationally and internationally recognized physicians whose collective reputation bring continuing business to the service via word-of-mouth recommendations have historically staffed the unit. Within this environment, new technology, competitive pricing, and operating efficiency are not deemed particularly necessary, and the service has largely forfeited opportunities to tap into the new departmental structure for assistance in modernizing operations. Consequently, goals to increase market share, enhance long-term profitability, or meet the needs of physician staff are not actively planned for.

The breast service is also handicapped by its own organizational design. Although physicians on the service report to the division chief, each operates his or her practice independently. While the advantage of this arrangement is physician autonomy, this delivery design has many weaknesses. The first is high staff costs. Each physician hires between one and three secretaries, whose responsibilities include reception, billing, filing, ordering supplies, and scheduling operations and physician time. In addition, some physicians hire physician extenders (a registered nurse, nurse practitioner, or physician assistant) to provide additional patient care. Little or no cross-utilization of functions exists—tasks are performed and passed on to the next compartment. The second weakness is procedural inefficiency. The senior secretary determines the charges for physician services; these charges are often arbitrary and have no relation to physician effort or practice costs. There is no strategy for the management of supplies/inventory, no standards of documentation for procedures, and no mechanism through which to monitor the quality of patient care. Third, the service staff is underdeveloped. Upon hiring, orientation to the EMC is perfunctory at best, and formal training in individual job responsibilities is nonexistent. Office practices are passed along through word-of-mouth, based on "the way we've always done it." The risk of perpetuating errors is therefore great. In 1997, it was discovered that a consistent error by a previous billing secretary had led to a large loss of revenue for one physician practice. The staff does not have a cohesive view of what needs to be done.

Staff development and formalized processes are needed to improve services and reduce mistakes in the breast service. Each office recognizes the need to take such steps, but lacks the necessary time. Heavy clinical responsibilities translate into physicians being, at best, disinterested managers, with all of the ramifications that term implies.

Weaknesses in the organization of the breast service have been exacerbated by a number of changes in physician personnel. Over a recent two-month period, the former service chief resigned and was replaced, one physician terminated her practice, and another has taken an indefinite leave of absence. This staff reduction will represent a significant decrease in service revenues. Two remaining breast surgeons are sharing the financial expenses of the unit. These two physicians have required the assistance of a recent graduate general surgeon to cover the overflow of patients. In addition, of three plastic and reconstructive surgeons integral to the functioning of a comprehensive breast center, one has left, a second plans to leave, and a third is inexperienced.

The unit can no longer function independently or comprehensively. The lack of reconstructive surgery undermines the service's stated mission as a comprehensive breast center, forcing patients to go elsewhere for these services.

External Issues: The Response to Change

In addition to internal pressures, the breast service is facing external pressures as well. Under the management of the previous chief, the service did not react to several environmental conditions that now make it less competitive in the local marketplace. Technical changes in the field have been rapidly advancing over the past two years to include a surgical procedure called sentinel lymph node biopsy and the use of the ABBI instrument for surgical treatment of breast cancer. As of yet, however, the breast service has not made a resource commitment in terms of dollars or personnel to these new procedures.

Second, the era of information systems technology has been ignored. The individual physician offices in the service continue to schedule appointments by hand. No integrated system, database collection, or outcomes measurement mechanism exists. Last, the service does not, to date, align itself with any insurance carrier. Provider shifts have taken place within the managed care industry, but the decision not to align endures. Breast service patients who decide to have surgery are informed by the secretary that they are responsible for investigating their own insurance benefits and for paying the remaining balance in its entirety. With the high costs of today's healthcare, many patients are actively seeking competent physicians within provider networks. Breast service physicians believe that the wave of managed care will pass, favoring the traditional fee-for-service model. Although this remains to be seen, it does not mean that care should not be managed efficiently and costs contained. Maintaining a position in the marketplace requires knowing what it costs to care for patients.

Another issue to consider is the reaction of patients to the delivery of care at the breast service. At present, enormous coordinated effort is necessary to take patients from scheduled appointments to the physician's consultation room, then into the hospital for surgery, and return them home satisfied with the services provided. Within this process are many pockets of inefficiency for staff and patients, resulting in delays and frustration at every point in the process. Historically, most patients have accepted office inefficiencies out of great loyalty to their surgeon. The contemporary woman who seeks care for breast disease has many choices in this marketplace. The question is, will the existing structure remain clinically respected and financially sound amidst the changing internal and external environment? Had the environment remained stable, the breast service might be able to perpetuate its existence with a low level of complexity. This possibility is no longer an option. The breast center must adapt to its environment and upgrade the complexity of its goals, strategy, and structure to maintain viability in the local marketplace. An organization with high complexity is more able to adapt to a changing environment, and adaptability is the key to survival.

Case Questions

1. What are the problems of the breast service?
2. What are the causes of these problems?
3. How do the goals of the physicians differ from those of the hospital management?
4. What should the service chief do in this situation?
5. What are the opportunities and constraints that face him?
6. How can he take advantage of these opportunities and overcome the constraints to implementation?

Short Case F
Managing a Difficult Workforce

Hila Richardson

Barbara Evans, patient services manager, arrives at her desk on Monday morning to find a telephone message that two nurses have called in sick. Just as Barbara is ready to arrange coverage, Emily Coe, RN, knocks on Barbara's door and asks to speak with her. Emily says she is quitting at the end of the week because "I can't handle all the case coordination work you make me do." Emily wants to know what she needs to do resign her job, and she wants to transfer her patients to another nurse as soon as possible.

When Emily leaves Barbara's office, Angela Johnson, the clinical director, calls to ask Barbara if she has done her case review for this week. Barbara knows this is the second week that she has not turned in her case review, and that if she misses this week, Angela is not going to like it. It could also influence Barbara's performance appraisal, raise, and bonus.

While Barbara is on the phone with Angela, her secretary hands her a message that "there are no per diem nurses available today," and another message that Ronda Clark, the regional administrator, called "to ask you about this week's case review."

Case Questions

1. What are the problems that Barbara faces?
2. What are the causes of the problems?

3. What part of these problems can Barbara control?
4. What options should Barbara consider?
5. What do you recommend that Barbara do now?
6. What should Barbara's supervisors do now?

Short Case G
Complaining Doctor and Ambulatory Care

Anthony R. Kovner

You are the assistant director for ambulatory services. An attending physician complains, "The clerks are no good in this clinic, and neither is the director of nursing." What do you say to him? Assume that the physician is an important customer.

Later during the week, he is still not satisfied. Now *you* are the problem. What do you do now?

Short Case H
Doctors and the Capital Budget

Anthony R. Kovner

You are the hospital CEO. Doctors on the capital budget committee can't agree on which equipment to recommend for purchase and for how much. They are way over budget. What do you say to them?

Short Case I
Doctors and a New Medical Day Care Program for the Terminally Ill

Anthony R. Kovner

You are the hospital CEO. Medical staff is opposed to the hospital's providing needed day care to the terminally ill, which is forecasted to break even financially. They say this is not what the hospital is supposed to do, and that it will actually or potentially compete with their business. What do you say to them?

Short Case J
Average Length of Stay

Anthony R. Kovner

You are the hospital CEO. Two of the doctors consistently keep too many of their patients in the hospital longer than the average LOS for several DRGs. They say their patients are older and sicker and that they're practicing higher-quality medicine. What do you say to them?

ADAPTATION

A hospital is a living organism, made up of many different parts having different functions, but all these must be in due proportion and relation to each other, and to the environment, to produce the desired general results. The stream of life which runs through it is incessantly changing; patients and nurses and doctors come and go, today it has to do with the results of an epidemic, tomorrow with those of an explosion or a fire, the reputation of its physicians or surgeons attracts those suffering from a particular form of disease, and as one changes so do the others. Its work is never done; its equipment is never complete; it is always in need of new means of diagnosis; of new instruments and medicine; it is to try all things and hold fast to that which is good.

—John Shaw Billings

Address on the opening of the
Johns Hopkins Hospital, May 7, 1889

COMMENTARY

Adapting the organization to external and internal pressures is a difficult challenge for the manager, particularly given the rapid rate of change in the healthcare environment. This section addresses the relationship between organization and environment, in which adaptation is the key issue.

The word "adaptation" suggests a view of organizational survival as dependent on a specific direction of change, that is, a change that leads to a closer fit between organization and environment. This close fit allows the organization to attract resources from society in exchange for a socially valued organizational output.

The key paradigm here comes from marketing. In quality improvement this is called customer-mindedness. Marketing has one central and powerful insight: it is easier to find out what people want and design the product or service to meet those preferences than it is to create a product or service and convince people they want it. Patients may seek healthcare when something hurts and the reason why is not known; they seek understanding and relief from pain. Medicine or surgery will hopefully provide quick and easy relief. Learning that one does not have a disease, such as cancer, is also valued by patients. It is much more difficult to convince people that they should control their blood pressure when it is not felt, and the benefits of doing so are to be gained far into the future.

Finding out what patients want and organizing to respond to those preferences is at the core of a customer-driven organization. Patient satisfaction surveys, focus groups, follow-up telephone calls after discharge, and community surveys are now widely used, and use of the Internet to supply customers and potential customers with information and choices is expanding rapidly.

Organizations vary in their sensitivity to environmental conditions and in the extent to which the environment impinges on internal operations. Healthcare organizations function in particularly complex environments, and failure to be responsive to a variety of conditions threatens their viability. Five aspects of the healthcare sector environment are especially important: competition, scientific technology, community service, funding, and workforce.

Competitive pressures are increasingly affecting the survival and growth of healthcare organizations. Since 1990, healthcare organizations have been characterized by mergers and acquisitions, some of which have resulted in the formation of some very large organizations, while others have already failed. Some organizations have suffered uncharacteristically large operating losses. Mergers have been both horizontal—of hospitals and hospitals—and vertical—of hospitals, home health agencies, group practices, and nursing homes. The managed care revolution has attempted to steer a large part of the American population into HMOs and other managed care networks that provide a broad scope of benefits to the employee at lower out-of-pocket costs than do providers outside these networks. HMOs are typically combinations of health plans, hospitals, and physicians—often competing with each other and with the remaining freestanding provider organizations—and subject to pressures stimulated by the preferences of large purchasers of healthcare for cost containment, together with quality and access. In some local markets, competitive pressures have been limited, and yet often intensified among fewer and larger organizations. As a result of mergers and acquisitions in many cities only two or three large systems have gained control of more than 80 percent of a local market.

The control of use by HMOs has given them bad press and some health insurers have said they want to be out of the "no" business of denying care to enrollees. A scientifically unproven treatment denied by the HMO may be seen as potentially life saving to a worried family. Self-pay and coinsurance put more of the cost consequences back onto the patient. Perhaps in the future more health insurance plans will have very large yearly deductibles (thousands of dollars) and require case management for the small percentage of all people needing costly complex care.

Scientific technology is one of the most important elements in the environment of nearly all organizations. Technology, to a large degree, determines an organization's internal structure. A medical clinic that diagnoses and treats individual patients uses different space and staffing patterns than does a screening unit that takes a standard array of diagnostic tests on dozens of patients a day.

As we can read every day in the newspaper, medical technologies are constantly changing. Effective drugs for mental illness introduced in the 1950s led to deinstitutionalization, community-based treatment, halfway houses, and an increase in homelessness. The growth of ambulatory surgery has reduced acute hospital admissions. Hernia surgery, which once called for a 20-day hospital stay, now routinely is an outpatient procedure, often at a freestanding ambulatory surgery center. The healthcare manager needs to be aware of the latest changes in technology. Advances in informatics and diagnostic technology are often heavily capital-intensive with benefits that are difficult to accurately forecast into the future. Already here are the paperless medical record, diagnostic laboratory and radiologic testing carried out at long distances (in the latter case using computer images rather than relying on film), and computer-assisted laser surgery. Digital radiology tests taken in the United States are being read by radiologists in Australia or India. Increases in the use of expensive drugs, which often have excellent health outcomes, are making sizeable dents in the budgets of many healthcare payers.

A third factor that makes patient care organizations highly sensitive to their environments is their "community service" character.[1] These services are provided on-site and in the community. Healthcare is said to be a "local" rather than a national product or commodity such as television sets or automobiles. Healthcare organizations are often identified with particular communities. As an institution serving a particular population, the organization is inevitably affected by the makeup of a community and its employers. In some communities, healthcare organizations, notably hospitals, have played leadership roles in working with other community organizations to improve health status and access to care and to control community healthcare costs. Some healthcare organizations are public institutions, whose goals may include, through law or charter, meeting the healthcare needs of all the individuals of a community service area.

There is controversy as to what medical care services should be available to all. Up until 1950, large cities provided charity hospitals that accepted patients regardless of ability to pay (and some still do). Medicare and Medicaid, introduced in 1996, are based on providing all with doctor and hospital care, although, under Medicaid, choice of provider is being restricted. The rising cost of health insurance has led to more people with no or inadequate coverage. There is growing interest in population-based healthcare and its measurement. This changes the view from excellent care for our patients to improved health status for the communities we serve. Excellent trauma care is not enough. What is the organization doing to reduce accidents to avoid the need for emergency care? What is the vaccination rate for all children in the community? What percentage of expectant mothers are seen early in their pregnancies? The demonstration of community benefit may be important in the future in justifying nonprofit tax status.

Healthcare organizations receive funding from a variety of sources. Much of their funding comes from government, and most of the rest often comes from other third-party payers, notably insurance companies. As part of this dependence on third-party funding, healthcare organizations are subject to a plethora of regulations and conditions, most of which are not under control through negotiation at the organizational level. Operational budgets are profoundly influenced for many organizations by the results of state budgets and legislation—for example, levels of Medicaid reimbursement (which many providers feel are set arbitrarily with no sense of the cooperative interacting of partners), reimbursement for bad debt and charity care, and for graduate medical education. Hospitals often feel powerless to collect from managed care companies, even after negotiating more or less successful rates of reimbursement. These companies are perceived to often arbitrarily (or again at least without the cooperative arrangements worked out by buyers and sellers who in some industries by some corporations are viewed as partners) withhold payments for certain days of services or treatments.

Healthcare organizations, as large (often the largest) employers in a community are subject to a variety of pressures. Healthcare costs are often viewed by many constituent groups, such as unions, as employment rather than health issues. The closing of healthcare facilities is often viewed as a serious blow to a community's attractiveness in the hiring of workers in companies which have nothing to do with healthcare. Healthcare managers must deal as well with the demands and preferences of tens of different types of employee groups as represented by unions and specialty societies. In some organizations, even the physicians have organized to be represented by a union. In other organizations, a specialty society has also become a union, such as a statewide professional nursing association engaged in collective bargaining.

Healthcare organizations function in a highly complex, volatile environment, and their responses to external pressures range widely, from pursuing acquisitions or merger, investing (or not) in highly intensive capital technology, saturation (or not) of community areas with satellite centers, to closing down services or units. Rapidly changing scientific technology, increased community expectations of service, competitive and purchaser pressures, and continuing demands from organized professional and labor groups necessitate environmental awareness and effective responsiveness on the part of the manager. This may require augmenting management support staff so that evidence can be generated and arrayed regarding best practices in other areas of the country or access to networks of experts and information as provided by organizations specially designed for this purpose. Managers may have little control over conditions external to their organizations, yet they must mold their organizations' internal operations and goals to be compatible with these forces. From the beginning, the context must be an integral part of the considerations in designing and developing the organization. Once established, the organization must constantly scan the environment to ensure that it remains sensitive to current developments and anticipates future trends.

Note

1. This is somewhat analogous to the economic concept of "social good," which is defined as a product that yields advantages to society in general as well as to the individual who purchases it, but whose side advantages are not evident in marketplace prices.

THE READINGS

Begun and Heatwole show how the cycling model of strategic planning facilitates adaptation. They address the shortcomings of traditional strategic planning in a dynamic environment. They emphasize continuous assessment of strategies based on feedback from benchmark analysis and stakeholder impact. Planning should include using multiple scenario and contingency plans developed in recognition of an uncertain future.

Strategic Cycling: Shaking Complacency in Healthcare Strategic Planning

Jim Begun and Kathleen B. Heatwole

From the *Journal of Healthcare Management* 44 (5), September/ October 1999

Executive Summary

As the conditions affecting business and healthcare organizations in the United States have become more turbulent and uncertain, strategic planning has decreased in popularity. Strategic planning is criticized for stifling creative responses to the new marketplace and for fostering compartmentalized organizations, adherence to outmoded strategies, tunnel vision in strategy formulation, and overemphasis on planning to the detriment of implementation.

However, effective strategic planning can be a force for mobilizing all the constituents of an organization, creating discipline in pursuit of a goal, broadening an organization's perspective, improving communication among disciplines, and motivating the organization's workforce. It is worthwhile for healthcare organizations to preserve these benefits of strategic planning, at the same time recognizing the many sources of turbulence and uncertainty in the healthcare environment.

A model of "strategic cycling" is presented to address the perceived shortcomings of traditional strategic planning in a dynamic environment. The cycling model facilitates continuous assessment of the organization's mission/values/vision and primary strategies based on feedback from benchmark analysis, shareholder impact, and progress in strategy implementation.

Multiple scenarios and contingency plans are developed in recognition of the uncertain future. The model represents a compromise between abandoning strategic planning and the traditional, linear model of planning based on progress through predetermined stages to a masterpiece plan.

The popularity and significance of strategic planning reside on a pendulum in the same manner as a host of other in-favor/out-of-favor management techniques. Strategic planning is alternately hailed as the savior or denounced as the false god of organizational management. As the pendulum swings, however, much of the contemporary literature portrays planning in a negative light, as it has become fashionable to attack formal strategic planning (Gray 1986, 89; Daft and Lengel 1998, 223). Recent empirical research on the effectiveness of strategic planning is also divided; numerous studies support its efficacy, but just as many cite no relationship with organizational performance (Boyd 1991; Bruton, Oviatt, and Kallas-Bruton 1995; Powell 1992; Sinha 1990).

This article will discuss both the negative and positive features of strategic planning. The negative concerns about strategic planning are related to the dynamic environment facing organizations in general, and more recently, organizations in the healthcare industry. Discussion of the positive and negative consequences of strategic planning and the environment in which planning in healthcare organizations must take place provides a framework for the use of a strategic cycling model. This model incorporates the positive features of planning and addresses the negative consequences to guide hospitals and other complex healthcare organizations through the turbulent environment.

Potential Adverse Consequences of Strategic Planning

Many legitimate concerns about the effectiveness of strategic planning have been voiced, particularly relating to the traditional, formal, linear method. There have been situations in which formal strategic plans have been more harmful than helpful to corporate organizations, and these issues translate to the healthcare industry. Six of the major negative consequences of strategic planning follow.

1. When "planning" is initiated by an organization merely to satisfy a regulatory body's requirement for a "plan," the effort becomes meaningless. No commitment is made on the part of key leadership, and no participation is given from those in the organization who will be responsible for implementing the plan. When the planning process becomes too bureaucratic, formalized, and irrelevant, creativity can be stifled and critical opportunities overlooked (Hax and Majluf 1991; Lenz 1985; Perry, Stott, and Smallwood 1993).

2. A bureaucratic planning process focused on top-down development may lack coordination and integration with other critical dimensions of the organization. The need for strategic integration includes not only the operational element of the organization and middle management, but other related functions such as financial resource management and information management (Hax and Majluf 1991; Henderson 1992).

3. One of the most common complaints regarding strategic planning is the lack of flexibility and responsiveness, particularly in a dynamic and rapidly changing environment. In many organizations, strategic planning has become so much of a science, with graphs, charts, statistics, and projections, that there is no accommodation for the art, intuition, and innovation that is so necessary if planning is to be effective (Luke and Begun 1994). Plans that are too rigid and detailed can inhibit flexibility and innovation (Aaker 1992; McDaniel 1997).

4. An interesting phenomenon that can be a significant negative consequence of planning is the automatic buy-in that can occur when a "masterpiece plan" is created. After creation of the masterpiece, the tendency is to try to make the plan work. Two factors are at work: (1) a fear of loss of face if plans change fosters an adherence to the plan even in situations where a change of course is clearly indicated (Mintzberg 1994); and (2) "organizations will generally tend to make changes closely related to their current strategies . . . to stay within their strategic comfort zone beyond which the organization does not wish to venture" (Shortell, Morrison, and Friedman 1992, 35).

5. Using the past to project the future is also a potential negative consequence of a formal planning process. The often-erroneous assumption that the future will follow past trends can lead to the development of flawed strategies. This emphasis on the past can lead to "the creation of strategies that are either repetitions of a largely irrelevant past or imitations of other organizations" (Wall and Wall 1995, 49). Ohmae (1982) refers to this flaw as "strategic tunnel vision," where the greater the need to broaden the vision, the more likely the tendency to narrow the focus, eliminating potentially viable options.

6. A final and deadly complaint against strategic planning is that too much attention and effort are placed on the development of the plan and strategies, and very little on implementation and monitoring. In many cases, the plan becomes the end of the process, not the spark to move the organization to change (Abell 1993; Curtis 1994).

The Positives of Good Strategic Planning

The listed adverse consequences are all legitimate complaints about the potential of strategic planning. Just as many positive consequences are associated with planning and these play a part in the success of many organizations. Following are several positive elements that are important to preserve as a new planning model is developed.

1. Strategic planning can provide an overarching direction or roadmap for an organization. As the various constituencies of the organization develop their individual objectives, the strategic planning process provides a framework so that efforts are coordinated with organizational strategies. The strategic planning process can help ensure that the key managers understand and are working in support of common organizational objectives (Hax and Majluf 1991).

2. Organizational discipline and control are also identified as positive results associated with a strategic planning process. The previous section identified the potential problems inherent in a process that "controls"; however, in any organization, particularly in unstable dynamic situations, a mechanism should be in place that forces the organization to envision the future, to look long term, and to be vigilant of potential opportunities and threats. In volatile settings, it is important to "find patterns in what appears to be a chaotic and constantly changing environment. The leaders will be the ones who are able to see order within the chaos . . . and who know how to use it" (Primozic, Primozic, and Leben 1991, 5).

3. Strategic planning can also provide the basis for an organizational decision-making process. Strategic planning provides the information and analysis needed to evaluate situations, opportunities, and strategies. A strategic planning process that encourages participation broadens the organization's perspective by considering divergent viewpoints and interpretations of possible strategies. The planning process is a catalyst through which an organization can develop consensus among the leadership on major strategies (Birnbaum 1990).

4. Improving overall communication among the various disciplines of an organization is another positive benefit associated with a strategic planning process (Langley 1989). The process educates the organizational team on the issues and choices faced by the organization, and can direct managers to think beyond their own departmental time frames and work with the organizational timelines in a focused and coordinated manner (Perry, Stott, and Smallwood 1993).

5. Another potential benefit of a strategic planning process is its motivational influence. Workers find the knowledge that their organization constantly assesses the dynamic environment and plans strategies to ensure organizational survival reassuring. The workforce is more secure in its future knowing that the organization is planning for whatever the future brings.

Planning in a Dynamic Environment

Many business organizations in the United States have discovered that the environment is changing too rapidly for a static, reactive planning process. Instead, attention has shifted to taking advantage of temporary gains, creating new products and markets, and staking out new competitive spaces (D'Aveni 1994; Hamel and Prahalad 1994; Moore 1996). The healthcare industry is following corporate America in facing a turbulent, uncertain environment. Healthcare is transitioning from a stable, comfortable, and complacent past to a confusing present and unpredictable future. All of the key aspects of the industry are experiencing dramatic shifts. A simple continuum analysis demonstrates the turbulence of the current healthcare environment. This continuum of the "Cs" (depicted in Figure V.1) highlights the challenges facing the healthcare industry.

Traditionally, patients and physicians were the "customers" of most healthcare organizations. Now, business and industry and insurers are major customers. In fact, in many instances, the desires of the patient and physician are secondary and the insurers dictate the hospital provider.

Control

In the past, most healthcare organizations held independent control of their strategies and futures. Now, most are part of systems or alliances—or are considering strategies to merge or partner. The individual healthcare organization must give up some control of its destiny and focus planning efforts on the partnership in addition to each member.

Capitation and Cost

The current reimbursement environment is schizophrenic, with varying degrees of managed care penetration causing a shifting mix of payment types

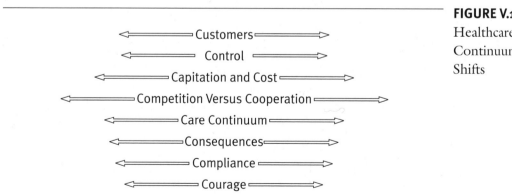

FIGURE V.1

Healthcare
Continuum
Shifts

from capitation to cost-based to percentage of charges. The future promises even more changes in reimbursement, and planning with future revenues and financial resources unknown will be challenging at best.

Competition Versus Cooperation

Most healthcare organizations face conflicting marketing strategies. The competitive environment has grown dramatically and organizations now face predatory attacks. At the same time, however, cooperative efforts among previous rivals are becoming commonplace.

Care Continuum

The care continuum refers to the paradigm shift from treating illness to focusing on wellness and prevention. This has been a relatively new focus for the healthcare industry. However, as the healthcare industry becomes increasingly responsible for the overall health of a defined population, the emphasis on improving health will become a primary focus.

Consequences

The "consequences" continuum acknowledges the many stakeholders that are now affected by any strategy developed by a healthcare organization. An organization's planning process must consider the consequences on other related organizations and constituencies. Equally important is the evaluation of the repercussions that strategies developed by these stakeholders will have on the healthcare organization.

Compliance

The recent increase in state and federal regulatory oversight as a means of quality control has had a dramatic effect on the healthcare industry, with increased scrutiny of the operation of healthcare delivery organizations. The public's confidence in the healthcare industry has been shaken as major accusations of fraud and abuse have been leveled at the industry. Strategies will not only need to address compliance, but also prove ethics and value.

Courage

All of these changes signal a need for healthcare leaders who have the skills to make the necessary changes—who have the vision and flexibility to lead and plan in turbulent times.

In summary, the healthcare industry is facing major changes. Changing customers, a changing product and mission, changing payment mechanisms, conflicting marketing strategies, more and different stakeholders, and a need for new leadership skills are just some of the major changes in the healthcare industry. The good news is that a dynamic and uncertain environment is not all bad. The fractious nature of the environment might prove to be the catalyst to shake the complacency from the current strategic planning process found in most healthcare organizations and encourage the development of more flexible, comprehensive models. The higher levels of tension and conflict can generate new perspectives (Stacey 1992, 39).

Strategic Cycling—A Planning Model to Shake Complacency

The previous discussion reveals that the process of strategic planning must adapt and evolve to be effective in the new healthcare environment. Although much of the current literature on strategic planning focuses on the negative qualities, the need for a process for appropriate future planning remains. In fact, most of the articles condemning strategic planning have created new terms such as strategic improvising, strategic processing, strategy application, issues management, and a wealth of other descriptive labels that still identify a thoughtful, proactive method or process to evaluate and set a course of action for an organization.

Much of the current literature on improving strategic planning focuses on a particular aspect or element of planning or addresses a specific complaint regarding a formal planning process. However, the previous discussion on the potential downsides of strategic planning and description of the environment in which healthcare organizations must chart their course indicates the need for a broader perspective. What is needed is a process that preserves the positive aspects of planning that are the "baby in the bathwater," while infusing the process with the flexibility and adaptability to not only respond to the rapidly changing environment, but to anticipate and thrive on it.

The strategic cycling model presented in Figure V.2 is a cycle or continuous process that provides a broad focus on critical issues that a healthcare organization should consider in planning strategically. The model differs from other contemporary frameworks in its emphasis on planning as a continuous feedback process rather than a set of stages that result in a relatively permanent and institutionalized plan (Ginter, Swayne, and Duncan 1998; Zuckerman 1998).

Overview of the Strategic Cycling Model

The strategic cycling model is arranged in a circular manner to avoid the linear and proscribed formal planning processes that create rigid, inflexible masterpiece plans. However, the model does not necessarily move in a clockwise manner. The arrows located in the center indicate the flexibility and responsiveness of the model, in which the process can react and adapt quickly

FIGURE V.2

Strategic Cycling
Model

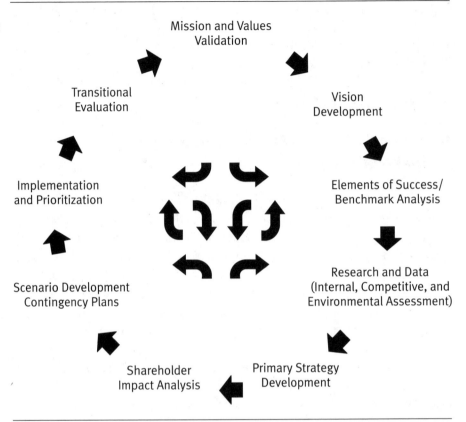

The diagram shows a circular cycle with the following elements arranged clockwise:

Mission and Values Validation

Vision Development

Elements of Success/ Benchmark Analysis

Research and Data (Internal, Competitive, and Environmental Assessment)

Primary Strategy Development

Shareholder Impact Analysis

Scenario Development Contingency Plans

Implementation and Prioritization

Transitional Evaluation

to changes in the environment. For example, an ongoing assessment of the competitive environment can detect threats that cause the leadership of the organization to develop a competitive strike contingency plan; or an analysis of the effect of certain strategies on a major stakeholder can create a need to reprioritize the strategies.

The strategic cycle is a process and not a plan. It represents a moving and flowing process of analysis and evaluation to continuously monitor the environment and adapt the organization. This cyclical or process emphasis with consideration of the relationships and contingencies must be included in a strategic planning process in these transformational times. Such a perspective facilitates systems thinking—a framework for seeing interrelationships and patterns that is often presented in terms of a continuous cycle emphasizing feedback effects (Senge 1990).

The elements of the strategic cycling process provide a broad framework to structure an approach to planning. The elements are general guidelines that should be violated to preserve innovation and creativity. Without some guidelines, however, the positive features of strategic planning dissipate. The elements of the strategic cycling model are described in more detail below.

Mission and Values Validation and Vision Development

The model uses the mission, values, and vision of the organization as the foundation for the process. However, if the mission, values, and vision become too abstract or, conversely, too specific with no room for interpretation, the planning process can become a rote confirmation of an obsolete direction. Strategic cycling calls for a revalidation of the underlying foundation of the organization. Missions are often believed to be carved in stone; however, the turbulent environment can dictate a necessary adjustment or even a major change in an organization's mission, values, and vision.

Elements of Success/Benchmark Analysis

The healthcare industry is just now beginning to catch up with industrial and corporate counterparts in the compilation, analysis, and dissemination of comparative performance data. Most healthcare organizations track trends in their own performance for a variety of financial and clinical indicators, but those data alone lack relevance in a broader sense. Mandated reporting requirements on both state and federal levels are now providing healthcare leaders with a wealth of comparative data. In most cases, the benchmark data are adjusted for differences in populations with regard to age and severity of care for more valid comparisons. Hospital "report cards" are becoming widely published for both consumer and payor review. Decisions regarding which provider to use are made based on the comparative data.

As part of the planning process, organizations must evaluate their comparative position in the market and determine the elements of success by which they will evaluate their own performance. The analysis identifies "best practice" hospitals and the scores on particular indicators that can become benchmarks or targets for the planning organization. Organizations that want to remain competitive must engage in benchmarking; "avoiding these comparisons is like burying your head in the sand" (Cleverley 1989, 33). This step in the planning process identifies measurable goals and keeps the organization continuously looking for benchmarks to improve its performance in relation to other similar organizations. The benchmark analysis not only alerts the organization to potential problem areas; it provides an opportunity to correct indicators before they are published in public reports.

Research and Data Analysis: Internal, Competitor, and Environmental Assessment

This element of strategic cycling is the standard bearer of traditional planning. In the past, strategic plans collected data and performed the infamous Strengths/Weaknesses/Opportunities/ Threats (SWOT) analysis. This element is still an important part of a planning process; however, rather than compiling a book of data, graphs, and trend lines that gathers dust on a shelf, the process of data assessment becomes an ongoing effort of monitoring and adjusting the organization in response to the analysis. A large amount of literature on environmental scanning, competitor analysis, and portfolio analytical tools suggests that these techniques continue to remain important in strategic planning (Drain and Godkin 1996; Ghoshal and Westney 1991). To avoid the negatives associated with this aspect of planning, focus should be placed on the use of the data and analysis to develop and implement strategies to prevent falling victim to the paralysis-by-analysis syndrome (Lenz 1985).

The means to create opportunities for product and service offerings that are not possible in the present environment and of "changing the environment to better suit the organization's goals" (Reeves 1993, 229) must also be considered. Possibilities for altering and creating new environments expand in uncertain times.

Primary Strategy Development

Although the term "strategy" in this element of strategic cycling is singular, the strategy development stage involves the development of multiple strategies. In this stage, the more scientific compilation of data and analysis combines with the less formal intuition and interpretation skills to develop workable strategies for the organization. An analysis of data and trends alone can lead to the development of erroneous strategies. The planning team must evaluate and interpret the data using experience and intuitive logic (Thomas, McDaniel, and Anderson 1991).

The coordination of the strategies among the various disciplines of the organization is a critical step in the process. This important activity solicits input and participation to avoid the problems discussed earlier in this article, where those responsible for implementation of the strategies had not been involved in nor did they believe in the validity of the strategies. Numerous anecdotal stories in the literature describe strategies that have been developed in direct conflict with other organizational directives. Clearly, one of the more important efforts involves integrating strategic development through the management team to all parts of the organization.

Shareholder Impact Analysis

Shareholders or stakeholders are "individuals, groups, or organizations who have a stake in the decisions and actions of an organization and who attempt to influence those decisions and actions" (Blair and Fottler 1998, 2). In the changing healthcare environment, shareholder impact analysis has become an even more critical aspect of strategic planning. Most healthcare organizations are now part of a system or alliance with other providers such as hospitals, physicians in PPO arrangements, and often with insurers to create a total product. Because of these vital relationships, planning becomes more complicated and the stakeholders must be considered in the planning process. In addition, the inter-relatedness among the stakeholders requires that the plans of these other individuals, groups, and organizations be considered as well. The concept of shareholder impact analysis is becoming a major focus in the planning literature. Whether called "linkage analysis" (Primozic, Primozic, and Leben 1991), "fostering generative relationships" (Lane and Maxfield 1996), or other creative terminology, the key is to evaluate relationships that can add value to the organization and to consider these potentially beneficial (or competitive) relationships in the development of organizational strategies.

Scenario Development/Contingency Plans

Scenario development and contingency planning are techniques that acknowledge that planning does not come with a crystal ball and that major assumptions can change with dramatic implications for the organization. Scenarios are "vehicles for helping people learn" (Schwartz 1991, 6). Obviously, an organization cannot anticipate all possible scenarios, nor do organizations have the time and financial resources to develop plans for all contingencies. The process of thinking about and planning for the unanticipated has the beneficial effect of moving leaders beyond their strategic comfort zone. The effort of scenario development and contingency planning leaves the organization better prepared for the unexpected. Scenario-based planning addresses one of the more serious negatives of strategic planning where only one possible "future" is considered.

Scenario-based planning can be very sophisticated, with computer models to run "what ifs," and the resulting analysis can be used to evaluate and develop possible actions in response to alternative situations that could arise (Georgantzas and Acar 1995). However, even if an organization does not have the computer or financial resources to simulate complex scenarios, a beneficial effect can be found in continuously evaluating and considering possible environmental changes or adverse conditions and thinking about the organization's options in response to these changes. This element of strategic cycling makes an organization more proactive and responsive, which will be a key factor of success in the turbulent healthcare environment.

Implementation and Prioritization

An often-cited negative consequence of strategic planning is that more effort goes into the development of a plan than into implementing it. One of the most important elements—it could be argued to be the most important element—of the strategic cycling process is the execution. Too often, the organization congratulates itself on the analysis, decisions, and creation of the plan, but rather than providing direction to a dynamic process of implementation, the "plan" is put on a shelf and forgotten. Implementation is one of the most critical aspects of the strategic planning process, but is often given little attention, which basically renders the "plan" useless.

Another important consideration in the implementation stage is the assignment of priorities. As resources are allocated to implementation of defined strategies, the allocation should be based on the strategies that have the most effect or are most critical—the top priorities for the organization. All of the key players in the organization must be committed and dedicated to the implementation of the strategies.

Transitional Evaluation

In the strategic cycling model, a continual evaluation of the implementation of the strategies completes the feedback loop. If strategies are not effective, the evaluation redirects the implementation process or redefines the strategy. Monitoring and evaluation provide for corrective action and put some control into the process. Evaluation and monitoring "make the planning effort a tangible reality rather than an academic exercise" (Birnbaum 1990, 221). In the model, the evaluation step can link back to any stage in the cycle to correct the implementation. If more data are needed, the process is flexible. If changes have taken place in the environment, then the scenario-development stage could provide possible alternative implementation efforts. Without an evaluation step, the planning process would be in serious contention to attain all of the negative results identified earlier in this article.

Conclusions

In the dynamic healthcare environment, strategic planning can be a vital and useful process to provide direction and guidance to a healthcare organization. But the possible negatives that can be associated with an ill-conceived process must be carefully considered. This article offers a strategic cycling model to broaden the planning perspective and address the potential drawbacks. The model takes into consideration the beneficial aspects of planning and focuses on a flexible, responsive, and proactive method of surviving the turbulent times. Although the current literature seems to focus on the downsides to strategic planning, a broader conceptualization of the strategic planning process provides real opportunities for healthcare organizations to face the uncertain future with confidence.

References

Aaker, D. 1992. *Developing Business Strategies*. New York: John Wiley & Sons.

Abell, D. 1993. *Managing with Dual Strategies: Mastering the Present, Preempting the Future*. New York: Free Press.

Birnbaum, W. 1990. *If Your Strategy Is So Terrific, How Come It Doesn't Work?* New York: American Management Association.

Blair, J. D., and M. D. Fottler. 1998. *Strategic Leadership for Medical Groups*. San Francisco: Jossey-Bass.

Boyd, B. 1991. "Strategic Planning and Financial Performance: A Meta-Analytic Review." *Journal of Management Studies* 28 (4): 353–74.

Bruton, G., B. Oviatt, and L. Kallas-Bruton. 1995. "Strategic Planning in Hospitals: A Review and Proposal." *Health Care Management Review* 20 (3): 16–25.

Cleverley, W. 1989. "How Boards Can Use Comparative Data in Strategic Planning." *Healthcare Executive* 4 (3): 32–33.

Curtis, K. 1994. *From Management Goal Setting to Organizational Results*. Westport, CT: Quorum.

Daft, R. L., and R. H. Lengel. 1998. *Fusion Leadership*. San Francisco: Berrett-Koehler.

D'Aveni, R. A. 1994. *Hypercompetition*. New York: Free Press.

Drain, M., and L. Godkin. 1996. "A Portfolio Approach to Strategic Hospital Analysis: Exposition and Explanation." *Health Care Management Review* 21 (4): 68–74.

Georgantzas, N., and W. Acar. 1995. *Scenario-Driven Planning: Learning to Manage Strategic Uncertainty*. Westport, CT: Quorum.

Ghoshal, S., and D. Westney. 1991. "Organizing Competitor Analysis Systems." *Strategic Management Journal* 12: 17–31.

Ginter, P. M., L. E. Swayne, and W. J. Duncan. 1998. *Strategic Management of Health Care Organizations*, 3rd edition. Malden, MA: Blackwell.

Gray, D. 1986. "Uses and Misuses of Strategic Planning." *Harvard Business Review* 64: 89–97.

Hamel, G., and C. K. Prahalad. 1994. *Competing for the Future*. Boston: Harvard Business School Press.

Hax, A., and N. Majluf. 1991. *The Strategy Concept and Process*. Englewood Cliffs, NJ: Prentice-Hall.

Henderson, J. 1992. "Aligning Business and Information Technology Domain: Strategic Planning in Hospitals." *Hospital & Health Services Administration* 37 (1): 71–87.

Lane, D., and R. Maxfield. 1996. "Strategy Under Complexity: Fostering Generative Relationships." *Long Range Planning* 29 (2): 215–31.

Langley, A. 1989. "In Search of Rationality: The Purposes Behind the Use of Formal Analysis in Organizations." *Administrative Science Quarterly* 34: 598–631.

Lenz, R. T. 1985. "Paralysis by Analysis: Is Your Planning System Becoming Too Rational?" *Long Range Planning* 18 (4): 64–72.

Luke, R., and J. Begun. 1994. "Strategy Making in Health Care Organizations." In *Health Care Management*, 3rd edition, edited by S. M. Shortell and A. D. Kaluzny, 355–91. Albany, NY: Delmar.

McDaniel, R. R., Jr. 1997. "Strategic Leadership: A View from Quantum and Chaos Theories." In *Handbook of Health Care Management*, edited by W. J. Duncan, P. M. Ginter, and L. E. Swayne, 339–67. Malden, MA: Blackwell.

Mintzberg, H. 1994. *The Rise and Fall of Strategic Planning.* New York: Free Press.

Moore, J. F. 1996. *The Death of Competition.* New York: HarperCollins.

Ohmae, K. 1982. *The Mind of the Strategist.* New York: McGraw Hill.

Perry, T., R. Stott, and W. N. Smallwood. 1993. *Real-Time Strategy.* New York: John Wiley & Sons.

Powell, T. 1992. "Research Notes and Communications—Strategic Planning as Competitive Advantage." *Strategic Management Journal* 13: 551–58.

Primozic, K., E. Primozic, and J. Leben. 1991. *Strategic Choices: Supremacy, Survival, or Sayonara.* New York: McGraw Hill.

Reeves, P. 1993. "Issues Management: The Other Side of Strategic Planning." *Hospital & Health Services Administration* 38 (2): 229–41.

Schwartz, P. 1991. *The Art of the Long View.* New York: Currency Doubleday.

Senge, P. 1990. *The Fifth Discipline.* New York: Currency Doubleday.

Shortell, S., E. Morrison, and B. Friedman. 1992. *Strategic Choices for America's Hospitals.* San Francisco: Jossey-Bass.

Sinha, D. 1990. "The Contribution of Formal Planning to Decisions." *Strategic Management Journal* 11: 479–92.

Stacey, R. 1992. *Managing the Unknowable.* San Francisco: Jossey-Bass.

Thomas, J., R. McDaniel, and R. Anderson. 1991. "Hospitals as Interpretation Systems." *Health Services Research* 25 (6): 859–80.

Wall, S., and S. Wall. 1995. *The New Strategists.* New York: Free Press.

Zuckerman, A. M. 1998. *Healthcare Strategic Planning.* Chicago: Health Administration Press.

Discussion Questions for the Required Reading

1. What is strategic planning?
2. Although strategic planning seems a good idea, in practice it may fall short or fail. Review the reasons for potential success and potential failure.
3. How would you use this understanding to improve management planning in the three cases that follow (Case 11, Case 12, and Short Case K)?

Required Supplementary Readings

Bigelow, B. and M. Arndt. "Great Expectations: An Analysis of Four Strategies?" *Medical Care Review* 1994, 51 (2): 205–233.

Center for Health Systems Change. (This organization tracks healthcare market changes in cities across the country and is an excellent ongoing resource for understanding current changes.) See www.hschange.org. Or, see Center for Studying Health System Change. "Market in Turmoil as Physician Organizations Stumble." In *Health Services Management: Readings and Commentary,* 7th edition, edited by A. Kovner and D. Neuhauser, 356–370. Chicago: Health Administration Press, 2001.

Kizer, K. W. "Health Care, Not Hospitals: Transforming the Veterans Health Administration." In *Straight from the CEO*, edited by G. W. Dauphinais and C. Price, 112–120. New York: Simon and Schuster, 1998.

Discussion Questions for the Required Supplementary Readings

1. Bigelow and Arndt review the problems and potentials of four strategies for hospitals in response to prospective payment. Compare the strengths and weaknesses of these strategies.
2. Kenneth Kizer led a remarkable effort to change the U.S. Government's Veterans Health Administration. This is an organization about which some observers would have said major change was impossible. What did Kizer do? How did he do it?
3. Healthcare change is not the same across the country. It differs by market area. What is happening in your area? What is it about your market area which would explain these changes? The Center for Studying Health System Change (see www.hschange.org) has been tracking such changes in a dozen market areas across the country. Pick an area that interests you and explain what is happening and why.

Recommended Supplementary Readings

Arndt, M., and B. Bigelow. "Reengineering: Deja Vu: All Over Again." *Health Care Management Review* 1998, 23 (3): 58–66.

Barnsley, J., L. Lemieux-Charles, and M. M. McKinney. "Integrating Learning into Integrated Delivery Systems." *Health Care Management Review* 1998, 23 (1): 18–29.

Begun, J. W., B. Zimmerman and K. J. Dooley. "Health Care Organizations as Adaptive Systems." In *Advances in Health Care Organizational Theory*, edited by S. S. Mick and M. E. Wyttenbach, 252–289. San Francisco: Jossey-Bass 2003.

Blair J. and J. A. Buesseler. "Competitive Forces in the Medical Group Industry: A Stakeholder Perspective." *Health Care Management Review* 1998, 23 (2): 7–27.

Blair, J. D. and M. D. Fottler. *Strategic Leadership for Medical Groups*. San Francisco: Jossey-Bass, 1998.

Burns, L. B., and J. C. Robinson. "Physician-Practice Management Companies: Implications for Hospital-Based Integrated Delivery Systems." *Frontiers of Health Services Management* 1997, 14 (2): 3–36.

Christensen, C. G., R. Bohmer, and J. Kenagy. "Will Disruptive Innovations Cure Health Care?" *Harvard Business Review* 2000, (Sept/Oct): 102–112.

Curran, C. R., K. W. Ruhn, M. Miller, A. Skalla, and R. D. Thurman. *Shaping an Integrated Delivery Network: Home Care's Role in Improving Service, Outcomes, and Profitability.* Chicago: Health Administration Press, 1999.

Evashwick, C. J. *Seamless Connections.* Chicago: American Hospital Publishing, 1997.

Feldman, R. D., D. R. Wholey, and J. Christianson. "HMO Consolidations: How National Mergers Affect Local Markets." *Health Affairs* 1999, 18 (4): 96–104.

Friedman, L. H. "The Unfocused Strategic Vision." *Managed Care Quarterly* 1997, 5 (4): 1–7.

Ginter, P. M., L. E. Swayne, and W. J. Duncan. *Strategic Management of Health Care Organizations,* 3rd edition. Malden, MA: Blackwell, 1998.

Griffith, J. R. "Managing the Transition to Integrated Health Care Organizations." *Frontiers of Health Services Management* 1996, 12 (4): 4–50.

———. *Designing 21st Century Healthcare.* Chicago: Health Administration Press, 1998.

Herzlinger, R. E. *Market-Driven Health Care.* Reading, MA: Addison-Wesley, 1997.

Jha, A. K., J. B. Perlin, K. W. Kizer, and R. A. Dudley. "Effect of the Transformation of the Veterans Affairs Health Care System or the Quality of Care." *New England Journal of Medicine* 2003, 348 (22): 2218–2254.

Levey, S., and L. Anderson. "Painful Medicine: Managed Care and the Fate of America's Major Teaching Hospitals." *Journal of Healthcare Management* 1999, 44 (4): 231–251.

Luke, R. D., J. W. Begun, and S. Walston. "Strategy Making in Health Care Organizations." In *Health Care Management: Organization Design and Behavior,* 4th edition, edited by S. M. Shortell and A. D. Kaluzny, 394–431. Albany, NY: Delmar Thomson, 2000.

Neumann, C. L., A. S. Blouin, and E. M. Byrne. "Achieving Success: Assessing the Role of and Building a Business Case for Technology in Healthcare." *Frontiers of Health Services Management* 1999, 15 (3): 3–28.

Olden, P. C., S. D. Roggenkamp, and R. D. Luke. "A Post-1990's Assessment of Strategic Hospital Alliances and Their Marketplace Orientations: Time to Refocus." *Health Care Management Review* 2002, 27(2): 33–49.

Walston, S. L., and R. J. Bogue. "The Effects of Reengineering: Fad or Competitive Factor?" *Journal of Healthcare Management* 1999, 44 (6): 456–77.

Wholey D. R., and L. R. Burns. "Understanding Health Care Markets: Actors, Products, and Relations." In *Advances in Health Care Organizational Theory*, edited by S. S. Mick and M. E. Wyttenbach, 252–289. San Francisco: Jossey-Bass 2003.

Zajac, E. J., T. A. D'Aunno, and L. R. Burns. "Managing Strategic Alliances." In *Health Care Management: Organization Design and Behavior*, 4th edition, edited by S. M. Shortell and A. D. Kaluzny, 307–329. Albany, NY: Delmar Thomson, 2000.

THE CASES

Adaptive capability involves organizational response to new conditions. Organizations must be innovative or proactive in responding to the pressures of competitors and regulators and to the expectations of various stakeholder groups, from customers to physicians. One indicator of adaptive capability is the presence of specialized units to carry out functions, such as strategic planning and marketing, that are concerned specifically with and held accountable for the adapting function.

Strategic planning can be conducted as a special unit, as part of a specialized unit, by management, or by some combination of the above and is an important area of managerial contribution. Top management sees to it that information is gathered and arrayed regarding the basic businesses of the organization. What is the current mission, nature of the services provided, nature of the population served and targeted to be served, the organization's competitive situation, and what are perceived obstacles to and opportunities for strategies to meet current objectives?

Milio (1983) reminds us that organizations have limited problem-solving capacities; they wish to avoid uncertainty by arranging negotiated environments, engage in problematic or biased searches for ways of adapting, act on the basis of limited knowledge, and select alternatives on the basis of past successes.

Obviously, decisions to adapt can be the wrong ones relative to organizational goal attainment and system maintenance. Even if the decisions can be shown, in hindsight, to have been technically appropriate, they may have been politically inappropriate. Managers may fail to integrate values of important stakeholders on those directions toward which the organization should focus effort to attain current mission and strategy. We are assuming, of course, that the healthcare organization already has a carefully worked out mission and strategy, one which it is constantly reassessing in terms of competitive and regulatory pressures and in terms of the preferences and expectations of stakeholders, such as physicians and nurses.

The three case studies in this section deal with questions of partnership and alliances and with changes in product focus and delivery. How these questions are answered and what strategies are selected may have consequences that are different for specific organizations and for specific managers. In the case of "The VNA of Cleveland," the CEO, Mary Lou Stricklin, is faced with a set of choices involving new relationships with local collaborators and competitors, some of whom may be seen by certain VNA stakeholder groups as threatening the core value upon which the organization was founded and has thrived for many years.

Similarly, Geraldine Patton, the CEO of the West Peoria Veterans Affairs Medical Center, must decide how her center should relate to managed care and to other VA facilities in the region. A task force has recommended that 8,000 patients be initially enrolled in the VA Community Integrated Service Network. A marketing plan that includes the endorsement of veterans service organizations may be undertaken to enroll veterans not currently using the VA, with the inclusion of new (and less seriously ill) patients being seen as critical to success. Other options are suggested, and the CEO must examine critically the assumptions underlying the three different points of view.

The third (short) case study raises the basic issues from a management perspective—that of a new chief of OB-GYN—testing our skills at developing an organized, coherent response.

Reference

Milio, N. 1983. "Health Care Organizations and Innovation." In *Health Services Management: Readings and Commentary*, 2nd edition, edited by A. R. Kovner and D. Neuhauser, 448–64. Chicago: Health Administration Press.

Case 11
In a State of Change: Veterans Affairs and HMOs

J. J. Donellan, A. R. Kovner, C. A. Milbrandt, J. Oliveri, B. L. Bell, D. Anderson, and P. J. O'Neil

The state of West Peoria leads the nation in healthcare reform. In each of the past three legislative sessions comprehensive healthcare reform laws have been passed. The legislation has brought about the following:

- The small employer insurance market has been restructured to enable more citizens to acquire health insurance coverage. Within two years all employers with more than 50 employees will be required to offer and subsidize coverage for employees and their dependents.
- A state-funded health insurance program has been created to cover those citizens who are unable to obtain private insurance and who do not

qualify for other government health programs. This program has been in effect for the past year and is offered on a sliding fee basis.

- In three years universal coverage for West Peoria will be implemented. At that time all West Peorians will be required by law to acquire a minimum "basic benefit" package.

With the advent of universal coverage most health providers will organize into integrated service networks (ISNs). Reimbursement rates for providers not participating in an ISN will be regulated by a state-run, all-payer system (a modified fee-for-service system) that will severely restrict reimbursement. ISNs will be licensed by the state and will be required to provide, at a minimum, the basic benefit package prescribed by law to anyone wishing to enroll.

Community ISNs (CISNs), a smaller version of an ISN, may begin enrolling patients immediately. Both ISNs and CISNs are required to make primary care services available within 30 miles of an enrollee's home. Secondary and tertiary services (with the exception of highly specialized services such as transplants, open heart surgery, and neurosurgery) must be available within 60 miles of an enrollee's home. Growth in ISN/CISN premium rates will be state regulated, and "report cards" comparing ISN and CISN performance on factors such as cost, quality, and customer satisfaction will be issued annually by the state.

HMOs and managed care plans have been developing in West Peoria since the 1950s. The market is dominated by managed care, with two-thirds of the state's eight million citizens enrolled in some form of managed care plan. Three HMOs now dominate the managed care market, covering 80 percent of the state's managed care enrollees.

Geraldine Patton was recently appointed director of the Dwight D. Eisenhower VA Medical Center in Peoria City (Peoria City VAMC). Patton was assigned to Peoria City by VA Central Office (VACO) for the specific purpose of developing and implementing a transition plan that will ensure VA's success in West Peoria's reformed healthcare market.

Peoria City VAMC is the largest of three VA medical centers in the state and is geographically located near the center of the state. The facility is five years old and is considered by many to be among the finest and most modern of the 163 VA medical centers nationwide. It currently consists of a 500-bed acute care hospital with medical, surgical, rehabilitation medicine, and psychiatric beds, and a 100-bed nursing home. It is a major teaching affiliate of the University of West Peoria Medical School. With the exception of transplant services, all primary, secondary, and tertiary healthcare services are available at the facility or through a sharing agreement with the university. These include a newly opened women veterans health program and a nationally renowned prosthetic and rehabilitation center. The Medical Center also manages a satellite outpatient clinic located 50 miles to the south of Peoria City. The veteran population of the state of West Peoria is 520,000. Peoria City VAMC treated 38,000 individual veteran patient cases during the past year.

Some management improvements are necessary at Peoria City VAMC. Length of stay for both medicine and surgery is three to five days longer than that found in comparable non-VA community and teaching hospitals. Waiting times for next available appointments are more than 30 days in many of the specialty clinics, and pressure to reduce overall government employment has forced staffing reductions in virtually all departments. A primary care program has recently been instituted, with approximately 25 percent of all outpatients enrolled in this program. Primary care has had a positive effect. Overall, waiting times for next clinic appointments have been reduced, and the satisfaction of patients served by a primary care provider has improved.

Two other VA medical centers are also located in West Peoria. The Lakeland VAMC is located 125 miles to the north of Peoria City, close to the state's northern border. This 150-bed facility offers primary and secondary health services to approximately 12,000 veterans and operates a specialized spinal cord injury program. The Leesville VAMC, located 90 miles to the southeast of Peoria City, operates a 350-bed acute and chronic care psychiatric hospital and a 250-bed nursing home. The hospital specializes in the care of chronic psychiatric patients, with specialized programs of excellence in substance abuse and post-traumatic stress. The nursing home operates at full capacity with a waiting list for admission. A small clinic at Leesville offers primary care services to approximately 10,000 veterans on an outpatient basis. Both the Lakeland and Leesville facilities were built in the 1930s; although some modernization has been done, they are both in need of considerable plant improvements. All three West Peoria VA medical centers are part of a referral network that also includes two VA medical centers in neighboring East Peoria, and one in the state of Tremont, located to the south of West Peoria.

Geraldine Patton appointed a task force from the Peoria City VAMC to analyze the current situation and present an action plan. The task force consisted of the chief of staff, Dr. Urban Grant (chairperson), several medical staff leaders, the associate dean for clinical programs at the University of West Peoria Medical School, the chief of medical administration and fiscal services, and leaders of three different veterans service organizations in the immediate community. Dr. Grant's task force reached consensus on establishing a VA-sponsored CISN based at Peoria City VAMC, with future plans to expand to a statewide ISN in conjunction with the Lakeland and Leesville VAMCs. The report included a financial analysis projecting that a benefit package providing comprehensive coverage meeting state criteria would cost $1,500 per enrollee under age 65, and $5,200 per enrollee age 65 and over (exclusive of supplemental services such as long-term care). For enrolled veterans not living near existing facilities, primary care and emergency services could be offered close to their home by shifting resources to set up multiple community clinics and by establishing contracts with community hospitals and providers.

The task force recommended that 8,000 patients be initially enrolled in the VA CISN (Community Integrated Service Network); 4,000 should come from Peoria City VAMC's existing patient population, and an additional 4,000 new enrollees should be sought. A marketing plan that included the endorsement of veterans service organizations would be undertaken to enroll veterans not currently using VA. The inclusion of new (and less ill) patients was seen as critical to success; the existing patient base of Peoria City VAMC was disproportionately skewed toward patients with multiple and chronic medical conditions.

The task force also recommended that Peoria City VAMC contract with MetroPru, a large health insurer in West Peoria, to do the actuarial work; to manage enrollment, billing, and collections; and to ensure that equivalent insurance options would be made available as a package to the dependents of veterans who chose to enroll. The cost of contracting with MetroPru to manage the plan was not factored into the report. The task force felt confident that the plan would be competitive in that it would offer health benefits to veterans not customarily available in other CISN/ISN packages (i.e., low-cost prescriptions and broad coverage for psychiatric benefits). Some legislative relief would be necessary, most especially from federal total employment ceiling restrictions. An additional funding stream would also be needed to meet the increased number of patients served. This could be accomplished either by an increase in funding to Peoria City VAMC by VACO based on new enrollment, or through legislative relief permitting Peoria City VAMC to retain insurance collections.

Ms. Patton discussed the task force recommendations with the directors of the Lakeland and Leesville VAMCs at a network meeting. They were less than enthusiastic. While Peoria City VAMC was well capitalized, the Lakeland and Leesville facilities simply did not have the physical plant and access to staff necessary to compete in the market. They questioned the urgency of such a drastic action, pointing out that many patients already elected to receive care by VA despite having other health insurance, including Medicare. In their opinion, the state reform agenda might in fact create a greater demand for VA care, noting that ISNs would likely exclude coverage of service-connected illness or injury, and offer only very limited psychiatric and long-term care benefits.

They suggested that rather than form an ISN or CISN, the medical centers specifically identify clinical areas of expertise and cost efficiency and aggressively market those services to health insurers. The insurers could purchase these services from VA for eligible veterans enrolled in their plans. They argued that those treatment areas not covered by the required "basic benefit" package where VA had specific expertise—such as prosthetic programs, long-term care, geriatric care, acute and chronic psychiatry, substance abuse, and post-traumatic stress disorder—would become a critical "safety net" for veterans, and an essential ingredient of the state program. Finally, they noted that their strategy would require little action in terms of redirecting resources and facility missions.

Ms. Patton is familiar with another option not yet presented, but one that she was involved in negotiating with the state of Columbia during her last assignment. Rather than trying to initially compete in the market as an insurer, VA could negotiate an arrangement directly with the state, whereby state payments and subsidies would be waived for any care provided to nonservice-connected veterans who met VA criteria for mandatory treatment and who elected to receive their care at a VA facility. Through such an arrangement, low-income nonservice-connected veterans eligible for state-funded health insurance could receive their care by VA under the auspices of the state plan but at no cost to the state. As category "A" patients, their care would be covered by federal appropriations rather than state payment. This was seen as a win-win arrangement in another state. Here the VA gained experience as a provider and administrator of a managed care plan in the early stages of state reform; the state realized savings by avoiding any costs associated with the care of low-income veterans receiving VA care.

Acknowledgments

The authors wish to thank Gary DeGasta, Brian Heckert, and Malcolm Randall for their ideas and suggestions and for their critical review of the case.

Case Questions

1. What criteria should Geraldine Patton use in choosing strategic options? Why choose these criteria?
2. What are the advantages and disadvantages of each of the three options? How do the options rate on each of the criteria that you recommended?
3. What do you recommend that Ms. Patton do? What is the rationale behind your recommendations?
4. How should Ms. Patton proceed in implementing your recommendations? What measurable objectives are reasonable for your recommendations?
5. What are the personal stakes involved for Ms. Patton in doing as you suggest? How can she maximize the upside potential and minimize the downside risks for her own career?

Case 12
The Visiting Nurse Association of Cleveland

Duncan Neuhauser

Mary Lou Stricklin, MBA, MSN, is chief executive officer of the Visiting Nurse Association of Cleveland (VNA). The home care market continues to change rapidly. Competition, DRG payment, HMO growth, the rising burden of indigent care, hospital-based home care programs, hospice, large growth of demand for home care, the explosion of specialized home care services, and the introduction of prospective payment for home care continue to affect this market. These rapid changes have led to a series of corporate reorganizations, and Stricklin is contemplating the next corporate transformation.

The year 2002 was the 100th anniversary of Cleveland's VNA. Throughout its history, the VNA has employed professional nurses with home care experience to provide care to the residents of the greater Cleveland area, which now has a population of approximately 1.2 million people. The mission and value statements for the VNA are shown in Figure 12.1.

Since then, the population has increased slightly and the economy has changed to services and regional distribution. In the 1990s, the economy was doing a bit better than the national average. Cleveland has a high per capita rate of philanthropic giving. The advent of Medicare and Medicaid in 1966 allowed for new revenue and expansion of the VNA. The original VNA board of trustees was largely composed of the wives of community leaders when one of the major board functions was to provide Christmas food baskets for

FIGURE 12.1
Today's VNA Mission Statement

Mission
To provide compassionate, innovative and effect community-based care that promotes health, independence and dignity to those we serve in Northeast and Central Ohio.

Vision
- To be the leader in innovative home care.
- To be the standard for quality care.
- To be the leader in community health planning and research.

Values
- We value personal dignity, the importance of integrity, honesty, and compassion.
- We are responsive to the needs of the community and our stakeholders.
- We value quality as a measurable outcome of emerging standards of performance.
- We value education and skill development of staff and clients.

needy patients. By the 1990s, the board was diverse by gender, ethnicity, and professional background.

1980: About the Only Game in Town

The 1980 organization chart of the VNA is shown in Figure 12.2. The core professional staff consisted of full-time salaried generalist nurses who worked out of four district offices to cover Cleveland and adjacent townships. The center office included administrative staff to coordinate several part-time social workers and physical therapists. Calls requesting care were handled by the district offices where nurses were assigned to respond. The nurses themselves decided whether or not a patient was able to pay.

FIGURE 12.2
The VNA of Cleveland Organization (1980)

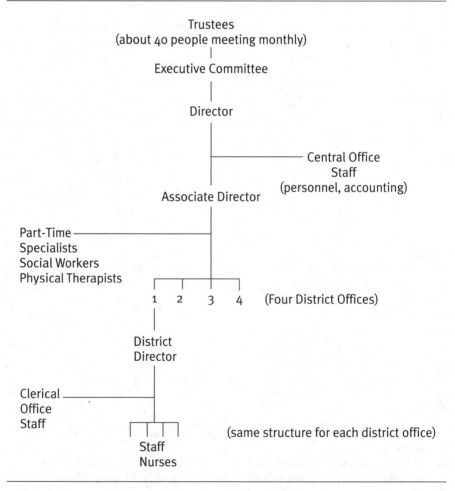

Reprinted with permission from the Visiting Nurse Association, Cleveland, Ohio.

Home care aide services were also provided by the VNA under contract from another voluntary organization, the Center for Human Services. Special contracts provided care for the elderly in several apartment complexes. All services were available during weekday working hours, and the agency was closed on weekends and holidays.

1982: Arrival of Competition

Ohio regulations made it easy to start a home care company, and more than 300 were created. The joke went that if you had a telephone and knew a nurse, you could start a home care agency. If costs could be kept down and full-pay patients selected, home care could be profitable. By 1982, competition for paying home care patients was growing. Others were content to let the VNA provide home care for those who could not pay. In 1984, VNA philanthropic gifts and endowment income yielded $190,000, plus United Way contributions of $540,000, out of a total of $5,000,000 in revenue. This allowed the VNA to provide care to all who requested it. However, the VNA needed mostly paying patients to survive.

This competitive situation led the VNA for the first time to ask the source of its patients and how the choice of home care provider was made. It turned out that 82 percent of patients came by way of hospital discharge and, of these, most came from a dozen of the area's largest hospitals. Typically a nurse, social worker, or discharge planner made the decision within the hospital. The choice of provider depended primarily on agency reputation, the ease of making a referral, and agency name recall.

Instead of being a passive receiver of telephone requests for services, the VNA decided to assign a staff nurse as contact person for each major hospital in addition to regular nursing care activities. Brochures, calendars, and small magnetized VNA symbols were distributed to promote name recognition.

The VNA organized a centralized intake service with one recognizable telephone number as an important step in making referrals easier. At the VNA the belief was that one competitor was giving away transistor radios to hospital-based referrers. After some discussion, the VNA decided not to follow suit.

By 1983, DRG payments had drastically shortened patient stay and emptied hospital beds. Now the hospitals were encouraging earlier discharge combined with home care. Hospitals began actively looking for new revenue-generating ventures and hospital-based home care became popular. By 1983, there was serious concern that the VNA's work would come to an end, as one hospital after another started its own home care program.

By 1984, a number of hospitals decided not to start their own programs, but rather to develop contracts with the VNA. The market again changed; no longer was it the individual nurse's or social worker's decision, but rather a hospital-based contract. One reason hospital contracting occurred was because hospital management was busy; the managers wanted to avoid a new program and save energy for higher-priority areas. By 1984, the VNA had contracts with eight hospitals, which accounted for about 35 percent of VNA's patients.

Early discharge drove the demand for increasingly complex home care requiring home care nurse specialists in intravenous (IV) management, pediatrics, mental health, hospice care, renal dialysis, and ostomy care, in addition to physical and occupational therapy and social work. This specialization and division of labor created economies of scale in home care. A small suburban hospital with paying patients and undifferentiated home care could prosper with small programs. Larger hospitals with more severely ill patients and high indigent care ratios found VNA contracting a better choice. Hospitals that started their own home care programs were unlikely to sell their program to nearby competing hospitals. Hospital contracts led to 24-hour service availability by the VNA rather than a 9-to-5 weekday organization. Hospitals wanted full-service agencies, so the VNA started homemaker services called "All for You." In response to these changes, the VNA reorganized in 1989.

1990 to 2000: Prosperity for a While

Between 1990 and 2000, the single not-for-profit 501(c)(3) organization became six organizations (see Figure 12.3). VNA's large group of trustees was divided into a smaller group of trustees with governance responsibility and a group of overseers—loyal supporters of the VNA with no line authority, but a right to advise and contribute. From 1990, the VNA organizations numbered five:

- *VNA Services* encompasses the bulk of the agencies' work; within this, Medicare is the largest payer.
- *VNA Care Plus* provides home aide assistance on a private basis (cleaning, food preparation, and personal hygienic care).
- *VNA Hospice* provides care for the terminally ill at home.
- *VNA Enterprises* is a small catch-all organization for receiving money for consulting and other services (for profit).
- *VNA Lines* provides IV solutions and other supplies needed in home care (for profit). This structure was active for several years before this market changed.

In the early 1990s, these organizations made surpluses; enough so that in 1995 the VNA could, with fundraising, move into a single new modern

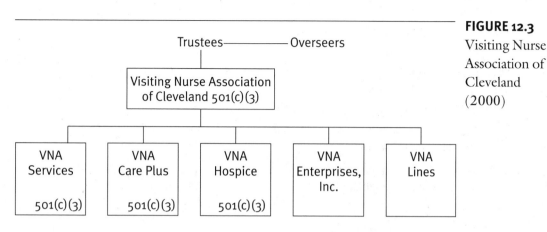

FIGURE 12.3
Visiting Nurse
Association of
Cleveland
(2000)

VNA Services

The VNA's full range of services and programs that help patients return to their optimal level of health are available in an eight county area of Northeast Ohio.

- Medical-surgical nursing
- Maternal and infant
- Pediatrics
- Personal care
- Enterostomal care
- Older adult
- Infusion therapy
- Rehabilitation services
  - Physical therapy
  - Occupational therapy
  - Speech-language pathology
  - Social work
  - Nutrition

- Behavioral health
  - Mental health services
  - Chemical dependency and ambulatory detox
- AIDS mental health
- Clozaril treatment
- Mental health management and support services

VNA Hospice

VNA Hospice and Special Care are programs for patients who are terminally ill. An interdisciplinary team provides compassionate care including:

- Skilled nursing care
- Pain and symptom management
- Respite care
- 24-hour crisis support
- Social work services
- AIDS care
- Residential/Nursing home care

- Home care aides
- Rehabilitation services
- Bereavement support
- Spiritual care
- Volunteer clergy, lawyers, companions, and Friendly Visitors

VNA Care Plus

VNA Care Plus, formerly All For You, Inc., provides 24-hour private duty nursing and personal care. RN, LPN, aide or homemaker services are available for short-term rehabilitation or long-term supportive care, meal preparation, companionship, respite care and child care.

(continued on next page)

FIGURE 12.3
(*continued*)

Services include the following:

- Private duty nursing
- Personal care
- Homemaker services

VNA Lines (For profit subsidiary)

VNA Lines incorporates nursing, pharmaceutical and supplies services for in-home and nursing home infusion therapy.

- Total parental nutrition
- Pain management therapy
- Chemotherapy and antiemetic therapy
- Antibiotic therapy
- Cardiac support therapies
- AIDS-related therapies

VNA Enterprises (For-profit subsidiary)

VNA Enterprises provides an expert team of home healthcare professionals who consult nationally and locally in the areas of administration, finance, operations, human resources management, MIS, fund development and program development.

Reprinted with permission from the Visiting Nurse Association, Cleveland, Ohio.

building in the center of the city near the expressway. By clearly separating out the possible for-profit activities, the nonprofit status of the whole organization could be preserved.

As of 1997, patients cared for by the VNA were paid for as follows: Medicare, 77 percent; Medicaid, 8.7 percent; commercial insurance and Blue Cross, 7.3 percent; other, 5.5 percent; and United Way, 1.5 percent. Reflecting the large Medicare component, most patients are over the age of 65. The VNA has 670 staff (full- and part-time) with a total revenue and expense of about $30 million.

The 40 separate Cleveland area hospitals of 1980 became four competing delivery systems by 1997, and only two by 1999. The two remaining systems are anchored by the Cleveland Clinic Foundation and University Hospitals of Cleveland, which are located a 15-minute walk apart. They have networks of community hospitals, group practices, HMOs, specialty services, and their own in-house home care programs. Cleveland's Metro Medical Center, the county hospital, had links to both systems but remained independent.

By 2000 the VNA had created a group of innovative new programs in association with other organizations. Special populations served included alcoholism, mental health, AIDS, bereaved families, and the elderly living in low-income housing (see Figure 12.4).

Today

Mary Lou Stricklin thinks of the VNA as an organized process of care through which patients pass (see Figure 12.5). This pathway is driven by mission,

FIGURE 12.4
Visiting Nurse
Association
of Cleveland

Innovations

Home Talk™

Through a joint venture with Telepractice in the fall of 1995, VNA introduced Home Talk™, a free telephone service for patients that improves access to their VNA clinician. Patients may choose from several options, including an on-line library with recorded health information. Home Talk™ supports the clinician's assessment of a patient's health status resulting in fewer readmissions to the hospital and unnecessary trips to the emergency room.

Ambulatory Detoxification Services

The VNA of Cleveland, Metrohealth, and Alcoholism Services of Cleveland are collaborating on an 18-month demonstration project to provide ambulatory detoxification services and chemical dependency care in home and community settings. This project is funded by a grant from the Cleveland Foundation.

Healthy Town

This program provides health promotion and disease prevention services to lower-income senior citizens and families with children at University Settlement and Collinwood Community Services Center, member organizations of the Neighborhood Centers Association. Funding is provided by the CAVS Charities and the Cleveland Foundation.

HIV/AIDS Mental Health

Through a grant from the AIDS Funding Collaborative, the VNA and the Free Clinic are collaborating to bring nursing care, social work, and consultative services to patients.

KID Connection

KID Connection nurses offer educational programs and consultation services for child care providers. These services help day care staff deliver high-quality care and meet state licensing requirements.

Vision on 22nd Street

To prepare students for community-based nursing, the VNA and Cleveland State University Department of Nursing formed an education-service partnership. A committee of community healthcare experts from both institutions developed new nursing curricula and began offering classes last fall. The program will educate over 200 nursing students within the next few years. Vision on 22nd Street is partially funded by the Cleveland Foundation.

Clozaril Management

Selected patients of the Mental Health program are participating in VNA's collaborative research study, funded by Sandoz Pharmaceuticals, to evaluate the effectiveness of Clozaril, and to implement the program in other areas of the country.

Camp TLC

VNA Hospice's Bereavement Camp TLC (Together Love Continues), is an annual day-long program helping children and family members who have lost a loved one to cope with their grief. The camp is underwritten by the Bicknell Fund.

vision, and values. Patients can be referred from nursing homes, physicians, hospitals, or networks. They proceed through admitting, scheduling, care, and community-based living. This process of care is supported by special services, quality control, and information systems provided by an administrative team.

Medicare, the dominant home care payer, has made several critical changes in order to control rapidly rising home care expenditures and monitor quality. Payment per visit has been changed to prospective payment, a fixed amount of money for a predefined type of patient. This has abruptly reduced the number of visits across the country. Secondly, a complex reporting system (OASIS) is required for each patient, put in place so that Medicare can monitor severity of illness and the outcomes of care (e.g., Were activity of daily living goals met for each patient? For example, can the patient now get dressed by herself?)

Fraud and abuse rules mean that unintentional reporting errors can lead to an expensive government review and harsh penalties. Complete and accurate records are essential. New privacy regulations have also required a full review of record systems to assure compliance. Good information management has become central to the VNA. So far, the VNA has done well in this area and is recognized for it.

FIGURE 12.5
1995: The VNA
Organization
as a Process

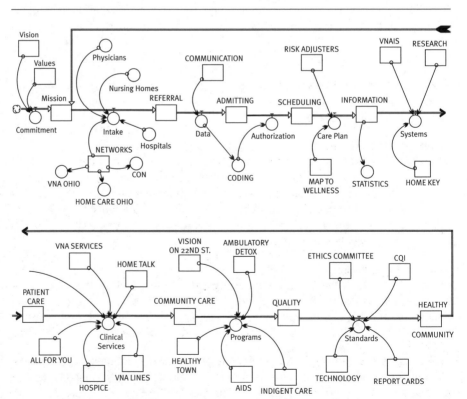

One consequence of these changes has been the shift of home care from a profitable small side item for a community hospital to a financially marginal business requiring substantial information management abilities and higher risk. These issues have caused many small agencies to go out of business. The VNA of Cleveland has been solicited by several small cities who have lost their local home care agencies. The VNA has opened operations in one small city with local philanthropic support. Even with this help, however, VNA faces new business start-up costs related to such horizontal expansion.

Medicare cost control has its largest impact on traditional skilled nursing care (VNA Services). VNA Care Plus, which provides less skilled housekeeping services in the home, is largely paid for out the patient's pocket, and has not been affected by prospective payment.

The nationwide nursing shortage has affected the VNA, which is finding it harder to recruit and retain professional nurses. It may, however, be to the VNA's advantage that many nurses prefer or enjoy home care to hospital-based nursing. Even if this is the case, Care Plus staffing poses other problems: these workers have competing job offers or they often live in the city while the clients are in the suburbs and transportation becomes a problem.

On a more positive note, Ms. Stricklin is excited about a new technology already introduced for a few VNA patients. A home monitoring device allows patients to record their own blood pressure, blood sugar, weight, or medication use. This information is transmitted to the VNA central office by cell phone technology for monitoring and as-needed contact, reducing the need for nurse home visits. This project is being done in partnership with a small local company that makes the monitors. Due to prospective payment substituting, such monitoring for a nurse visit does not affect Medicare revenue.

For the first time, the VNA has created a physician home care service called "VNA House Calls" in partnership with several primary care physicians backed up by advance practice nurse practitioners. Contracted physicians and nurses make house calls for patients, often frail elderly people who have difficulty getting to the hospital. This program has received favorable publicity and apparently fills a need.

The Future

Ms. Stricklin is very pleased with her core management team and sees many new challenges ahead of the VNA. What should the VNA's priorities be?

- Implement cost and quality control for the existing business, particularly for the Medicare part of the business, which is being squeezed for funds now and probably well into the future. For the first time, the VNA is

FIGURE 12.6
VNA of Cleveland— Current Corporate Operating Structure

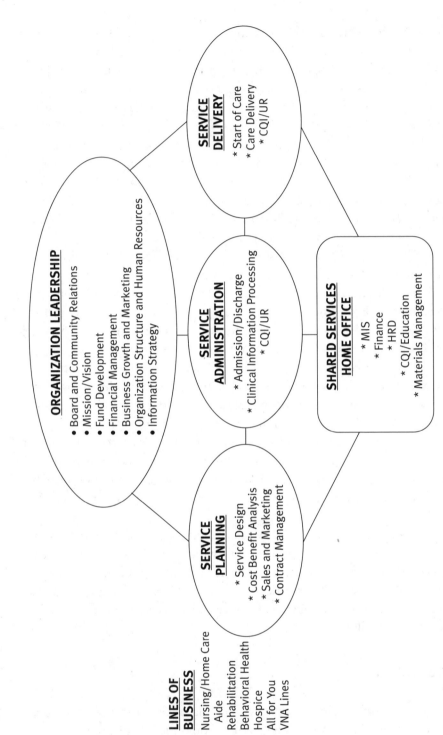

MIS - Management Information Systems, HRD - Human Resources Development, CQI - Continuous Quality Improvement, UR - Utilization Review getting regular national comparative performance data that can be used to measure outcomes of care and patient satisfaction.

- Expand horizontally by moving to new nearby communities in need of home care services. The VNA's current corporate headquarters structure could support such expansion. Figure 12.6 shows the current grouping of activities carried out by corporate staff.
- Grow VNA Care Plus, which is not federally regulated like Medicare.
- Provide back-office services for other home care agencies unable to cope with the new demands for information.
- Start a research center to seek funding to study the data being collected.

Case Questions

1. In which direction should the VNA go?
2. How should the VNA board be brought along to agree with the change recommended?
3. How can staff morale be maintained in the face of uncertainty?
4. Who are the stakeholder groups whose expectations Ms. Stricklin must manage to succeed in implementing your recommendations?
5. What are the personal stakes involved for Ms. Stricklin in doing as you suggest? How can she maximize the upside potential and minimize the downside risks for her own career?

Short Case K
New Chief of OB-GYN: The Next 3 Years

Anthony R. Kovner

Since Dr. Mikhail has taken over as chief of OB-GYN at North Heights Medical Center in New York City, the following has occurred: a slight increase in deliveries, a significant expansion of primary care centers and visits, a large increase in abortions, a large increase in research grants, improvement in facilities, and an improvement in patient service. However, patient revenues have decreased slightly because of improvements in health for preemies, and use of the preemie nursery has decreased significantly. North Heights serves a low-income diverse population and is a large hospital and health system with a $200 million budget.

The following discussion has occurred among a group of consultants brought together by Dr. Bright, the medical director.

Dr. Strong: The service needs to increase its share of the market. St. Brennan's hospital represents a threat in this regard and Washington Hospital represents an opportunity.

Dr. Light: There is a leakage in primary care away from North Heights. Hire an outreach worker to find out the reasons for the leakage and do something about it.

Dr. Bright: Dr. Mikhail should increase marketing efforts including advertising.

Dr. Quick: Dr. Mikhail should continue to present strategy. Deliveries are down in the Bronx, and market share is slowly increasing.

Dr. Rough: Dr. Mikhail should reduce full-time staff and produce the same number of deliveries with a smaller budget.

Dr. Clever: Dr. Mikhail should alter his research strategy and develop grants aimed at interventions which will increase the number of deliveries.

Case Questions

1. What are the key facts in the situation?
2. What are the problems and issues?
3. What should Dr. Mikhail do and why?

ACCOUNTABILITY

Let's not be too hasty; speed is a dangerous thing.
Untimely measures bring repentance.
Certainly, and unhappily, many things are wrong in the Colony.
But is there anything human without some fault?
And after all, you see, we do move forward . . .
—C. P. Cavafy

COMMENTARY

O rganizations receive resources from society based on the acceptability of their products or services to their users and purchasers. If health services are perceived as acceptable, then the organization is meeting the expectations of purchasers, employers, or patients, all of whom have an interest in organizational performance. Of course, expectation levels can be changed— for example, by communicating to patients or employees what specifically the organization is promising them in terms of performance in return for their patronage or willingness to work.

According to Pointer and Orlikoff (2002), the boards of trustees (directors) of healthcare organizations have five functions: formulating the organization's vision and key goals and ensuring that strategy is aligned with vision and goals; ensuring high levels of management performance; ensuring high-quality care; ensuring financial health; and ensuring the board's effectiveness and efficiency. The CEO is the board's agent, on site.

Primary accountability in health services organizations is shifting away from focusing on physicians, who know best which services patients should receive and how, to customers or potential customers, based on a trajectory of the patient. For an example of the context for building organizational supports for change, see Figure VI.1, which is taken from the Report of the Committee on Quality of the Institute of Medicine, *Crossing the Quality Chasm* (2001).

Healthcare is increasingly purchased wholesale, rather than retail, by purchasers or their agents, who will pay providers for specified benefits at specified amounts. Agents for wholesale purchasers exchange increases in patient volume for price discounts, assuming that retail customers are satisfied with quality and service, given a sufficient choice among providers.

Healthcare managers are concerned with production costs on the one hand and customer preferences on the other, a situation that American business organizations have faced for years. Two factors are vital in applying the concept of accountability: (1) a specification of organizational performance that is mutually agreed upon in advance by stakeholders; and, (2) the capability of managers to control the resources and behavior necessary to achieve such specified performance objectives.

FIGURE VI.1
Making Change
Possible

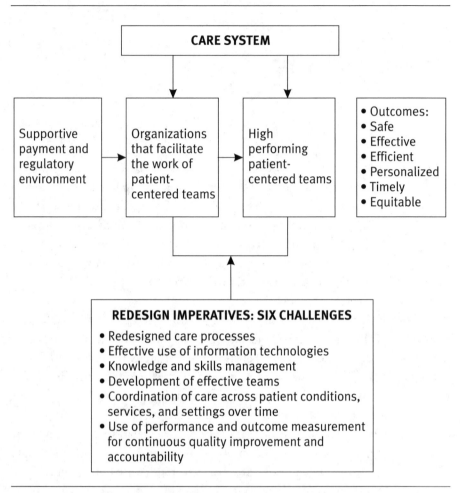

CARE SYSTEM

Supportive payment and regulatory environment

Organizations that facilitate the work of patient-centered teams

High performing patient-centered teams

- Outcomes:
- Safe
- Effective
- Efficient
- Personalized
- Timely
- Equitable

REDESIGN IMPERATIVES: SIX CHALLENGES

- Redesigned care processes
- Effective use of information technologies
- Knowledge and skills management
- Development of effective teams
- Coordination of care across patient conditions, services, and settings over time
- Use of performance and outcome measurement for continuous quality improvement and accountability

SOURCE: Committee on Quality, Institute of Medicine. 2001. *Crossing the Quality Chasm: A New Health System for the 21st Century.* Washington, DC: National Academy Press.

Expectations of Organizational Performance

Stakeholders assess levels of organizational performance in a variety of ways. Increasingly, organizations are using "balanced scorecards" as strategic management systems. As posited by Kaplan and Norton (1996), measures are linked from four perspectives: (1) financial, such as return on investment; (2) customer service; (3) internal business processes, such as the hospital readmission rate for the same illnesses; and (4) learning and growth, keyed to employee's morale and suggestions. This framework can easily be adapted to the expectations for performance on the part of stakeholder groups such as physicians or consumers. For example, physicians are concerned that the hospital makes a sufficient surplus to finance capital equipment, while consumers want a high level of customer service, as manifested in a same-day appointment system for ambulatory care.

To meet consumer expectations for service, managers can undertake marketing studies to find out what patients say they like and do not like about the organization's services. Physicians can be regularly surveyed too for likes and dislikes. Managers can set up special units to advocate for patients or physicians. Managers can reorganize work so that fewer persons provide more services for each patient or physician. Managers can reevaluate organizational routines regularly in terms of impact on patient outcomes or convenience of physicians. Special units or committees can be organized for quality improvement.

The manager can tour the facility regularly; talk with physicians, nurses, and patients; and observe how services can be improved and made more convenient. The manager can make it easier for patients or physicians to complain by establishing a hotline to her office or to that of another manager. The manager can analyze patient and physician complaints, their resolution, and follow-up, and can talk to complainants personally. The manager can let patients and physicians know what service levels they should expect and what behavior is expected from them. Similar sets of activities can be conducted to improve employee perceptions and employer accountability.

The manager can report regularly as well to other stakeholders—such as purchasers and employee representatives—on performance, plans, and problems. Members of such constituencies can be included on policy-making and advisory committees. Management information systems can be developed to gain access needed for planning and evaluating services; information should include population served, population using various services, quantities of services, cost of service, quality of service, and patient satisfaction. Summaries of reports of regulators and accreditors can be shared with constituent groups. Organizational goals and performance can be analyzed, as can information on trends in turnover, overtime, and absenteeism; fundraising; profitability; and new capital equipment. The process of decision making itself can be examined and improved, either as a process, given certain ends, or as a structure, as to the inclusion of constituent groups who are affected by organizational policy. By making itself more formally accountable, the leadership incurs substantial costs in terms of management time spent on the process, dollars spent on information systems upgrades, and conflict raised by difference as to present and future direction. But the leadership may also reap substantial benefits: plans that are more acceptable to constituents, and therefore more feasible to implement; greater commitment from key clinicians to organizational goals; and a sharper focus on the organization's mission so that goal attainment is more easily obtained and justified to employees and customers.

Stakeholder Claims on the Organization

Organizational performance can be improved (or negatively affected) by governmental legislation. For example, the Omnibus Budget Regulation Act enacted by Congress in 1987 was, at least in part, responsible for a decline in the use of physical and chemical restraints and rates of urinary incontinence and catheterization. In New York State, the government publishes a consumer's guide to Medicaid Managed Care in New York City, ranking health plans according to the quality of care provided to children and adults and according to patient satisfaction with access and service. Such guides are also available to the public in magazines, such as *Consumer Reports*, and over the Internet.

Managers may have less control over accountability than they do over control systems, organizational design, professional integration, or organizational adaptation, because they lack influence over external groups that have their own expectations and interests regarding organizational and managerial performance. And health services is particularly challenging for managers because of the difficulties in specifying organizational performance in measurable terms and in isolating the contribution of a delivery system to an improvement in health status for a community or a population. These difficulties complicate reaching agreement among organizational leadership, internal stakeholders, and external groups as they seek to influence each other's expectations and behavior.

Managers can, however, be successful in affecting stakeholder expectations. The Mayo Clinic is an example of a healthcare organization that has been successful in this regard. According to Berry and Bendapudi (2003), this organization manages a set of visual and experiential clues so that stakeholders recognize that care is organized around patient needs rather than around doctors' schedules or hospital processes. The Mayo workforce is hired because they embrace the organization's values. These values are emphasized through training and reinforced in the workplace.

To encourage collaboration among professionals, physicians at Mayo are paid on salaries; sophisticated internal paging, telephone, and videoconferencing are used; and electronic medical records have been implemented. Facilities themselves are designed to relieve stress, offer a place of refuge, create positive distraction, convey caring and respect, symbolize competence, minimize crowding, facilitate way finding, and accommodate families (Berry and Bendapudi 2003).

Managers can ensure that key stakeholders are identified and that their expectations and satisfaction levels are regularly measured. For objectivity in this regard, measurement should usually be done by external organizations explicitly organized for this purpose, such as *Consumer Reports* magazine, that rates goods and services.

References

Berry, L. L., and N. Bendapudi. 2003. "Clueing in Customers." *Harvard Business Review* 81 (2): 100–104.

Committee on Quality, Institute of Medicine. 2001. *Crossing the Quality Chasm: A New Health System for the 21st Century.* Washington DC: National Academy Press.

Kaplan, R. S., and D. P. Norton. 1996. "Using the Balanced Scorecard as a Strategic Management System." *Harvard Business Review* 74 (1): 75–85.

Pointer, D. D, and J. E. Orlikoff. 2002. *Getting to Great: Principles of Health Care Organization Governance.* San Francisco: Jossey-Bass.

THE READINGS

The required reading for Part VI, Accountability, is "A New Health System and Its Quality Agenda," by Don Detmer. Detmer urges that healthcare organizations offer sufficient support so that clinicians can seriously pursue safety and quality initiatives. He suggests that executives can influence organizational performance in four key areas—leadership, people, culture, and infrastructure. Detmer does not discuss what consumers and patients want and what they are willing to pay for, or of how consumers and patients and their advocates and representatives can influence health services organizations to be more responsive their concerns.

A New Health System and Its Quality Agenda

Donald E. Detmer, M.D.
Excerpted from *Frontiers of Health Services Management* 18 (1),
Fall 2001

> "[W]e cannot wait any longer to address the serious quality of care challenges facing our nation. A comprehensive and strong approach is needed now."
> —Kenneth I. Shine, M.D.,
> President, Institute of Medicine

> "You must be the change you wish to see."
> —M. Ghandi

It is time for profound changes in healthcare. Despite the good results that the U.S. health system produces for many individual patients, it could and should do better. Given available knowledge and technology as well as the vast resources devoted to the health sector in this country, patients may reasonably expect to receive consistently high-level performance from healthcare organizations and professionals. Yet, we observe large quality variations across providers, a lower population health status than other nations despite higher spending per capita, long lag times in dissemination of new knowledge, and missed opportunities for critically ill patients to participate in clinical trials (thereby reducing potential gain for individuals as well as for contributions to medical knowledge) (Anderson 1997; Balas and Boren 2000; Chassin et al. 1986; Lara et al. 2001; Schuster, McGlynn, and Brook 1998; Weiner et al. 1995).

Moreover, the healthcare sector faces growing pressures that will further tax its capabilities and inhibit its ability to meet growing consumer demands. For example, recent workforce shortages among some health professional disciplines (e.g., pharmacists and nurses) are forcing provider organizations in some markets to subject patients to long waiting times or to curtail services (Appleby 2001; Jaklevic and Lovern 2000). Healthcare organizations were designed to serve and health professionals were trained to treat acute care, but today chronic care is the predominant need, with population health management not far behind. Obtaining and using information technology continues to be problematic for healthcare organizations, despite success with this area in other industries. In the name of privacy, taking full advantage of information technology may be hampered by restrictive regulation and legislation that limits access to patient data for legitimate research. In addition, reimbursement and other incentive mechanisms have not kept pace with the changing practice of medicine.

Fundamental changes are needed in healthcare delivery processes, payment mechanisms, information infrastructure, patient communications, and health education of the public. Without such changes, we are likely to experience a mixture of substantial cost escalation, service deterioration, irrational decision making, uneven outcomes in the treatment of individuals, a demoralized health workforce, marginally satisfied patients and loved ones, and little improvement in the health of our population. These factors signal the compelling need to attend to the complicated task of building a true healthcare system. Needless to say, this represents a formidable challenge in light of the existing structure of healthcare resources, the nation's tradition of pluralism and preference for incremental market-based programs blended with an array of internal and external regulations, and the culture of autonomy that has heretofore pervaded the profession of medicine.

Nevertheless, the current configuration of healthcare resources (i.e., facilities, personnel, processes) must be converted from a collection of organizations and people working on similar tasks to a true system in which the components are aligned by a shared goal, motivated by consistent incentives, and supported by a common infrastructure. This conversion does not imply that the United States either needs or wants a monolithic, national health system. It does, however, require focused, productive action by the public and private sectors alike at national, regional, and organizational levels. Only through the concerted effort of health professionals (including administrators), organizations (including providers, insurers, and foundations), and government (including local, state, and federal) within the context of a coherent national framework can the cacophony that characterizes the current health system be harmonized.

What exactly should the health system of the twenty-first century look like and how do we get there? Two recent reports from the Institute of Medicine (IOM) Quality of Health Care in America Committee offer the nation substantial initial guidance on improving our healthcare system (IOM 1999a, 2001). The starting point for the reports was the need to improve safety and quality. However, the group concluded that improvement requires changing systems of care (rather than further stressing current systems of care), thus the reports provide a vision for a new healthcare system and a range of actions to initiate threshold improvements in quality. Reaching these goals will require that healthcare become increasingly driven by the right combination of values—including a commitment to the care of individuals as well as the total population, to care based on scientific evidence, to the use of information technology, and to respect for the values and preferences of individuals involved in care (Blue Ridge Group 1998).

A Health System for the Twenty-First Century

Patient safety is an important dimension of quality patient care but does not encompass the complete set of quality issues. The Quality of Health Care in America Committee's second report, *Crossing the Quality Chasm: A New Health System for the 21st Century*, takes a broader view on how the healthcare delivery system can be designed to innovate and improve care. The report is "a call for action to improve the American health delivery system as a whole, in all its dimensions of quality, for all Americans" because "healthcare harms too frequently and routinely fails to deliver its potential benefits" (IOM 2001, pp. 1–2). It presents a new view on the purpose and aims of the healthcare system, how patients and their clinicians should relate, and how to design care processes to optimize responsiveness to patients' needs. In so doing, it paints a picture of what healthcare could and should be in this nation.

As first advanced by the President's Advisory Commission in 1998 and adopted by the Quality of Health Care in America Committee, the purpose of the healthcare system is to continually reduce the burden of illness, injury, and disability and to improve the health and functioning of the people of the United States. The system should be guided by six aims. At all times and for all people, the delivery system should be designed to be

1. Safe (avoid injuries to patients from care that is intended to help them);
2. Effective (provide services based on scientific knowledge to all who could benefit and refrain from providing services to those not likely to benefit);

3. Patient centered (provide care that is respectful of and responsive to individual patient preferences, needs, and values, and ensure that patient values guide all clinical decisions);
4. Timely (reduce waits and sometimes harmful delays for both those who receive and those who give care);
5. Efficient (avoid waste, including waste of equipment, supplies, ideas, and energy); and
6. Equitable (provide care that does not vary in quality because of personal characteristics such as gender, ethnicity, geographic location, and socioeconomic status).

To achieve these aims, healthcare organizations will need to redesign their systems, so the IOM study committee developed a set of redesign rules to aid them in that task. In so doing, the committee noted that other complex social systems (e.g., the Internet) have succeeded through use of shared aims and general directions.

Three additional attributes of a twenty-first century health system that were not emphasized by the IOM project committee have been addressed in other IOM reports and by other groups. First, health professionals and organizations should manage the health of the population within their regions in addition to the healthcare of individuals (Blue Ridge Group 1998). Thus, they must view the determinants of health broadly, identify health risks to populations, communicate those risks, and work with their communities to address specific needs that undermine the health of that community or region. Population health management requires an information infrastructure to support data gathering and analysis, integration between public health and medical systems, and willingness of local communities to assume responsibility for, work with health professionals on, and allocate resources to improving the health of their population.

Second, patients must be willing and able to assume greater responsibility for managing their own health. Healthcare professionals and organizations need to educate patients to become better consumers of healthcare. Equally important, insurers and purchasers need to adopt reimbursement mechanisms that provide incentives to patients to adopt healthy behaviors.

Third, essential, effective health services should be available to all citizens. Thus, the issue of universal coverage must remain on the nation's health agenda. Several organizations, including the American College of Physicians, the American Hospital Association, and the Association of Academic Health Centers (AHC), seek to keep this issue before the American political leadership. For example, in January 2001 the AHC board of directors adopted a policy seeking to reduce the uninsured population by 5 million individuals for each session of Congress, and in collaboration with other organizations, the AHC has established the Academics for Access to Health Care Initiative

(Bulger 2001). In addition, the IOM is currently exploring the various dimensions of uninsurance and underinsurance in a series of studies, because inaccessible care is clearly not quality care.

Framing a New System

Two basic premises underpin the six aims, the ten redesign principles, and the three additional attributes for our future health system. First, we must view healthcare from a systems perspective and design each component of the future healthcare system to support our ultimate goal of reducing the burden of illness and improving the health and functioning of the U.S. population. Second, evidence-based decision making is sensible for all areas of healthcare, not just in clinical circumstances. Thus, payers, administrators, policymakers, and regulators should all be making decisions in the context of the six aims and the ten redesign principles with the best available knowledge and information. In general terms, all healthcare organizations—from delivery organizations to payers to regulators to researchers and others—should use available knowledge and evidence to identify areas that offer opportunities for high-yield returns on improving quality and safety, develop realistic change plans, monitor progress, apply learned strategies where appropriate, revisit change plans when and if unsuccessful, and share findings broadly.

In pursuit of patient safety and consistently high-quality healthcare services, the IOM committee recommended an extensive list of actions for a wide range of groups. These recommendations can be classified in terms of four interdependent changes that in combination create a culture and build necessary systems for safety and quality. These changes must occur at the industry, organizational, and individual levels.

First, leadership within the health sector and healthcare organizations must commit anew to safety and quality as high-priority issues and demonstrate their importance through allocation of sufficient resources to achieve measurable improvement. Second, the healthcare environment must institute clear incentives for organizations and professionals to pursue quality and safety. Third, the structures and processes of the healthcare industry (e.g., information infrastructure and knowledge management) must support organizations and professionals in their pursuit of quality. Fourth, in many instances, healthcare organizations and professionals will need to acquire new skills and technological capabilities and modify behaviors to achieve consistently high-quality performance.

Leadership for the Health Sector

Building this new health system will require at least two kinds of leadership (Blue Ridge Group 2001). First, healthcare needs innovative transformational leadership to move our current system to one that meets the expectations described above. Innovative transformational leaders use "new stories about the nature of problems and solutions that permit people to conduct tasks of significant change" (Couto, forthcoming). These leaders attempt to raise the level of a group's practices to its values and in so doing increase the amount of a group's social capital (i.e., the communal bonds and moral resources that members of a community invest in one another).

Healthcare needs leaders who can help a wide range of constituents manifest the huge potential of a health system that is driven by the six aims. These leaders need to build a common understanding and foster willingness to change so that organizations and individuals alike begin to act in a manner consistent with the vision. Ultimately, leaders will need to convince many different stakeholders that the new system will be worth the costs they will bear individually.

Second, healthcare needs transactional leadership. Articulating a clear vision that motivates a wide range of constituents is only part of the change process; healthcare also requires individuals who are able to get things done through the use of tangible processes and behaviors. These leaders must be able to manage both the conflict and collaboration that inevitably accompany change. They must be technically adept and possess strong interpersonal skills or emotional intelligence so that they can "inspire, empower, and exert broad influence" rather than exercise centralized control (Blue Ridge Group 2001; Henry and Gilkey 1999; Goleman 1998). These individuals will build the necessary infrastructure for change through technology investment, legislative and regulatory actions, research funding, educational programs, or partnerships among different kinds of organizations. Through their actions, these leaders will cultivate a culture of ongoing learning and a climate for change and enable the transformation from vision to reality for a health system driven by quality.

The report on medical errors specifically recommends that a clear focal point for leading national efforts to advance patient safety be established. No such focal point is urged for quality. Given the more diffuse responsibility for creating and maintaining momentum on system quality, it becomes even more important that individual healthcare delivery organizations and health professional organizations make redesign for quality a priority within their own institutions so that incentives are generated and change occurs.

Incentives for Quality and Safety

Well-designed external incentives are needed to create a climate in which safety and quality improvement is a priority and ultimately becomes a matter of routine performance (IOM 2001). The set of possible incentives (i.e., regulations, liability conditions, reimbursement mechanisms, as well as licensing and certification criteria) is created by a combination of public and private organizations with different levels of influence exerted by individual organizations and varying degrees of coordination among the organizations. Each kind of incentive presents challenges that must be addressed so that the combined effect is an environment that promotes rather than thwarts pursuit of quality.

For example, despite the fact that some states use the Joint Commission on Accreditation of Healthcare Organizations (Joint Commission) guidelines as part of their licensure requirements, these requirements and their enforcement vary across states, resulting in differing levels of performance by healthcare delivery organizations (Brass 2001). In addition, few licensure standards currently focus on safety, and those that do exist are not fully implemented (IOM 1999a). Differences exist among states in requirements for mandatory reporting of serious adverse events and variations in reporting formats that make analysis of data more difficult. Greater emphasis on patient safety issues is also needed as part of the process of licensing and certifying healthcare professionals.

Current reimbursement mechanisms often penalize healthcare providers who improve quality by reducing use of reimbursable services. Purchasers and health plans could exert substantial influence by modifying payment practices that fragment the care system and by establishing incentives to improve quality. With better design, the liability system could be a much stronger motivator for improving and maintaining safety and quality. Consideration must be given, however, to ensuring that fear of litigation does not inhibit collection of essential information that will enable organizations to identify and eliminate safety problems. Regulation of health professionals often hinders innovative and less costly approaches to care delivery (e.g., scope of practice of nonphysician clinicians). State regulatory bodies would be wise to evaluate current regulations in terms of the six aims of quality.

Enhanced Industry Capabilities

Although it has not yet reached its full potential, information technology affects virtually all dimensions of healthcare, including consumer health, clinical care, administration, financial transactions, public health, professional education, and research (National Research Council 2000). Moreover, it has a pivotal role to play in safety and quality improvement efforts (e.g., process redesign, coordination of patient care, communication among team members and with patients, increased use of evidence-based medicine, and patient access to clinical knowledge). Thus, a robust information infrastructure is a critical component of safety and quality improvement and must become a higher priority for the entire health sector. While *Crossing the Quality Chasm* calls for a renewed effort to build an information infrastructure, it offers limited guidance on how to do so.

According to the National Committee on Vital and Health Statistics (NCVHS), an information infrastructure is a framework that connects distributed data and delivers information to individuals when and where they need it so they can make informed decisions (NCVHS 2000). A health information infrastructure includes technologies, standards, applications, systems, values, and laws that support all facets of individual health, healthcare, and public health. The health information infrastructure is not an attempt to collect personal health data from individuals or providers or to create a centralized government database to store personal information. Rather, it will provide a means of capturing, storing, communicating, processing, and presenting information upon the request of authorized users.

As currently envisioned, this national health information infrastructure (NHII) will support three key users and therefore encompasses three different but related dimensions (NCVHS 2000). The personal health dimension will support the management of individual wellness and healthcare decision making through access to a personal health record and information relevant to personal health. The healthcare provider dimension is intended to enhance the quality and efficiency of healthcare services. It is encounter based, focuses on an individual's health patterns, includes information captured during the care process, and can be linked to clinical knowledge to guide decision making. The community health dimension supports public health. It will include statutorily authorized data in public health systems; it could also include anonymous population data for use in research.

Many of the components of such an infrastructure exist, but legal, organizational, cultural, financial, and technical barriers remain to be addressed before it reaches its full potential and can be reliably used by the entire health sector (Detmer 1997; NCVHS 2000; President's Information Technology Advisory Committee 2001). The investment needed to secure such an NHII for our healthcare system is large, but its wide-reaching benefits surely qualify it as a public good. However, healthcare organizations will likely not invest sufficiently in the information infrastructure given current financial constraints. Moreover, even if such investment did occur, existing policies for security and connectivity would not allow the benefits of an NHII to be realized fully. Hence, a genuine need exists for a federal program of support that provides between $7 and $10 billion over a five- to seven-year period to address the range of issues associated with building the NHII (Detmer 2000). Both the NCVHS workgroup on a national health information infrastructure and the President's Information Technology Advisory Committee have helped to articulate the need for and tasks involved in building the NHII (NCVHS 2000; President's Information Technology Advisory Committee 2001). Their work provides an important framework for NHII development but represents only the beginning of a long-term process.

For example, the national effort must ensure development of workable standards (including content, format, and security) for computer-based personal, patient, and population or community records. It must also include establishing an ongoing process for standards development and quality control. Mechanisms are needed for assessing and ensuring safety in the development and use of information technologies (e.g., clinical decision support) so that the systems intended to eliminate certain errors do not introduce new kinds of problems (Fox and Das 2000). Other countries that have built or are building an NHII provide models and useful lessons for efforts in the United States (Detmer 2000; NCVHS 2000). Therefore, the research agenda should include a study of international experiences.

In addition to being able to access patient data when and where it is needed, healthcare professionals need to be able to find and apply evidence (i.e., relevant knowledge) as part of the care process. This implies that raw information has been converted into useful knowledge (e.g., results of multiple research studies synthesized), that healthcare professionals and organizations have easy access to current scientific knowledge, and that they have the skills or tools with which to assess the relevance of knowledge. Efforts to capture, share, and deploy both tacit and explicit knowledge to meet specified goals are generally known as knowledge management (Blue Ridge Group 2000). Knowledge management is becoming increasingly important to the success of organizations throughout the economy but has particular relevance in healthcare where the volume of knowledge that professionals and even patients must navigate is large and rapidly growing. From the perspective of the health industry, knowledge management comprises efforts to increase the knowledge base; improve knowledge dissemination mechanisms; implement or strengthen reporting or monitoring capabilities and use; and modify curricula for undergraduate, graduate, and continuing education to provide the workforce with needed skills and knowledge. Similar knowledge management tasks are relevant for healthcare organizations, particularly those seeking to distinguish themselves in the marketplace by providing patient-centered and even customized services (Blue Ridge Group 2000).

A knowledge infrastructure is essential to the consistent, appropriate application of knowledge to healthcare delivery. Parts of this infrastructure already exist but must be strengthened through public-private efforts. According to the IOM, such an infrastructure should initially focus on priority conditions and include ongoing analysis and synthesis of the medical evidence, delineation of specific practice guidelines, identification and sharing of best practices in the design of care processes, enhanced dissemination efforts to communicate evidence and guidelines to the general public and professional communities, development of decision-support tools to assist clinicians and patients in applying the evidence at the point of service, goals for improvement in care processes and outcomes, and development of quality measures for tracking progress, especially with regard to priority conditions.

Such an infrastructure can be enhanced in a variety of ways. Reporting and monitoring systems play a role in the regulatory environment but also are critical to building a robust knowledge base on patient safety and other quality dimensions. They also serve an important function in measuring progress toward specified goals. Purchasers and regulators can require accountability through measures for each of the six aims. Healthcare consumers should be informed about the six aims, why they are important, and how to interpret levels of performance of the systems they use or could use. Funding agencies can promote research on new designs for the care of priority conditions. Moreover, as is beginning to happen, training and ongoing licensure and certification should reflect the need for lifelong learning and the evaluation of baseline competencies and performance data on care that has been actually delivered, including patient outcomes.

Organizational Responses

What can individual healthcare organizations do to improve patient safety and quality and contribute to the transformation of the overall healthcare system? First and foremost, organizations must offer sufficient support so that healthcare professionals committed to a new vision of care can seriously pursue safety and quality through innovative initiatives, including new policies and procedures and ultimately better routine care processes. Although healthcare professionals have the most direct effect on patients, the combination of all organizational components determines how well the institution performs. Executives can influence their institution's safety and quality performance terms in four key areas—leadership, people, culture, and infrastructure.

Organizational Leadership

Like all profound organizational changes, leadership commitment and action constitute the most critical elements of the effort to improve safety and quality. It must be palpable if an organization is to succeed across the range of needed initiatives, which include but are not limited to the development of an organizational health information infrastructure. If such leadership is lacking, pockets of improvement may occur as a result of efforts of committed healthcare professionals, but such initiatives will be difficult to sustain and are unlikely to spread and become indigenous to the culture. Executives, governing boards, and clinical leaders collectively must make "a serious, visible, and ongoing commitment" to creating systems of care that consistently deliver high-level quality (IOM 1999a, p. 12). Such commitment can begin with the incorporation of the purpose of healthcare, the six quality aims, and the ten redesign principles into the organization's mission and goals accompanied by a strategy and work plan that delineates how the goals will be accomplished.

Commitment must be followed by action in the form of clear assignments for and expectations of safety oversight and quality improvement (e.g., assign responsibility for management and improvement in risky systems). Executives can send a strong message about the importance of safety and quality by assuming responsibility for developing a meaningful safety program for their institution. They may choose to do so by initially focusing on implementation of proven medication practices and systems (see "Medication Safety" below). Action must also take the form of allocating resources (both human and financial) to analysis and system redesign (e.g., medication safety programs or process simplification) as well as to an institutional infrastructure (such as information technology and knowledge management resources) that supports safe, high-quality care. For patient safety, executives must oversee development of a systems orientation to safety, rather than an orientation that finds and attaches blame to individuals. Yet, they must also attend to the issue of identifying and dealing with unsafe practitioners and related staff.

Performance measures for individuals, units, and the organization as a whole need to become a natural part of daily work so that the degree to which performance is consistent with best practices and the degree to which patients benefit from services is clear, and low performance can be identified and remedied. Both boards and executives can reinforce the importance of safety and quality by requiring frequent aggregate reports on performance and improvement efforts. In addition, executives can walk through potential or identified hazardous areas, design and incorporate safety and quality improvements into annual business plans and performance reviews, and champion best practices originating both within and outside their organization. Of particular importance for organizational leaders is the need to anticipate and prepare for potential patient safety and quality erosion issues during organizational changes (e.g., reorganizations, mergers, or other changes in staffing, responsibilities, workload, and relationships among caregivers).

Of increasing importance for organizational leaders is their interaction with their external environment and targeted efforts to shape their environment (Blue Ridge Group 2001). This task applies to safety and quality improvement as well. For example, executives can involve community physicians in safety programs, seek incentives to demonstrate continuous quality improvement in patient safety from purchasers, initiate regional communication on safety and quality issues among healthcare organizations, and communicate their workforce needs to health professional schools as well as professional and credentialing organizations. They can also ensure that their organization participates in efforts to identify problems in the field with drugs (i.e., postmarketing surveillance) and work with healthcare consumers to enable them to become more informed patients and better prepared healthcare consumers.

Healthcare executives can turn to their professional organizations as partners in quality. Professional organizations such as the American College of Healthcare Executives, the American Hospital Association, and others cannot only respond to but help to build momentum for safety and quality initiatives in a variety of ways. For example, they can relate to the recommended Center for Patient Safety, represent their members at national forums on the issues, participate in efforts to define voluntary reporting and increase the knowledge base about patient safety and quality, disseminate information about leading efforts to their members, and establish a permanent committee dedicated to patient safety. Executives can also work with licensing and credentialing groups regarding the addition of patient safety issues to examinations. Professional organizations can recognize exceptional performance or innovations in each of the six aims through annual awards established in honor of past champions of such work.

People

Three important dimensions of the healthcare professional workforce must be assessed in the context of an organizational initiative to improve safety and quality. First, executives need to ensure that the organization has the right mix of workers to perform the work that results from system redesign in pursuit of the six aims. This will require organizations to examine with their professionals the current scope of work so that clinician time is optimized to provide care effectively and efficiently and benefits from ongoing technological developments (Christensen, Bohmer, and Kenagy 2000). In some instances, this will require executives and clinical leaders to overcome institutional and financial structures and customs. It may also lead to changing state laws and regulations, modifying accreditation and credentialing requirements, and negotiating new reimbursement rates or models.

Second, organizational leaders must ensure that workers possess the right set of skills to function in an organization driven by safety and quality. Thus, in addition to necessary clinical skills, all healthcare professionals must demonstrate proficiency in knowledge management and evidence-based medicine, and some healthcare professionals will need to possess expertise in population health management and systems analysis and redesign. This will likely prove to be an evolutionary process as innovative practices become diffused among healthcare organizations and healthcare professionals learn new skills to keep pace. Healthcare delivery organizations can turn to health professional schools and organizations for undergraduate, graduate, and continuing education programs that enable professionals to develop needed skills.

Furthermore, valuable lessons and approaches from other industries and other countries may be transferred to American health settings.

Third, healthcare professionals need to work effectively as team members. Health professional training should seek to increase understanding of effective teams and incorporate more opportunities for various disciplines to work together. This goes beyond the usual "motherhood and apple pie" statements on the importance of teamwork. Teamwork means that each player knows who comprises the team, what the roles and responsibilities of each team member are, and how their performance can both help and hinder those with whom they work. Increasingly, this means convincing the patient, and at times his or her loved ones, to play a key role as a team member or even team leader. To achieve this level of performance all team members need easy, timely access to requisite tacit and explicit information and knowledge. Furthermore, they must be supported in creating and recreating processes that minimize errors and enhance the other five dimensions of quality.

The organization must motivate staff via clear priorities, performance measures, and incentives. The team as well as the coach need to know how they are doing, and they must celebrate their successes while they openly and collectively analyze their shortcomings. Team leaders need to encourage all team members "to internalize the need to be alert to threats to patient safety and to feel that their contributions and concerns are respected" so that they will be willing to report adverse events and other quality deviations (IOM 1999a, p. 156). All of these efforts must be complemented by recognition of and efforts to supplant the traditional hierarchy in the practice of medicine and autonomy ingrained in clinicians (particularly physicians) as part of their training, with a commitment to measurable aggregate performance (Schwartz et al. 2000).

Culture

Safety and quality programs with clearly defined objectives, personnel, and budgets are necessary but not sufficient to achieve dramatic changes. Ultimately, healthcare professionals deserve to work within a culture committed to safety and quality. Patients and staff alike should experience reinforcement of these organizational priorities in virtually every interaction they experience with the systems and professionals of the organization. Achieving such an environment requires that personnel view the entire organization as a system and the search for improved safety and quality "as a lifelong, shared journey" (IOM 1999a, p. 144). Thus, underlying a culture of safety and quality is a learning environment that maintains an ongoing process for discovery and clarification of safety and quality issues and application of design principles and existing or new knowledge to eliminate system problems (see Figure VI.2)

FIGURE VI.2
Safety
Improvement
Cycle

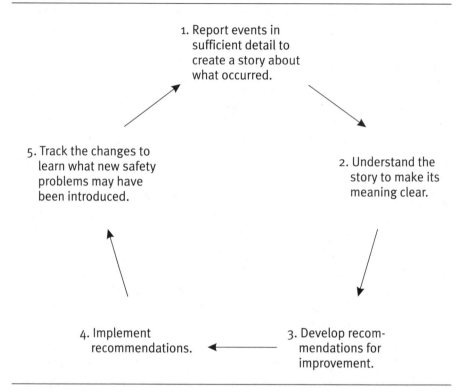

1. Report events in sufficient detail to create a story about what occurred.

5. Track the changes to learn what new safety problems may have been introduced.

2. Understand the story to make its meaning clear.

4. Implement recommendations.

3. Develop recommendations for improvement.

Based on information from Institute of Medicine. 1999. *To Err Is Human: Building a Safer Health System*, edited by L. T. Kohn, J. M. Corrigan, and M. S. Donaldson. Washington, DC: National Academy Press.

The learning environment is supported by availability of resources (including an information infrastructure as discussed in the "Infrastructure" section below) to monitor and evaluate errors or other deviations in quality and to implement solutions to identified shortcomings. The learning environment promotes communication among staff, including reporting of errors, hazardous conditions, or other barriers to quality. It also promotes innovation (e.g., through special units established to analyze performance data that can then be used in decision making) and shared learning through collaboration and benchmarking. The learning organization also seeks to contribute to the overall learning of the industry through participation in voluntary reporting systems.

Infrastructure

Two elements of organizational infrastructure are particularly important for safety and quality improvement—design of care processes and availability of a robust information infrastructure. Organizations bear ultimate responsibility for the design of their systems and should strive to incorporate well-known design principles into their environment. In addition to the ten redesign principles offered by the IOM, healthcare organizations would benefit from familiarity with design principles that have emerged from other industries.

For example, processes must realistically respect human limits. Jobs can be designed to avoid reliance on memory by using forcing functions that guide the user to the next appropriate action or decision, structuring critical tasks so that errors cannot be made, simplifying key processes, and standardizing work processes across units. Trial and error can help balance the workability of such programs.

Organizations can and should expect the unexpected by examining new technologies and processes for threats to safety or quality and redesign them prior to the incidence of harm. Experts with specialized knowledge of technical systems can test and retest vulnerable systems to anticipate potential problems. Organizations can also plan for recovery in the event of adverse events. Recovery preparation may include keeping antidotes for high-risk drugs up to date and easily accessible, establishing procedures that are standardized across units to respond to adverse events, setting equipment to default to the least harmful mode in a crisis, and conducting simulation training.

An organization's information technology infrastructure supports healthcare professionals and patients by facilitating communication, reducing potential errors, making staff more efficient, and in some instances increasing clinician availability to patients through electronic consultations and e-mail. It can also support patients by providing them with direct access to organizational resources (such as clinical knowledge sources or electronic scheduling), thereby extending the accessibility and perhaps the attraction of the institution. Although improved communication can result from simple methods such as repeating oral instructions or using color-coded wristbands to alert staff of allergies, healthcare organizations also must take advantage of the benefits offered by information technology. They must develop a plan for effectively using information technology, allocate resources to technology acquisition and implementation, and provide support for staff during system transitions. Moreover, progress toward a national health information infrastructure would benefit individual health organizations through the removal of barriers that currently impede their efforts to implement a robust information infrastructure as well as through the resources that will be available via the NHII. Therefore, healthcare organizations would be well served to provide vocal support for federal investment in an NHII program.

The combination of automating clinical information and making it readily accessible to patients and the care team in the form of computer-based patient records and providing access to clinical and organizational knowledge is an extremely powerful lever for improving each dimension of quality (Bates et al. 1998; McDonald 1976; Teich et al. 2000). For example, automated reminder systems can improve compliance with practice guidelines. Information technology can facilitate patient access to clinical knowledge and improve timeliness through Internet-based communication and immediate access to test results. Prompt availability of both clinical data and decision-support systems can improve efficiency by reducing unneeded tests. Support of evidence-based medicine can ensure consistency in clinical decisions across patients. Moreover, institutional learning benefits from standardized data sets available for internal analysis that can be compared to regional or national data.

Intermountain Health Care (IHC) provides an example of what is possible through the combination of robust information systems and system redesign (Detmer 2000). Based on past experience in improving patient safety and quality (e.g., through computer-based adverse drug event alerts), IHC's process redesign is based on the premise that cost savings will come through quality improvement (Grandia et al. 1995). IHC focuses on risk assessment and problem avoidance rather than on systems for detection. Organizational leadership recognizes that practice variations are endemic and emphasizes getting the system right rather than focusing on an individual caregiver. The organization is driven by the beliefs that patient experiences are central to their systems and that quality can constantly be improved (Gardner 1995).

Determining where to focus system design involves analysis of variables such as patient volumes, costs per case, perceptions of risk, and damage to health if not done right. Initially, IHC identified 600 candidate processes, of which 62 accounted for over 90 percent of inpatient care. Fifteen acute and 15 chronic disease processes accounted for almost 80 percent of all outpatient disease-specific care processes. Areas identified for process improvement include adverse drug events; iatrogenic infections; deep venous thrombosis with risk of pulmonary embolism; decubitus ulcer prevention and treatment; patient strength, agility, and cognition; blood product transfusions; and sentinel events such as wrong-side surgery. Once flagged for redesign, processes are evaluated in terms of key measures, critical process steps, major clinical outcomes, data definitions, and audit standards. For example, when patients are identified upon admission as meeting established criteria for being at risk for falling out of bed, an order for raising bed rails is automatically generated, thereby providing clear direction, addressing all potential fall risks, and freeing physicians and nurses to attend to more complex issues.

Medication Safety

Improving medication safety is likely to be a high priority for system redesign for many healthcare organizations because the potential harm to patients is great, and knowledge about how to prevent the most common kinds of errors is well known. Although some of these improvements depend on investment in and implementation of information systems, some of the changes do not require sophisticated technology or substantial resources. Thus, most healthcare organizations can implement a limited set of strategies in the near term that are likely to yield positive results.

Conclusion

The dramatic successes in healthcare over the past century both allow us and compel us to raise our sights and create a consistently sound healthcare system. Profound changes are needed throughout the health sector—at the system, organizational, and individual levels—so that we ultimately have delivery that is safe, effective, patient centered, timely, efficient, and equitable. It is critical that the development of our new health system be shaped by both private and public sectors. A great deal of work has yet to be done by the federal government to provide the foundation for a health system driven by safety and quality. The private sector has an equally important role to play in urging the federal government to act promptly and build upon the framework established by the public sector. National professional associations and healthcare delivery organizations can help to accelerate the process and should be prepared to support patients and clinicians who seek to align themselves with organizations that embrace safety and quality as priorities sooner rather than later.

Leaders of individual organizations will contribute to the transformation of our healthcare system in tangible and important ways. They can translate the larger system vision into a vision for their organization. They can prepare their organization for forthcoming changes by promoting a culture of change and experimentation as well as making needed investments in information technology and knowledge management capabilities. They can offer genuine support to nascent leaders within their ranks who are willing and capable of becoming champions of these efforts. They can equip all healthcare professionals within their institutions with the skills needed to navigate the new health system. They can ensure that their institution is ready and willing to do the same for patients and citizens.

In addition, leaders of these organizations can help to shape the future health system through institutional pilot projects with purchasers, payers, other provider organizations, and patients. They can build on existing community relationships to lay the groundwork for needed changes in the health behaviors of the population in their community or region. They can work with their professional organizations to advance a culture of safety and quality throughout the industry, including creation of supportive incentives and better policy formulation and regulation. Finally, they can advocate the need for federal investment in a national health information infrastructure worthy of the name.

Ultimately, progress at this frontier of health services management will depend on innovations in practice and shifts in culture initiated and enabled by healthcare leaders and their professional organizations as they build upon the aims, recommendations, and concepts offered by the IOM reports on safety and quality. In ten years we should be able to look back and see that genuine progress has been made. We owe it to ourselves as professionals to see that the decade is one of progress on these issues. Most importantly, we owe it to our patients and to society.

Acknowledgment

The author gratefully acknowledges the able support of Elaine B. Steen, M.S., in the preparation of this article.

References

Appleby, J. 2001. "Shortage Boosts Salaries, Safety Concerns." *USA Today*, March 15.

Anderson, G. F. 1997. "In Search of Value." *Health Affairs* 16 (6): 163–71.

Balas, E. A., and S. A. Boren. 2000. "Managing Clinical Knowledge for Health Care Improvement." In *Yearbook of Medical Informatics*, 65–70. Bethesda, MD: National Library of Medicine.

Bates, D. W., L. L. Leape, D. J. Cullen, N. Laird, L. A. Petersen, J. M. Teich, E. Burdick, M. Hickey, S. Kleefield, B. Shea, M. Vander Vliet, and D. L. Seger. 1998. "Effect of Computerized Order Entry and Team Intervention on Prevention of Serious Medication Errors." *Journal of the American Medical Association* 280 (15): 1311–16.

Blue Ridge Group. 1998. *Promoting Value and Expanded Coverage: Good Health Is Good Business.* Washington, DC: Cap Gemini Ernst and Young U.S. LLC.

———. 2000. *Into the 21st Century: Academic Health Centers as Knowledge Leaders.* Washington, DC: Cap Gemini Ernst and Young U.S. LLC.

———. 2001. *In Pursuit of Greater Value: Stronger Leadership in and by Academic Health Centers.* Washington, DC: Cap Gemini Ernst and Young U.S. LLC.

Brass, H. 2001. "A Question of Quality." *Health Affairs* 20 (2): 255–62.

Bulger, R. 2001. Personal communication.

Chassin, M. R., R. H. Brook, R. E. Park, J. Keesey, A. Fink, J. Kosecoff, K. Kahn, N. Merrick, and D. H. Solomon. 1986. "Variations in the Use of Medical and Surgical Services by the Medicare Population." *New England Journal of Medicine* 314 (5): 285–90.

Christensen, C. M., R. B. Bohmer, and J. Kenagy. 2000. "Will Disruptive Innovations Cure Health Care?" *Harvard Business Review* (Sept/Oct): 102–12.

Couto, R. A. Forthcoming. *To Give Their Gifts: Community, Leadership, and Health.* Nashville, TN: Vanderbilt University.

Detmer, D. E. 1997. "The Future of IAIMS in a Managed Care Environment: A Call for Private Action and Public Investment." *Journal of the American Medical Informatics Association* 4:S65–S72.

———. 2000. "Information Technology for Quality Health Care: A Summary of United Kingdom and United States Experiences." *Quality in Health Care* 9 (3): 181–89.

Fox, J., and S. Das. 2000. *Safe and Sound: Artificial Intelligence in Hazardous Applications.* Menlo Park, CA: American Association for Artificial Intelligence.

Gardner, R. 1995. Personal communication.

Goleman, D. 1998. *Working with Emotional Intelligence.* New York: Bantam Books.

Grandia, L., A. Pryor, D. F. Willson, R. M. Gardner, P. J. Haug, S. M. Huff, B. R. Farr, and S. H. Lam. 1995. "Building a Computer-Based Patient Record System in an Evolving Integrated Health System." In *The First Annual Nicholas E. Davis CPR Recognition Symposium Proceedings*, edited by E. B. Steen, 5–33. Schaumburg, IL: Computer-Based Patient Record Institute.

Henry, J. D., and R. W. Gilkey. 1999. "Growing Effective Leadership in New Organizations." In *The 21st Century Health Care Leader*, edited by R. W. Gilkey, 101–10. San Francisco: Jossey-Bass.

Institute of Medicine (IOM). 1999a. *To Err Is Human: Building a Safer Health System*, edited by L. T. Kohn, J. M. Corrigan, and M. S. Donaldson. Washington, DC: National Academy Press.

———. 2001. *Crossing the Quality Chasm: A New Health System for the 21st Century.* Washington, DC: National Academy Press.

Jaklevic, M. C., and E. Lovern. 2000. "A Nursing Code Blue: Few Easy Solutions Seen for a National RN Shortage That's Different from Prior Undersupplies." *Modern Healthcare* (Dec. 11): 42–47.

Lara, P. N., R. Higdon, N. Lim, K. Kwan, M. Tanaka, D. H. M. Lau, T. Wun, J. Welborn, F. J. Meyers, S. Christensen, R. O'Donnell, C. Richman, S. A. Scudder, J. Tuscano, D. R. Gandara, and K. S. Kit. 2001. "Prospective Evaluation of Cancer Clinical Trial Accrual Patterns: Identifying Potential Barriers to Enrollment." *Journal of Clinical Oncology* 19 (6): 1728–33.

McDonald, C. J. 1976. "Protocol-Based Computer Reminders, the Quality of Care and the Non-Perfectability of Man." *New England Journal of Medicine* 295 (24): 1351–55.

National Committee on Vital and Health Statistics (NCVHS). 2000. *Toward a National Health Information Infrastructure: Interim Report.* [Online article.] http://ncvhs.hhs.gov/nhii2kReport.htm.

National Research Council. 2000. *Networking Health: Prescriptions for the Internet.* Washington, DC: National Academy Press.

President's Information Technology Advisory Committee. 2001. *Transforming Health Care Through Information Technology.* [Online article.] www.ccic.gov/pugs/pitac_hc_9feb01.pdf.

Schuster, M. A., E. A. McGlynn, and R. H. Brook. 1998. "How Good Is the Quality of Health Care in the United States?" *The Milbank Quarterly* 76 (4): 517–63.

Schwartz, R. W., C. R. Pogge, S. A. Gillis, and J. W. Holsinger. 2000. "Program for the Development of Physician Leaders: A Curricular Program in Its Infancy." *Academic Medicine* 75:133–40.

Shine, K. I. 2001. "Foreword." In *Crossing the Quality Chasm: A New Health System for the 21st Century*, xii. Washington, DC: National Academy Press.

Teich, J. M., P. R. Merchia, J. L. Schmiz, G. J. Kuperman, C. D. Spurr, and D. W. Bates. 2000. "Effects of Computerized Physician Order Entry on Prescribing Practices." *Archives of Internal Medicine* 160 (18): 2741–47.

Weiner, J. P., S. T. Parente, D. W. Garnick, J. Fowles, A. G. Lawthers, and R. H. Palmer. 1995. "Variation in Office-Based Quality: A Claims-Based Profile of Care Provided to Medicare Patients with Diabetes." *Journal of the American Medical Association* 273 (19): 1503–08.

Discussion Questions

1. How serious and extensive are the safety and quality problems Detmer refers to in the American health system?
2. If they are serious and extensive, why hasn't more been done by American health services organizations to satisfactorily meet consumer and patient expectations for safety and quality?
3. What are the opportunities and constraints facing managers seeking to improve safety and quality in healthcare organizations?
4. How should patients and consumers and their advocates and representatives be involved in holding health services organizations formally accountable for their quality and safety performance?
5. How do the incentives under which health services organizations operate impact quality and safety performance in healthcare management?

Required Supplementary Readings

Batalden, P., J. J. Mohr, E. C. Nelson, S. K. Plume, G. R. Baker, J. W. Wasson, P. K Stoltz, M. E. Splaine, and J. J. Wisniewski. "Continually Improving the Health and Value of Health Care for a Population of Patients: The Panel Management Process." *Quality Management in Health Care* 1997, 5 (3): 41–51.

Herzlinger, R. E. "Let's Put Consumers in Charge of Health Care," *Harvard Business Review* 2002, 80 (7): 44–55.

Weil, P., and R. Harmata. "Rekindling the Flame: Routine Practices That Promote Hospital Community Leadership." *Journal of Healthcare Management* 2002, 47 (2): 98–110.

Young, D., D. Barrett, J. W. Kenagy, D. C. Pinakiewicz, and S. M. McCarthy. "Value-Based Partnering in Health Care: A Framework for Analysis." *Journal of Health care Management* 2001, 6 (2): 112–133.

Discussion Questions on the Required Supplementary Readings

1. How realistic is population-based health to the management of primary care practice?
2. What are the pros and cons of Herzlinger's approach to consumer sovereignty in healthcare?
3. What strategies should hospitals consider in managing relationships with other community organizations?
4. To what extent should non-profit boards and CEOs be accountable to the communities their hospital serves?

Recommended Supplementary Readings

Anderson, G., and J. R. Knickman. "Changing the Chronic Care System to Meet People's Needs." *Health Affair* 2001, 20 (6): 146–160.

Berry, L. L., and N. Bendapudi. "Clueing in Customers." *Harvard Business Review* 2003, 81 (2): 100–104.

Cleary, P. D., S. Edgman-Levitan, T. W. Milmer, W. McMullen, J. D. Walker, and T. L. Delbanco. "Patients Evaluate Their Hospital Care: A National Survey." *Health Affairs* 1991, 10 (4): 254–267.

Evans, R. G. "Healthy Populations or Healthy Institutions: The Dilemma of Health Care Management." *Journal of Health Administration Education* 1995, 13 (3): 453–472.

Ford, R. C., M. D. Fottler. "Creating Customer-Focused Health Care Organizations." *Health Care Management Review* 2000, 25 (4): 18–33.

Institute of Medicine. *"Crossing the Quality Chasm."* Washington DC: National Academy Press, 2001.

Kenagy, J. W., D. M. Berwick, and M. F. Shore. "Service Quality on Health Care." *Journal of the American Medical Association* 1999, 281 (7): 661–665.

Kindig, D. *Purchasing Population Health.* Ann Arbor: University of Michigan Press, 1997.

Malvey, D., M. D. Fottler, and D. J. Slovensky. "Evaluating Stakeholder Management Performance Using a Stakeholder Report Card: The Next Step in Theory and Practice. *Health Care Management Review* 2002, 27 (2): 66–79.

Scott, G. "Accountability for Service Excellence." *Journal of Health Care Management* 2001, 46 (3): 152–155.

Studnicki, J., F. V. Murphy, D. Malvey, R. A. Costello, S. L. Luther, and D. C. Werner. "Toward a Population Health Delivery System: First Steps in Performance Management." *Health Care Management Review* 2002, 27 (1): 76–95.

Walshe, K. "Nursing Home Regulation: Lessons Learned for Reform." *Health Affairs* 2001, 20 (6): 128–144.

Weiner, B. J, J. A. Alexander, and H. S. Zuckerman. "Strategies for Effective Management Participation in Community Health Partnerships." *Health Care Management Review* 2000, 25 (3): 48–66.

Weech-Maldonado, R., and S. B. Merrill. "Building Partnerships with the Community: Lessons from the Camden Health Improvement Learning Collaborative." *Journal of Healthcare Management* 2000, 45 (3): 189–205.

THE CASES

Accumulating evidence suggests a significant misallocation of medical care resources relative to improving the health of the American people. At a time when nutrition, health education, and even literacy among low-income groups is relatively neglected, there are too many hospital beds, too much surgery, and too few medical specialists available to low-income patients. Who is accountable? What are the consequences to the manager of pursing organizational accountability?

When a patient reports his experience, such as in "A Personal Memorandum on Hospital Experience," how is the manager to know whether his complaints are justified? When the manager knows complaints *are* justified, what can she do to resolve them satisfactorily? It takes time to complain, and patient expectations regarding remediation may be low. To what extent should the manager make it easier for patients to voice their responses to care, or help develop and share organizational goals that will limit and focus patient and consumer expectations?

Obviously, if services are being provided satisfactorily, management need not get involved. This is seldom the case, however, because of scarce resources and high patient expectations. Quality and service will not usually improve significantly unless leadership gets importantly involved in the process. Management should have responsibilities for improving quality and service, and physicians and nurses should be accountable to top management for performance.

Of course, in some organizations, physicians and nurses are formally accountable for patient care only to their peers and to patients. Often, however, the manager sees something wrong or patients complain to her. The manager can respond directly to certain problems, such as uncleanliness, lack of information systems, or lack of translators. Other problems, such as physician or nurse rudeness, malpractice, and lack of physician visits to patients, can be referred to departmental chiefs or nursing management. The manager can communicate with patients by survey or interview to find out how they perceive services and how services can be improved.

As a rule, patients do not wish to get involved with organizational functioning. They want things to run smoothly. Patients expect to be treated equitably compared to other patients. They expect not to be harmed by physicians, nurses, and others. For many patients, their time is valuable, and they expect it to not be wasted. Patients want to be relieved of pain. They expect appropriate access to care, and some want explanations of their problems and the treatment options open to them with probable related costs and benefits. Patients wish to be treated with dignity and with respect for their privacy. They wish to pay a fair price. How patients feel about the care they receive varies by factors such as demographic and provider characteristics, patient condition, and services offered.

Managers expect patients to return to the facility for services, to complain if they feel they are not properly treated, to make decisions about their own healthcare, to expect only the possible from providers (e.g., certain illnesses are not curable, sufficient staff are not always available), to respect the rights of other patients and providers, and to respect the facility's equipment and supplies.

These expectations seem reasonable. Why then don't those who work in healthcare organizations behave as patients expect, and vice versa? First, there is the lack of formal accountability of physicians, when they are not employees of the organization. Or hospital trustees may only pay lip service to improving quality, rather than backing management initiatives which are resisted by physicians. Consumers may lack price or consumer information to make informed choices, or providers may be extremely limited under specific insurance plans. Inpatients do not usually complain because they remain dependent on the good will of providers while hospitalized. Many patients prefer not to make decisions about treatment but rather to trust the physician's judgment. When providers are paid primarily on their costs, they may lack an incentive to be efficient. When physicians are paid fees for service, there may be an incentive to provide extra services rather than extra time with patients. When physicians are paid on salary or by capitation they may have a tendency to see fewer patients in the office. Physicians and patients are human beings, as are managers, who all have their own failings and strengths.

When service breaks down, what options are open to patients and consumers? Patients may take or threaten to take their business elsewhere. They may complain, in the case of a physician, to the departmental chief, a manager, or to a member of the board of trustees. Letters, such as the "patient memorandum" in the case study are few and far between, especially in that detail. Patients may form organizations (as in chronic care facilities) to advocate for their rights. Patients can sue to recover costs from a provider's malpractice. Patients can lead healthier lives so that they are less dependent on the healthcare system or they can raise their threshold tolerance for pain and discomfort. Consumers can control organizational performance by obtaining positions on governing boards and reporting back to their constituencies. Government regulatory agencies, national accrediting agencies, and large purchasers can represent consumers and patients in holding providers accountable for meeting minimally adequate standards of care.

Managers are paid to help the organization attain goals and to obtain a level of resources and productivity necessary for system maintenance (which is what Ken Wherry is attempting to do in the case study "Whose Hospital?" as CEO of Brendan Hospital). Stakeholders in healthcare organizations include trustees, managers, physicians, other health professionals, nonprofessionals, patients, other payers, accreditors and regulators.

Vendors and volunteers also have a stake in organizational performance. We believe that accountability is blurred unless some mutual agreement is specified among stakeholders on mission, goals, satisfactory ways of measuring goal attainment, and of ways to change organizational goals. Some of the consequences when such specification does not occur are shown in "Whose Hospital?"

An alternative to formal accountability is mutual adjustment. Rather than establishing goals, interest groups confront each decision on its merits and its effects upon them. Should a hospital purchase or lease a CT scanner, provide services to the chronically ill, or purchase several physician practices? If a significant minority of the ruling coalition objects to a new policy direction, then such a new direction may be stymied until consensus can be achieved.

To whom is the healthcare organization accountable? How is it accountable? How can its level of performance be ascertained by those who wish to hold it accountable, or by those who are concerned with demonstrating that it *is* accountable?

The two long cases in Part VI deal with accountability from different perspectives. "A Personal Memorandum on Hospital Experience" is written from the patient's point of view (but can be considered as well from the perspective of prospective patients and taxpayers). "Whose Hospital?" is written from the manager's point of view, and involves trustee and physician stakeholders. The short cases in Part VI deal with the conflicts of interest between the manager and the organization in "The Conflicted HMO Manager" and the management of diversity in a nursing home in "The Great Mosaic."

Case 13
A Personal Memorandum
on Hospital Experience

Elias S. Cohen

Recently, I spent some 17 days in a hospital of very fine repute, indeed, one of the finest medical centers of the East. While there I underwent two surgical assaults on my system and had sufficient time to do some observing from a patient's point of view.

I occupied a semiprivate room and enjoyed the company of one roommate during my entire stay. My roommate was a man 72 years of age, in the hospital receiving treatment for metastatic carcinoma of the esophagus. While he had been in this country for some 30 years, his command of the English language was not good; indeed, he was most comfortable speaking in his native German. He was fully ambulatory and received cobalt therapy daily. His esophagus was somewhat obstructed so that it was necessary for him to subsist on a bland and liquid diet.

In contrast to my own situation he was very much alone. His wife had passed away four months earlier. They had been childless. A dog which they had had for 16 years had died about five or six months before his wife passed away. He had a sister in New York, a brother in Florida, and a brother in Australia. His sister visited him once a week, and he received mail at least every other day.

This, then, was the environment in which I resided while recovering from two operations performed a week apart. These observations are in no way meant to suggest that the situations I encountered were the case in all situations, or were necessarily typical throughout this one hospital. I was stimulated, however, by this experience to reflect upon the meaning of hospital care for some patients and the impact of various aspects of hospital operation on the consumer of hospital service.

On Admissions

I had been told that I was to be at the hospital at 10:30 a.m. to be admitted for hospitalization. I arrived shortly before that only to learn that hospital admissions were scheduled for 11:00 a.m. I was asked to have a seat in a very pleasant lounge, and I thereupon waited for about an hour before I was called by an admitting clerk. The admitting clerk took the usual information and received the customary authorizations for treatment, waivers, etc. She was most pleasant and told me that it would probably be some time before the room would be ready. In this case she suggested that I might want to go down to the snack bar and have a cup of coffee and otherwise relax. I took her advice, and about 45 minutes or an hour later my name was called and I was escorted to my room.

Upon arriving at the room I found that the bed was not made, the floor was not swept; indeed, it was visibly dirty. I was told I might want to go up to the lounge and wait, which I did. Subsequently I returned to the room and found the bed had been made. The floor was still dirty. I asked the nurse if I should change into pajamas and was told to do so. At no point did anyone tell me what the routine might be that first day or ask if

I had any anxieties about my hospital admission. There appeared to be no awareness of this by anyone on the floor. It would seem to me that there are a number of patients who arrive at their hospital room quite anxious about what is going to happen, perhaps somewhat awed and afraid of this new environment, who could benefit substantially by having a nurse come in, introduce himself, and explain what the general routine for that particular day might be, including the request for specimens, the taking of blood, when the physician would visit, some explanation about meal service, and some offer to explain whatever the patient might not understand. It may be thought that the very nice brochure that the hospital had prepared was sufficient. However, I would venture that the personal contact, and whatever suggestion of reassurance might be offered, would be helpful to many patients.

On Design

I was struck by the severe inadequacies of design in this facility. The room, which had been designed for two beds, as manifested by the two fixtures for piped-in oxygen, the recessed cubicle curtain rods, and the two call bells, was decidedly undersized. I learned this, to my discomfort, upon my return from surgery on two occasions when an inordinate amount of jockeying and bumping of the surgical litter took place to put it next to the bed. To make room for the litter, several pieces of furniture had to be moved: my roommate's bed, my bed, my roommate's bedside table, and one of the two easy chairs in the room. The only pieces of furniture in the room that were *not* moved were the other easy chair and the two bedside cabinets.

Apart from this inconvenience, I would point out that my bed was generally no more than a foot and a half away from my roommate's. The other side of my bed was about three to four feet away from the adjacent wall. My bed was the one located closest to the door. If I, or a guest, were sitting in the easy chair located at the foot of my bed, it was impossible for anyone to pass between without either bumping my bed or asking the individual to move his chair. While the hospital has very liberal visiting hours, it would have been impossible for my roommate and me to have had more than one visitor at a time.

It was equally surprising to find the toilet fixtures in the bathroom without any kind of adjacent hand rails. Indeed, there were no hand rails of any kind in the corridors or any place else that I was able to observe. These deficiencies in room size and design are all the more surprising when one considers that this building was constructed within the last five years.

The lounge on this floor, which is the only place where a person can go if he wants to walk outside of his room, was located at the extreme end of the floor. Its design and furniture layout were such that it was virtually impossible for two or three people to gather in a knot to talk. It is a large room with some couches and chairs placed around the periphery with a television set at one end. There is nothing there to invite three or four ambulatory patients to sit in a small group, or for a patient who may have a couple of visitors to go to the lounge and sit in a way that the three people might face each other. The lounge is windowless and dimly lit. It seemed, in all respects, a place that would tend to deaden socialization or the opportunity for patients to converse together. Indeed, as some of my comments below will indicate, many things in this hospital seemed to conspire to keep patients very much alone.

For the lonely patient, and particularly the elderly patient who may be facing a terminal illness or an illness that threatens to change his lifestyle, loneliness can be a very destructive force. With increasing numbers of elderly making use of our hospitals, I would venture the suggestion that just as we encourage nursing homes to take into account the social needs of their patients, so we must encourage our hospitals to recognize the social needs of their patients.

On Medical Surveillance

I could not help but be enormously impressed with the medical surveillance extended to me and to my roommate. Our physicians and the residents assigned to us were in to check with us no less than twice a day and more typically three and four times a day. The residents gave every appearance of competence, concern, and conscientious attention. They were alert and were careful to explain what they were about to do, what it was that was going to happen to us, etc. They were ready to answer questions.

I must comment, however, on one instance concerning my roommate. In the course of making the diagnosis of cancer of the esophagus, it was necessary to insert an instrument into his esophagus to secure a sample of tissue. He told me if he had to undergo it again he would prefer to die.

One day when his physician was inquiring about how he was eating and whether the food was adequate and whether he was able to swallow, he complained that he was having difficulty. His physician explained that the cobalt treatments might tend to inflame the esophagus somewhat, cause swelling, and thereby make swallowing a difficult procedure. However, if it became too difficult, the physician went on to explain, it would be a small thing to insert a plastic tube through which he could be fed. It was evident, almost at that moment, that my roommate equated the insertion of this plastic feeding tube with the examination he had undergone earlier. He had no opportunity then and there, and he was not quick enough, because of his language problem, to complain about this possibility. All through that day the man worried himself almost into a great state of anxiety. Finally, in the evening he could bear it no more and he asked the nurse to call a physician. When the physician came, one of the residents, he told the resident that he would not permit the insertion of a plastic tube. The resident said, "I thought you didn't understand it when your doctor told you about it," and he then went on in a very calm, kind, and humane manner to explain to my roommate that this would be a very simple and painless procedure that had no relationship to the examination he had undergone earlier. This came as a great relief to my roommate, but he had spent a day torturing himself over the chance and, indeed, innocent remark of his physician.

The point here is that physicians must take great care, particularly with the elderly, the uninformed, and with those who perhaps have language difficulties, to explain in some detail what it is they might do, how much pain may be involved, how difficult the situation is, etc.

Perhaps the thing that is worse even than pain in a hospital is not knowing. It is the not knowing when something is going to happen, or the not knowing what is going to happen, how much it will hurt, how long it will hurt, what has been done to you, why your body is or isn't reacting in a certain way, what the chances are that things will get better or not get better, how serious some development is, what medication is supposed to do, etc., that is difficult to endure.

On Nursing Service

Perhaps the most noteworthy comment I can make on the nursing service is its variability in the face of extraordinarily conscientious supervision, hard work, dedication, and attentiveness to duty. The level of discipline appeared high—and I use the word discipline in the sense of adherence to routines, safeguarding the issuance and handling of medications, recordkeeping, shift-to-shift reporting on each and every patient, etc.

1. The numbers of staff seemed to be adequate but certainly not excessive.
2. All staff were uniformly pleasant, jovial, and apparently interested.
3. The nursing assistants did their work well and with dispatch.
4. Nurses receiving additional training were very good.

Thus, it is so surprising in retrospect the neglect with which I was treated on my return from surgery the first time. I was brought back from the recovery room about 1:30 p.m. From that time until 9:15 the following morning, with the single exception of responses of nurses to give me painkilling shots, I received no attention from any nurse—despite the fact that the room was beastly hot and my wife and I had complained about the heat. Because of the heat I was drenched most of the time with perspiration, particularly through the night during which I endured the discomforts of a Foley catheter. Nobody washed my face or offered a cool washcloth, nobody suggested or advised me that I might have a pain shot sooner than I had requested it. Nobody, in fact, even inquired as to whether they could do anything to make me more comfortable. No one came in to straighten a sheet. No one offered to change the position of my legs although it was difficult, if not impossible, for me to move them without some help.

Early in the evening of the day of my first operation, I was visited by a member of my staff who is a registered nurse. In talking with me, she observed that the IV fluid was infiltrating. She brought this to the attention of an orderly, who recognized the situation for what it was immediately, and advised the nurses who subsequently called a physician to reinsert the IV. It appeared this had been infiltrating for some time. Apparently the IV had not been adequately checked.

During that first afternoon and night following surgery I think I had more attention and time from physicians than I did from nurses. On that day and the day or two following, but at no other time during the rest of my 17 days of hospital stay, I found the response to the call button singularly bad. It was not uncommon to wait 20 minutes or more for someone even to come over the enunciator system to ask what it was I wanted. In that first day or two following surgery it was not uncommon to wait an additional 15 minutes or so after I had made my wants known. I think this bothered me most when I asked for some relief from pain. It wasn't the waiting so much as the feeling that perhaps they were insensitive. I am sure that this is not correct. It would have made waiting much easier if someone had answered the enunciator and had said, "It's going to take us ten or fifteen minutes to get to you. We're in the midst of trying to give somebody a treatment," "We're in the midst of preparing our medications," or, "Everybody is out in the rooms trying to serve the patients," or something of that sort. At least I would have known that they were trying, which I am sure they were.

As it turned out, on the second day after surgery I had a chance encounter with the field representative from the State Department of Public Welfare, which supervises and approves the hospital. She was making rounds with a representative from the administrator's office and she encountered me quite by accident. I explained to her what I had found at the hospital and what my experience had been. Following that encounter the nursing service visibly improved. I don't say this to suggest that there was a connection. Frankly, I do not think there was. I don't know what the problem was the first day because as I was better able to get about, I observed the nursing activity on all shifts. They were busy, conscientious, dedicated, and very serious about taking care of medications, checking orders, and passing on bits of information to each shift. I can only guess that there is some problem somewhere in the systems review that could make it possible for a postoperative patient not to get some kind of regular checking every hour or two, and some kind of special attention, or at least inquiry, as to well-being and comfort.

One final little note, which perhaps should have some cross-reference to housekeeping. On the Sunday before I was discharged I happened to make use of a urinal during the night. Having partially filled the vessel, I placed it on the floor next to my bedside cabinet. Monday morning I was amused to find the housekeeping service sweep around this partially filled urinal. Members of the nursing staff came and went without paying any attention to it. On Tuesday morning I observed the same thing with the housekeeping staff, and through Tuesday another three shifts of the nursing service passed over the urinal's presence. On Tuesday evening, a female visitor carefully averted her eyes from this partially filled urinal until I pointed it out to set her somewhat at ease, explaining that I was then in the midst of an experiment. I was discharged from the hospital Thursday morning and at about ten o'clock I confessed to the nurses on duty that I had not said anything to anybody about this partially filled urinal, which had stood there since Sunday night, but that I felt compelled to do so at this juncture since it might conceivably upset any patient who followed me into that room if that urinal was still there. The nurses were visibly upset by this. It was certainly not my intent to upset them and it was not a perverted sense of whimsy that led me to leave the urinal there. It does indicate, however, that there is some confusion about responsibility between the nursing service and the housekeeping service or else the nursing staff is either unobservant or embarrassed. I can't believe either of the latter and must confess being baffled as to how this could occur.

It is, indeed, difficult to understand the variation of level of service among this group of bright, alert, pleasant, and conscientious professionals. Indeed, I would not hesitate to employ any of them to pursue duties in my office or in any institution for which I might have some responsibility. How and why these things can occur is a matter that deserves considerable study. Indeed, it is a matter that requires more study than chastising. My guess is that a look at the work of the nurses would indicate some fault or deficiency with the systems that have been designed for them to follow.

On Food Service

The food service at this hospital had an error incidence of between 20 and 30 percent, which is almost beyond belief. Certainly no less than one in five meals, and more likely one in three meals, was served with either small or great errors. These errors included no meal being served at all despite the fact that no stop had been ordered; dry toast being served my roommate, who was on a very strict liquid diet; failure to include part of my roommate's meal, although his caloric intake was a matter of grave concern to the physicians; minor absurdities such as soup being served to both of us with no spoons on either tray and none available on the floor; the use of a palatized system for keeping hot things hot with a palate omitted from under the plate; or the sending up of a plate with a hot palate under it and nothing on the plate; and on to inappropriate silverware, no silverware, the almost unbelievable use of picnic-type plastic ware for eating, etc.

One obvious difficulty, in my opinion, lay in the nature of the form used for selecting menu items. While this form was adequate for telling the cooks what they had to prepare on the following day (it was a mark-sensed form that could be run through an IBM machine to calculate how many portions of each item were necessary), its layout was such that anyone trying to check the trays on a trayveyor system against the form would either go blind or out of his mind after looking at about ten of these.

Another problem, I believe, lay in the inadequate communication between the floor dietitians and the kitchen dietitians. While my own situation was not terribly important so far as diet was concerned, that of my roommate was. He was on a very strict liquid diet. He was losing weight steadily. This was a matter of considerable concern to his physicians. It was not until his physician complained bitterly about the inattention to his patient's food that the dietary service made some sincere attempt to develop foods my roommate might conceivably enjoy. Some of the choices that they gave him can only be described as almost vile. While taste is a personal matter, it is hard to believe that anyone who has ever tasted liver baby food would try to offer this as being a tasty dish. Despite the fact that my roommate had indicated he could not abide a bacon flavor in blended eggs, he was served blended eggs with bacon. I had to protest this kind of neglect and oversight to two dietitians and a physician before I felt any impression had been made in the dietary service.

I cannot believe that an error rate anywhere close to that which the dietary service produced would be tolerated for as long as 24 hours in the hospital's pharmacy or in their central supply, or if operating rooms were inappropriately prepared for scheduled procedures with improper tools, or instruments, available for the surgeon. I would feel that the situation in the dietary service in this hospital is so bad as to represent a virtual crisis because it is so close to almost total breakdown. I have no doubt that there are patients being hurt, and seriously hurt, because of this high error rate. I observed this with my own roommate who, because of errors in one day, suffered a higher weight loss than any other day during the time that I was there. How much of his weight loss was caused by error, lack of imagination, or lack of concern on the part of the staff, is hard to assess, but I am convinced that some of his weight loss must be ascribed to the inadequacies of the dietary service.

On Housekeeping

Perhaps the best and worst that might be said about the housekeeping service, at least so far as my room was concerned, is that it was lackadaisical and unenthusiastic. I only saw people dry-mopping the room during my stay. At no time was the floor of the bathroom wet-mopped, much less the floor of the room I was in. I did observe walls and the corridors and some other rooms being scrubbed down. This appeared to be on some kind of schedule. However, so far as room cleaning was concerned, it was not much.

I would comment on one other minor point. My room was located just outside the service closet. Housekeeping personnel apparently gathered there at 7:30 in the morning to pick up their supplies preparatory to emptying wastepaper baskets or doing whatever they had to do. They made no effort whatsoever to modulate their voices. The gathering was apparently a noisy, social occasion. They frequently called to each other halfway down the hall and at that hour this was somewhat disturbing.

On Social Services

My experience leads me to believe that, at least in this hospital, a new approach to hospital social services may be called for. It is insufficient to rely on the patient to ask for help from social services. The plain fact of the matter is that most patients are not aware of what a social worker can or can't do for them. On the other hand, a social services department has much to offer many patients who need help from a professional social worker. This is going to become increasingly more the case as older people avail themselves of the benefits of Medicare. Take my roommate, for example. This man was hospitalized for treatment of what he knew might be a fatal illness. He was very much alone despite contacts with some relatives and had recently suffered the loss of his spouse. He was a man who, like one-third of all people 65 and over, spoke with a foreign accent and who might have increasing difficulty with English as tension, stress, and anxiety levels increased.

My roommate said to me one day, "I suppose my whole life will have to change now. I will have to get a nurse or a housekeeper in to live with me. I will have to get somebody to prepare my food. Maybe I won't be able to drive any more." He discussed the provisions of his will with me indicating some anxieties about what his relatives might think about this or that provision. He was not a poor man by any means—indeed, he was quite well-off. He had some plans to go to Florida in the fall and then to Israel in the spring to visit a nephew. He was concerned about approaching his physician about what he could or couldn't do. This man was a bundle of anxieties. Many of these

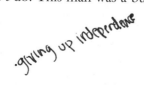

giving up independence

things could have been anticipated from his admission form and by some kind of routine communication from the nurses to the social services department.

However, I doubt that there was any provision for communication except in terms of the most overt kind of cry for help from the patient. My roommate was a man who could have benefited from some effort to find him a chess partner. He had brought a chess board and chess pieces and a chess book with him. This was something that meant a great deal to him. He, unfortunately, in me drew a partner who not only did not know how to play chess but, for whatever reasons, did not want to learn. No volunteer came to play chess, no group workers appeared to help this lone person. I wonder how many others on other floors were as ambulatory as he and who were as alone and as anxious, who put up not only with days and days of worry and anxiety, but perhaps with weeks. When I left the hospital he was completing his third week, and would probably be in the hospital a fourth. His days had very little to fill them after his 15 or 20 minutes of treatment and fewer minutes than that of attention from his physician.

I have one other comment that probably is not relevant to social services but does have something to do with accommodating non-medical, non-nursing patient needs. As noted, my roommate was alone and had very few visitors. Rather than wear the unironed hospital pajamas, he changed during the day into pajamas of his own. However, he had no one to make arrangements for the laundering of these pajamas. He was an extraordinarily meticulous and neat individual and this concerned him. It was only when my wife suggested that she would take the pajamas to the laundry and I would arrange for a friend to pick them up that any provision was made for this at all. It is not sufficient to rely on informal methods for this kind of service. It is also insufficient to expect the inarticulate to call for this kind of service or request it on their own. Hospital staffs must be somewhat more sensitive than they appear to be to these kinds of non-medical, non-nursing service needs.

I believe that social services departments in hospitals must look beyond their traditional concerns and begin to look at these elderly, lonely patients who may be facing a health situation that will introduce major changes in their lives, their relationships, and their lifestyles. Much of this can be picked up in very simple ways. However, the relationship that a social worker enters into will not come easy, as those who work in the field of aging can attest. But the older person is captive and has time, and social service has a great deal to offer in helping him and perhaps his family adjust to altered modes of living, the prospect of death, and of diminished energy and ability.

As a first step, I would urge hospitals to take a hard look at the characteristics of the older people who are coming through their doors, regarding well their length of stay, their marital status, the number of visitors they have, ascertaining on whom they rely, and trying to ferret out what it is that concerns them about their hospitalization.

No one should mistake the purpose of this memorandum. <u>It is not to criticize or complain.</u> I went to this hospital because I sought out a particular surgeon. I secured excellent medical care and, for the most part, excellent nursing care. My goal was to correct a bodily defect through surgical intervention. This goal will have been achieved. Despite what deficiencies may have existed that I have described above, measured in terms of the goal established, one must report success. However, not all cases are that simple and in not all cases are the results so direct. In some cases those good results are achieved only at the cost of a certain amount of anguish and aggravation. Perhaps this memorandum can serve to avoid some of that anguish.

Other cases, however, will not "succeed," and failure may be ascribed to failures in the system. This memorandum is in part addressed to that possibility. Beyond that, I think that all of us have some duty to try to improve on what may already be a reasonably good operation. Here again, this is among my prime purposes in writing all of this down. My main hope is that this memorandum will serve some <u>constructive purpose.</u>

Case Questions

1. How do you feel about the level of patient care given in this medical center? How do you think the patients feel? The doctors? The managers?
2. What are some of the problems with patient care in this hospital? What are the most important problems that the manager can do something about?
3. What are the causes of these problems?
4. As the hospital CEO, what would you do, if you had received this memorandum?
5. How would you have solved the problems to which the memorandum refers?
6. What organizational factors would constrain implementation of your recommended solutions?
7. How would you, as the CEO, overcome these constraints?

Case 14
Whose Hospital?

- Blurred accountability
- Ken Wary manager attempting to
  ★ predict�ion

Anthony R. Kovner

Tony DeFalco, a 42-year-old electrical engineer, and president of the board of trustees of Brendan Hospital in Lockhart, East State, wondered what he had done wrong. Why had this happened to him again? What should he do now? The trustees had voted, at first 10 to 6 and then unanimously, to fire Don Wherry, the new chief executive officer. Brendan Hospital had hired Wherry, who had been DeFalco's personal choice from more than 200 candidates, just 18 months before. DeFalco had told the trustees that he shared the burdens of managing Brendan Hospital with Wherry, that there was no way of dissociating Wherry's decisions from his own decisions. So in a way, DeFalco pondered, the board should have fired him, too.

Tony DeFalco had lived in Lockhart all his life, and he loved the town, commuting one-and-a-half hours each day to his office at National Electric. Lockhart was one of the poorest towns in the poorest county in central East State, with a population of about 50,000, of which 30 percent were Italian, 25 percent Puerto Rican, and 10 percent Jewish. The leading industries in town were lumber, auto parts manufacturing, and agriculture.

On June 7, 1979, Joe Black, president of the Brendan Hospital medical staff, had called Tony DeFalco, telling him that some doctors and nurses had met over the weekend and that they were going to hold a mass meeting at the hospital to discuss charges against CEO Wherry. DeFalco had called Wherry immediately in Montreal, Canada, where Wherry was giving a lecture to healthcare administration faculty about the relationship between the chief executive officer and the board of trustees. Wherry was as shocked as DeFalco had been and returned immediately to Lockhart. That night DeFalco and Wherry went to a hospital foundation meeting near where the mass meeting was being held in the hospital cafeteria.

DeFalco and Wherry had been planning the foundation meeting for several months now. It had been scheduled and rescheduled so that all eight of the prominent townspeople could attend. The key reasons behind forming the foundation were to enlist the energies of community leaders in hospital fundraising, thereby freeing the hospital board for more effective policy-making, and to shield hospital donations from the state rate-setting authority. Brendan Hospital had held a successful first annual horse show the previous fall, netting $10,000 and creating goodwill for the hospital, largely through the efforts of DeFalco and two dedicated physicians who owned the stable and dedicated the show and all proceeds to the hospital. Because this was a very important meeting, and because they had not been invited to attend the mass meeting, DeFalco and Wherry decided to attend the foundation meeting. There, they elicited a great deal of verbal support for the foundation, and for DeFalco's leadership. The community leaders were familiar with the problems of employee discontent in their own businesses and with the political maneuverings of former Brendan medical staffs. It would all calm down, no doubt. The wife of the town's leading industrialist said she appreciated DeFalco's frankness in sharing the hospital's problems with them.

But, of course, everything was not yet calm. The mass meeting was held and a petition signed to get rid of Wherry. The petition was signed by half the medical staff and by half the employees as well. A leadership committee of four doctors and nurses demanded Wherry's immediate resignation, and it was rumored that if the board didn't vote Wherry out, the committee wanted the board's resignation as well. Brendan Hospital was being site-visited for JCAHO accreditation that Thursday and Friday. A board meeting was held on Wednesday afternoon, before the site visit. After much discussion, a decision emerged to meet with the staff and employee representatives on the following Monday. The accreditation site visit somehow went smoothly.

The four doctor and nurse representatives met with the board on Monday afternoon, stating that they could not speak for the others. They delivered the petition to DeFalco, who read it to the trustees. The petition stated that the undersigned demanded Wherry's resignation because he was "incompetent, devious, lacked leadership, had shown unprofessional conduct, and had committed negligent acts." The representatives would not discuss the matter at that time. They had been delegated only to deliver the petition. Thus, DeFalco scheduled another board meeting for the following Wednesday afternoon to hear all the charges by all the accusers and to allow Wherry to confront his accusers, 13 days after the mass meeting of June 8.

The meeting of June 22 was attended by eight physicians, 18 registered nurses, 5 department heads, a laboratory supervisor, one dietary aide, and the medical staff secretary. (For an organization chart of Brendan Hospital see Figure 14.1.) All but one of the 18 hospital trustees were in attendance, including Wherry, who was a member of the board. The meeting was held in the tasteful new boardroom of Brendan Hospital, complete with oak tables and plush burgundy carpeting. The committee's presentation is summarized as follows.

The Accusers' Charges

Perrocchio: The most important thing we have to discuss today is patient care. That's why all of us are here. Many of us are not here because we have a personal gripe, but because we want to do what's best for the patient.

Tully (department head): Mr. Wherry humiliated and intimidated three department heads, Mr. O'Brien, Mrs. Williamson, and Mr. Queen.

Pappas (department head): There is a bad morale problem in the laundry.

Patrocelli (supervisor): Laboratory morale is low. There are too many people in other departments and not enough personnel in our department. Companies who deliver to us have put us on COD.

Fong (department head): Mr. Wherry humiliated Mr. Queen.

Frew: There has been a problem in staffing new areas of the hospital. We were told that these would be adequately staffed. I realize they haven't opened yet.

FIGURE 14.1

Brendan Hospital Organizations Chart, Board of Trustees

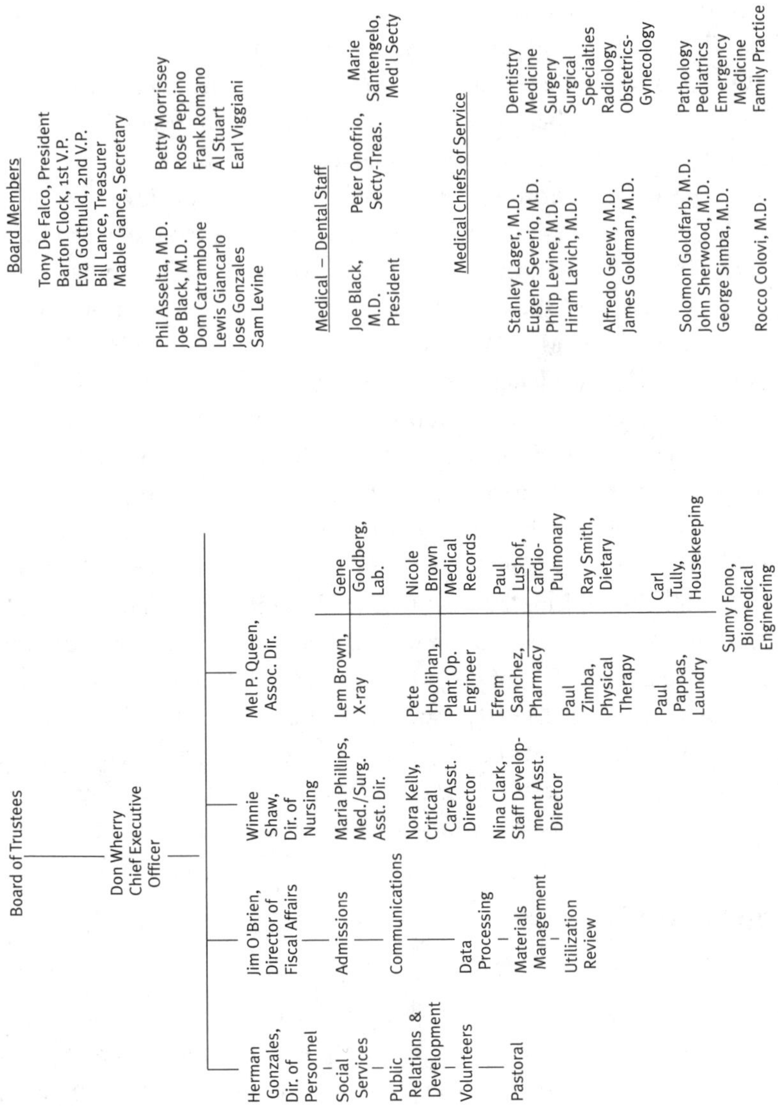

Board Members

Tony De Falco, President
Barton Clock, 1st V.P.
Eva Gotthuld, 2nd V.P.
Bill Lance, Treasurer
Mable Gance, Secretary

Phil Asselta, M.D. — Betty Morrissey
Joe Black, M.D. — Rose Peppino
Dom Catrambone — Frank Romano
Lewis Giancarlo — Al Stuart
Jose Gonzales — Earl Viggiani
Sam Levine

Medical – Dental Staff

Joe Black, M.D. President — Peter Onofrio, Secty-Treas. — Marie Santengelo, Med'l Secty

Medical Chiefs of Service

Stanley Lager, M.D. — Dentistry
Eugene Severio, M.D. — Medicine
Philip Levine, M.D. — Surgery
Hiram Lavich, M.D. — Surgical Specialties
Alfredo Gerew, M.D. — Radiology
James Goldman, M.D. — Obstetrics-Gynecology
Solomon Goldfarb, M.D. — Pathology
John Sherwood, M.D. — Pediatrics
George Simba, M.D. — Emergency Medicine
Rocco Colovi, M.D. — Family Practice

Board of Trustees
Don Wherry, Chief Executive Officer
Mel P. Queen, Assoc. Dir.

Herman Gonzales, Dir. of Personnel — Jim O'Brien, Director of Fiscal Affairs — Winnie Shaw, Dir. of Nursing

Under Herman Gonzales, Dir. of Personnel:
Social Services
Public Relations & Development
Volunteers
Pastoral

Under Jim O'Brien, Director of Fiscal Affairs:
Admissions
Communications
Data Processing
Materials Management
Utilization Review

Under Winnie Shaw, Dir. of Nursing:
Maria Phillips, Med./Surg. Asst. Dir.
Nora Kelly, Critical Care Asst. Director
Nina Clark, Staff Development Asst. Director

Under Mel P. Queen, Assoc. Dir.:
Lem Brown, X-ray
Pete Hoolihan, Plant Op. Engineer
Efrem Sanchez, Pharmacy
Paul Zimba, Physical Therapy
Paul Pappas, Laundry
Gene Goldberg, Lab.
Nicole Brown, Medical Records
Paul Lushof, Cardio-Pulmonary
Ray Smith, Dietary
Carl Tully, Housekeeping
Sunny Fono, Biomedical Engineering

Tontellino: Several months ago a nursing survey was sent around by Mr. Wherry, and we all sent in our responses. We have received no response from Mr. Wherry about the survey.

Carter (RN): We need more help on the floors.

Greenberg: Insensitivity is the problem. The administrator, as you can see from all the comments made so far, is insensitive to the people who work in the hospital.

Santengelo (medical staff secretary): The director of volunteers' salary should have been explained to the rest of us. Employees should continue to get the Christmas bonuses. It means a lot to many of them. Mr. Wherry has created a whole lot of unnecessary paperwork. I don't feel he heard what we were telling him.

Lafrance (RN): There has been a lack of communication between administration and employees. Mr. Wherry actually has asked people to give him the solution to a problem they presented to him.

Shaw (RN and former director of nursing): Mr. Wherry used four letter words in his office with me. He called one of our attending physicians a . . .

Levari (RN): When there was a bomb scare, Mr. Wherry came to the hospital and stayed for 20 minutes. Then he left before the police came, which I definitely think was wrong.

Leon (RN): It took Mr. Wherry ten months to call a meeting with the head nurses. Problems in nursing have to be solved around here by the nursing department.

Kelly (RN and assistant director): The problem has been lack of communication. I was humiliated when I presented a memo to Mr. Wherry about increases in operating room expenses. He said he couldn't understand what was in the memo, although it was right in front of him. His whole manner was rude.

Phillips (RN and assistant director): When the state inspector came on one of her inspections, she said that Mr. Wherry should be dumped.

Santengelo (medical staff secretary): He told Dr. Burns one thing and me another when we needed extra help in my office.

Bernstein (RN): Mr. Wherry was evasive and showed a lack of concern. He asked me for my suggestions. I told him to put an ad in the paper to get more help, and it was in the next day. Nurses were not present at administrative meetings.

Brown (department head): Mr. Wherry said Dr. Black would also have to sign an x-ray equipment request for $100,000. That is poor leadership.

Ferrari (RN): I didn't like the tone of his response when I called him at home to ask about treating a Jehovah's Witness in the emergency room. When we call Mr. Queen, the associate administrator, we nurses never experience that kind of problem.

Lashof (department head): I felt intimidated by Mr. Wherry. The hospital has a morale problem that interferes with patient care.

Brown (department head): He said to me "If you can't handle the problem" (we were having in x-ray) "I'll find someone who can."

Charlotte (RN): I've had a problem with my insurance and the personnel department still hasn't gotten back to me for three weeks now. I am divorced and I have a little girl, and it's really creating a hardship for me. I don't understand why Mr. Gonzales, the personnel director, hasn't gotten back to me. I've called him about it many times.

Lafrance (RN): Mr. Wherry sounded upset and annoyed when I called him at home about the electrical fire in maternity.

Gerew: The problem is communication. Mr. Wherry promised something and he didn't deliver. I have been working here for three years trying to develop a first-class radiology department. How can we cut costs and improve service in the outpatient department? I asked for help from fiscal affairs and I didn't get any.

Lavich: The family no longer has any confidence in its father. There was a unanimous vote of no confidence for Mr. Wherry in my department.

Greenberg: Mr. Wherry has a repressive style. There has been a tremendous turnover of personnel in the nursing department since he became the administrator.

Mendez: There is poor morale at the hospital. The nurses are upset. Mr. Wherry used derogatory language concerning foreign medical graduates. This was in the student administrative resident's report on what to do about the emergency room. Let's remove what is causing the problem.

Black (president of the medical staff): Department heads should be on board committees. No one came around and told department heads that they were appreciated. People at Shop-N-Bag make more money than nurses. Our medical people want to be appreciated, too.

Frew: Tony DeFalco, the board president, is seen as being in Mr. Wherry's pocket. There must be accountability for the situation that arose. I have no personal grievance. Accountability starts at the top.

Black: Dr. Fanchini was behind a good deal of what I was doing. A lot of critical things have happened, making for a crisis situation. Dr. Simba was hired to head up the emergency room, without adequate participation of the medical staff. Dr. Fanchini resigned as a board member. Dr. Burns resigned as president of the medical staff because of his personal problems. Mr. Wherry said that Dr. Severio was not really a cardiologist. The radiologists at Clarksville Hospital asked for emergency privileges. What made the medical staff unhappy was when Mr. Wherry said we weren't going to get a CT scanner and when he said that there were no problems in nursing morale. At the meeting of the medical executive committee held this Monday night, June 20, the committee reaffirmed our lack of support for Mr. Wherry, giving him a vote of no confidence by a vote of ten for the motion, one against, and one abstaining.

Listening to the doctors and nurses, DeFalco felt as if he was a spectator watching a Greek tragedy. The committee representatives left the boardroom. DeFalco remembered when the board had met in the old private dining room only two years before, voting to dismiss the previous administrator of 22 years, Phil Drew, because Drew allegedly hadn't kept up with the times, some doctors said he had sexually harassed several of the nurses, and the hospital wasn't doing well financially. Drew had been a good man, and Tony DeFalco had promised himself that he would do everything in his power to prevent this from happening again.

Wherry's Defense

"First I'd like to go through the state of the hospital, as it was when I got here," Wherry began nervously. And yet DeFalco thought Wherry seemed perfectly assured of himself, confident in the rightness of his cause. That was probably one of the things the doctors held against him. Don had attended Princeton undergraduate and Harvard Business School, and had worked for a government regulatory agency in hospital cost containment before taking the Brendan job.

Wherry: There was bad leadership in the nursing department and in several other departments, a lack of medical staff leadership, and few competent department heads. Nursing is a difficult occupation. Morale is always a problem in this department. These are young people with children; they are working evenings, nights, and weekends; and the work is physically, emotionally, and administratively demanding. The doctors at this hospital are like doctors in other hospitals like Brendan, fearful of anything that threatens to affect their livelihood or freedom. I can understand that. But there is a small, embittered group with axes to grind against me. [For a list of 1978 Brendan Hospital goals and accomplishments, see Table 14.1. For 1979 Brendan Hospital goals, see Table 14.2.]

I have been busy with the finances of the hospital and in improving external relationships with the Latinos, state officials, and other groups. Mel Queen, the associate administrator, has been busy with the new construction and the move into our new $5 million wing.

	1978 Goals	1978 Accomplishments
TABLE 14.1 Brendan Hospital 1978 Goals and Accomplishments (from 1978 Annual Report)	1. Stablize hospital finances	• $75,000 surplus • Improved Medicaid and Blue Cross reimbursement • Expenditures reduced in line with lower than expected occupancy
	2. Increased fundraising	• Modernization fund pledges on target • Successful first annual horse show
	3. Improve hospital morale	• Regular employee-administration meetings • Regular publication of *Brendan News*
	4. Improve quality of nursing care	• High patient evaluations in survey • New director of nursing recruited
	5. Organize department of emergency medicine	• Department organized and Dr. George Simba recruited as chief
	6. Establish effective management information and control system	• Implemented auditors' recommendation • Evaluating new data processing alternatives
	7. Increase communication with Spanish-speaking community	• Several meetings held with Hispanic leaders • Increased Hispanic staff in patient areas, including social services
	8. Increased accountability of medical departments for quality assurance	• Board resolution requiring annual reports • Joint conference committee and trustee seminar for better communication between medical staff and trustees
	9. Increased community participation in long-range planning	• Four community members added to long-range planning committee • Wide distribution of annual report with attendance encouraged at annual meeting
	10. On schedule, on budget, fully accredited new wing	• New wing scheduled to open in April 1979 • Building is roughly within budget and on schedule

TABLE 14.2
1979 Brendan
Hospital Goals
(from 1978
Annual Report)

1. Stabilize hospital finances and improve cash flow
2. Improve board, administration, and medical staff communication
3. Increase hospital involvement of Spanish-speaking community
4. Fill administrative vacancies and recruit needed medical staff
5. Increase pediatric and obstetrical inpatient occupancy
6. Accomplish complete availability of new wing by April and obtain full hospital accreditation
7. Establish quality assurance programs for all professional departments
8. Establish productivity and efficiency goals for all hospital departments
9. Develop an operational long-range plan, including time and dollar estimates for new programs
10. Continue to contain increases in hospital costs

We've had a new director of nursing on board for five weeks now, and I wish that everyone would have just given her a chance. Dr. Burns' resignation as president of the medical staff didn't help me any, and I have had a director of personnel, Gonzales, with acute personal problems, which has been a problem for me, too. Next, it's quite unusual for someone to have to defend himself on the spot to a list of specific charges that I have been waiting for these past 13 days and just now have been made aware of. I think the way this whole thing has been handled by the doctor and nurse ringleaders is disgraceful. The charges they have made are largely not true and could not be proven even if they were true. Even if the charges are true to a substantial extent, there is still not sufficient reason for your discharging me, certainly not suddenly as they are demanding you to.

The doctors are out to get me because I'm doing the job you've been paying me to do, what I'm evaluated on, and for which I received a very good evaluation and a big raise at the end of last year, presumably because I was doing a good job. (For Wherry's evaluation, see Appendix 14.1; for DeFalco's raise letter, see Appendix 14.2.) Certainly none of you have told me to stop doing what I have been doing to assure quality, contain costs, and improve service. During the past year I gathered information for the medical staff on a new reappointment worksheet so that reappointments aren't made on a rubber stamp process every two years. I pointed out the problems that the low inpatient census in pediatrics would create in retaining the beds in the years to come. I obtained model rules and regulations for the medical staff and shared these with the president, Dr. Black. I questioned the effectiveness of the tissue committee, which hasn't been meeting, and when it has met, whose minutes are perfunctory. I questioned the performance of the audit committee after our delegated status under PSRO was placed in question by a visiting physician, Dr. Lordi. I suggested we explore mandated physician donations to the hospital, as was passed and implemented two years ago by another East State hospital. When patients made complaints about doctors I took these up with the respective chiefs of departments. I investigated the assertion by a lab technician that tests were being reported and not done by the laboratory. I questioned and had to renegotiate remuneration of pathologists and radiologists, all with knowledge of the president of the board, Mr. De-Falco, and I have done nothing without involving the medical executive committee.

I have been involved in the lengthy and frustrating process of getting support from other hospitals for a CT scanner and in justifying financial feasibility of the CT scanner at this hospital. I have suggested ways to recruit needed physicians into Lockhart and have shared with the staff other approaches used by East State hospitals, such as a guaranteed income for the first year. I followed up a trustee's question about the appropriateness of fetal monitoring with the chief of obstetrics and gynecology, and worked out a satisfactory response to poor ophthalmology coverage in the emergency room with the chief of ophthalmology. I became involved in trying to convince one of our three pathologists not to resign because of a run-in with the chief of pathology. I have to get after physicians who do not indicate final diagnosis or complete their charts on time, because this delays needed cash flow for the hospital. I suggested that the hospital develop a model program for providing day hospital and other care to the elderly and chronically ill, and sought the cooperation of State University in designing a research protocol to measure the need for such services. This action was resented by several members of the staff, although we have not gone ahead with the State research program pending staff approval, or, if they disapprove, I said we would not go ahead with it.

I initiated a study of how we can prevent malpractice at the hospital, conveyed board disapproval of radiology equipment, which we had scheduled to buy but couldn't afford because other radiology equipment broke down in an unforeseen way. There are several very difficult physicians on the medical executive committee who have never gotten along with any administrator or with other physicians. I am the one who has to discuss with the surgeons and the radiologists ways to decrease costs in their units when these costs are way above the state medians and we have to reduce them or face financial penalties.

As far as nursing goes, here is a list of what I have done: I have met with all shifts, with head nurses, with supervisors, and regularly with the director and assistant directors. I hired a new director and fired an old assistant director whom the nurses said showed favoritism, lied to them, and overpromised. This was opposed, by the way, by Dr. Fanchini, former director of obstetrics and gynecology. I hired an expert nursing consultant to help us develop appropriate goals and ways of meeting these goals. I was in the process of obtaining the services of an operations research consultant, at no cost to the hospital, to help us with our scheduling problems. We implemented a study done by an administrative resident on improved staffing and scheduling. I pointed out all the problems of authoritarian leadership, lack of adequate quality assurance programs, and lack of appropriate scheduling and budgeting to the previous nursing director, which is why she had to be demoted. Mrs. Shaw always tried to do her best, but she lacked the proper education and skills. I obtained 15 additional approved nursing positions, including one additional full-time RN in inservice and an additional $80,000 for inservice, from the state rate-setters, something that no one has been able to do at this hospital for the past eight years. Our expenditures in nursing are already above the state median. I obtained a staffing plan from another hospital for the director of nursing and influenced her to distribute a questionnaire to all nurses to better find out their feelings and ideas.

I could go through each of the charges made by the people assembled here, but it won't really prove anything. Yes, I did call a doctor a . . . in my office. Yes, I did leave the hospital after the bomb scare before the police came, but only after I was convinced that it was a scare. I had a meeting to go to in Urban City, and I called one hour later to see that everything was all right. I think it is significant that none of the department heads supposedly humiliated by me showed up at this meeting. You have asked me to resign, but I'm not going to resign. That would not solve the hospital's problems. Firing me will not solve the bad nursing morale here or the doctor distrust. It will show the doctors and nurses and the community who runs this hospital. Is it the board of trustees or some doctors and nurses (the nurses are mainly being used by the doctors)? Whose head will these doctors be asking for the next time they want to get rid of somebody? The bond issue set for next month that could refinance our debt on the new wing will not go through if you fire me. And we shall have a $355,000 payment to make in August which will be difficult to meet.

"Does anybody have any questions?" DeFalco asked the other trustees. There were a few questions, but nothing significant, no major contradictions of anything Wherry had said. A vote was taken to clear Wherry of the charges without rebuttal, and this passed 7 in favor, 5 against, with 4 abstentions. Then the trustees asked Wherry to leave the room and told him that they would make a decision.

That evening, after dinner with his wife and teenagers, DeFalco watched a baseball game on television. He couldn't get his mind off that Friday night board meeting, the vote 10 to 6 against Wherry, and the ultimate unanimous vote to dismiss him with two months' severance. During the previous week, DeFalco had made it his business to discuss the Don Wherry situation with the other 16 trustees (Wherry and he made 18). As best as he could recollect, the following was the essence of their comments to him.

Board Comments

Clock (age 55, life insurance salesman, first vice president of the board, former mayor, and DeFalco's long-time confidant): I have been one of Don Wherry's strongest supporters since he got here and before he got here. I was a member of the search committee that selected Don, as you remember. I still like Don personally, really I do, but it has become obvious to me, at least, that Don can no longer manage the hospital. Whether Don is right or wrong, the docs don't like him. (Wherry told DeFalco that Clock sold a lot of life insurance to a lot of doctors.) Don's biggest mistakes have been in not firing Mel Queen, the associate administrator, who never has supported him properly, and Winnie Shaw, the ex-director of nursing whom he should never have kept around and I told him so.

Gotthuld (age 50, second vice president of the hospital board, president of the board of Preston College, and wife of a beer distributor): I have been spending one or two weeks out of every month in Vermont, you know, George, where we bought a distributorship, and last year Sam and I spent six months on a luxury liner trip around the world. So I really don't know what's going on that well. As chairman of the executive committee, we gave Don a good evaluation and if he isn't acting properly as chief executive officer, then at least part of the fault is ours. I see no reason to fire Don abruptly because of these alleged charges.

Lance (age 45, president of a local lumber company, treasurer of the hospital, and chairman of the buildings and grounds committee): I have always been one of Don Wherry's closest friends, although he may not admit it now. I think Don could do an excellent job managing a university hospital, but that he definitely cannot do the job here at Brendan and that we should get rid of him now. Don might care more than anyone else, certainly more than I do, about the welfare of the hospital employees, but Don just hasn't communicated that to them.

Gonce (65 years old, RN, secretary of the hospital, recently returned for the board meeting from University Hospital in Urban City where she was recovering from a heart attack): Tony, you know I fought bitterly against Don Wherry's coming to Brendan in the first place, voted then for Mel Queen, the associate administrator to do the job, and I vote for him now to do a better job than Don Wherry. Don should be working for the government somewhere, not in a small town. Mel Queen will make an excellent administrator of Brendan Hospital. We should have given it to him in the first place.

Giancarlo (age 60, president of a local canning firm, newly elected to the board in January): I don't know much about the facts of the situation, Tony; I like Don Wherry personally, but obviously the doctors and many of the employees are unhappy with him. They must be listened to. It doesn't seem that anything they are complaining about is new or isolated.

Gonzales (age 40, secondary school teacher, was one of Don Wherry's strongest supporters): I see what Don has done to meet with all the Latino leaders without any crisis, to hear out our problems and respond to us. Don has reorganized and improved services in the emergency room, hired a Spanish-speaking social work assistant, increased the number of minority supervisors. I am not that impressed, really, by these charges. There's no meat to them. I think this is just a bunch of doctors trying to get rid of Don as they got rid of Mr. Drew, the last CEO, and I do not think the board should bow down to them this time.

Peppino (age 34, senior bank vice president): Knowing Don Wherry as I do, I can understand a lot of the charges and sympathize with those making the complaints. Don Wherry is cold and authoritative, and if he knows so much, maybe that isn't what the job needs anyway. Mel Queen can run the hospital perfectly well, I'm convinced of that. And if the doctors are going to stop admitting patients as they threaten to do, they must feel very strongly about Don Wherry. It's important to calm the doctors down and get on with business as usual, and the sooner the better. Don Wherry will have no problem finding a job somewhere else. Maybe he was going to leave Lockhart anyway after a few more years.

Black (age 45, president of the medical staff): We have to get rid of this guy. He's nothing but trouble. I tried to work with him, but the guys don't like him. Maybe it's because he went to Princeton or something. He gives the guys this feeling that he feels superior to us. He's the big time administrator and we're the lowly doctors. We'd much prefer Mel Queen running the hospital. We don't have to put up with this Wherry guy, and now's the time to get rid of him.

Romano (age 50, president of a lumber company, newly elected to the board in January): I feel the way Lew Giancarlo does. I never thought being elected to this board would involve all these problems, and I'm certainly spending more time on this darn hospital than I would like to be spending. It's a tough thing for this Wherry guy. I like Don personally, but I really think we're going to have more problems with him than without him.

Levine (age 45, attorney, newly elected to the board in January): I think this is disgraceful what we're doing to Don. I don't like the way the whole thing was done, even if Don has made mistakes. You don't treat an employee this way, certainly not the chief executive officer. But I don't think that Don has handled it right, either. He should have gone to the mass meeting and defended himself. He should have organized people to speak on his behalf. That's the advice I would have given Don as a lawyer. And I think it's a darn shame this has to happen. It doesn't have to happen really, if someone would only stand up and fight for Don and his cause. I'm doing the best that I can, but I've only been on the board a short time, and I feel I'm therefore limited in what I can do.

Morrissey (age 47, housewife): Don and his wife Sue are personal friends of mine, but I can't let that get in the way of making the right decision for the hospital. Don is certainly a brilliant guy who cares about people and doesn't want to see the patient or the consumer taken advantage of. He wants to do all the right things and he has done a lot of the right things. The hospital is a safer, warmer, financially sounder place than it was when Don took over. I'm certainly going to vote for Don. I'm sorry, but I don't feel I know enough to be really energetic about this.

Viggiani (age 60, owner of a large real estate firm and chairman of the county Democratic Party): I think it's a terrible thing what they're doing to Don. It's just like with the other guy, Phil Drew. This guy has always been there when we needed him. He works night and day. If anything's the matter, then it must be our fault because this guy has been doing what we've been telling him to do. He hasn't done anything without telling the doctors and us first. I think it's a disgrace.

Asselta (age 70, general practitioner): The staff just doesn't like him. I like Don Wherry. I know he's been trying to do the right thing. I've tried to help Don, after I made sure of him, every way I can. You know my wife has been very sick and I haven't been able to attend to hospital affairs lately as I would like. I guess I'll go along with the majority, either way.

Goldman (age 61, chief of ob-gyn, newly elected to the board in January): I don't think the man knows how to manage the hospital, asking the employees to come up with the solutions to their own problems. That's bad management. Our group is against him.

Catrambone (age 50, director of a large funeral home): Tony, I'm only sorry I won't be at the meeting to speak for Don. There's a right and a wrong, and I can tell the difference. Ask yourself who is right and who is wrong and you've got to vote for Don Wherry. I happen to think he's a pretty fair manager to boot. I wish you would count my vote. Since my open heart surgery, I've got to be in Rochester, Minnesota, for my annual heart examination.

Stuart (age 41, senior vice president of the same bank of which Mrs. Peppino is assistant vice president.) [Don Wherry had told DeFalco that Stuart and Peppino were against him because he gave all the bank business per finance committee recommendation to a competing bank.]: I don't like Don Wherry. I never have. I served with him on the personnel committee and we were usually in disagreement. Don always made me feel somehow that I was ignorant, that he felt himself superior to me. This is not how he should have acted. And I'm sure a lot of the employees feel the same way about Don that I do.

APPENDIX 14.1

Summary of CEO Evaluation (November 25, 1978)

	Rating 1–5 (1 is high, 5 is low)	
	Self	Avg. Trustee
I. Goal Achievement		
1. Stabilize hospital finance	1	2.7
2. Increase fundraising	3	3.6
3. Improve hospital morale	3	4.9
4. Improve quality of nursing care	1	3.7
5. Organize emergency room department	1	2.9
6. Establish an effective management information and control system	2	2.1
7. Maintain on-schedule, on-budget west wing building program	3	2.3
8. Establish plan for utilization of west wing and integration with total hospital operations	3	2.1
9. Increase communications with the growing Spanish-speaking community	1	3.1
10. Increase accountability of medical departments for quality assurance	1	3.1
11. Prepare to obtain three-year hospital accreditation upon completion of west wing	3	1.9
12. Increase community participation in hospital long-range planning	1	2.2

CEO Remarks:
1. CEO is goal-oriented.

(continued on next page)

2. He needs to spend yet more time developing consensus and persuading key stakeholders and earning their respect.

Trustee Remarks:
1. Many of these "specifics" are difficult for an outside director to judge.
2. I think CEO's contributions are acceptable except in items 3 and 4, where they should have been significantly greater.
3. Morale is a question.
4. CEO is doing a fine job for Brendan.
5. CEO's capability is great for achieving all goals. Sometimes his motives are not understood, and some obstacles are not of his doing.
6. The answers to some of these questions are based more on perceptions than actual knowledge.

President's Remarks:
I agree that the CEO is goal-oriented. He has attained goals we have given him about as well as anyone could reasonably expect.

II. System Maintenance   2   3.5

CEO Remarks
1. Given what the CEO was hired to do, a certain amount of distrust is inevitable.
2. The CEO tries dilligently to establish regular and continuing dialogue with all key hospital groups and individuals.

Trustee Remarks:
1. Greatest weaknesses in this category are in maintaining adequate commitment of employees to organizational goals and developing adequate trust between management and medical staff.
2. The board is not made aware of exactly the number of employees needed and the department that has this need. There seems to be a feeling of unrest among the administrative staff (department heads). Trust between management and medical staff is currently very poor.
3. CEO's capabilities are limitless, but I feel he has developed a schism between himself and the medical staff.

4. Small areas of difference need to be cleared by better communication and understanding of mutual problems. Main problem area is with doctor contracts.
5. I suspect that the only positive factor in the above list would be "maintaining adequate administrative and control systems."

President's Remarks:
1. Our "hospital system" has undoubtedly provided sufficient patient care of adequate quality at reasonable cost. I therefore believe the trustee evaluation to be too low in this area.
2. A mistrust of the administration by the medical staff does exist. I am also apprehensive about the "team play" of the administrative staff. We must address these problems in 1979.

III. Relationships with Important External Publics   1   2.1

CEO Remarks:
The hospital had done well with licensing, regulatory, and reimbursement agencies, and with other provider agencies during 1978. The CEO speaks frequently to consumer organizations and volunteer groups as well and has been well received.

Trustee Remarks:
1. The CEO had done an especially good job with third-party payers.
2. This is definitely the CEO's strongest area.
3. Excellent record.

President's remarks:
I am pleased with the CEO's accomplishments in this area.

IV. Management Roles
1. Interpersonal   3   3.6
2. Informational   1   2.4
3. Decisional   1   2.8

CEO's Remarks:
The CEO is intelligent and quick. He works long hours and is subject to constant pressures. He cannot possibly talk at length continously with 18 trustees, 40 key doctors,

(*continued on next page*)

APPENDIX 14.1

(*continued*)

20 department heads, and other key personnel outside the hospital. He must try harder to be cheerful, quiet, friendly, and low-key.

Trustee Remarks:

1. I think the CEO has done a good job in 1978, especially in view of what he walked into.
2. The CEO has weakness in providing motivation, also in recognizing disturbances of uneasiness within the hospital personnel, and in dealing with incompetent or unproductive personnel.
3. The CEO seems to be seeking many changes. His method for achieving this isn't always productive. The CEO has great potential but doesn't seem to implement it well.
4. I'm not too sure if CEO is handling personnel adequately. Morale has not improved within the hospital.
5. The CEO has done and is doing an outstanding job. I am proud to work with him and would give him even higher marks if possible.
6. The CEO is excellent on a one-to-one basis. He handles groups well. He is anxious to please and to get cooperation.

President's Remarks:

1. Changes in staff personnel in 1978 have hampered the efficiency and effectiveness of this group. When stability of this group occurs, provided the right group has been chosen, improvement in hospital management will be most evident.
2. The dissemination of information is exceptional.
3. I have confidence in the decisions that are being made. I am not sure about their method of implementation.

V. President's Summary:

1. Areas of evaluation:
   The CEO has exceeded my expectations. In sum total, I am extremely pleased with his accomplishments.

2. Strengths:
   Planning, establishing priorities, dealing with regulatory agencies, understanding and articulating hospital organization, financial management, intelligence, creativity, ability to negotiate, potential, sincerity, and directness.

3. Weakness:
   Impatience and aloofness (coldness).

4. Uncertainties:
   Evaluation of personnel, evaluation of situations, employee motivation, and nonpeer and subordinate relationships.

5. Recommendations:
   Attempt to gain trust and respect of medical staff.
   Improve trust and respect of employees in presence of others.
   Refrain from reprimanding employees in presence of others.
   Work toward having assistant responsible for day-to-day operation of hospital.
   Continue to attempt to improve morale.
   Improve patience; realize that few people can match intelligence quotient.
   Continue to develop administrative staff.

6. Conclusion:
   The CEO has performed well in 1978. He has acceptably attained his goals. As a new manager, he has been severely tested by the board of trustees, medical staff, and employees and has withstood their challenge. I believe his inherent intelligence will allow him to correct any and all identifiable deficiencies.

   The CEO's self-evaluation was extremely accurate. It is comforting to know that he has the ability to correctly assess his strengths and weaknesses.

   The following elements will be necessary for his continued success:
   1. Constructive advice and support by board of trustees.
   2. Trust of medical staff.
   3. Melding of administrative staff into stable, competent, and qualified team with common objectives.

APPENDIX 14.2
Letter from
Tony DeFalco
to Don Wherry
on January 10,
1979

Personal and Confidential

Mr. Don Wherry   January 10, 1979
Brendan Hospital
Lockhart, East State

Dear Don,

The Board of Trustees of Brendan Hospital, on January 8, 1979 unanimously approved a 10 percent increase in your annual salary along with a $500 increase in automobile allowance for 1979. The above increases will result in a per annum salary of $57,750 and an automobile allowance of $2,300. Your receipt of this letter provides you with the authority to make the stipulated adjustments effective January 1, 1979.

Our board believes that you have done an outstanding job as our chief executive officer and hopes that the above increases have fairly rewarded your effort.

Very truly yours,

Tony DeFalco, President
Brendan Hospital, Board of Trustees

Case Questions

1. How do you feel about what happened to Ken Wherry?
2. Do you feel the board was justified in acting as it did?
3. What could Wherry have done to prevent being fired? What could the board have done to have prevented this? Should the medical board have acted any differently?
4. Should Wherry have resigned as the board wished him to?
5. Whose hospital is Brendan Hospital? What are the consequences of this being the case, for consumers, patients, managers, physicians and trustees?

Short Case L
The Conflicted HMO Manager

Anthony R. Kovner

Bill Brown built up University Hospital's HMO over ten years so that now it had 100,000 members, and his boss Jim Edgar decided to sell the insurance part of the business (retaining the medical groups) because University wasn't in the insurance business. Bill was asked to recruit some bidders, one of whom, Liberty National, Jim came to prefer because of its financial strength and excellent reputation. In the process of working with Liberty National, Bill learned that it wanted to hire him, after the sale, to be the president of its regional HMO activities. Bill told Jim what was likely to happen in this regard. The deal was subsequently approved by Bill's board (of the HMO) and by Jim's board (of the hospital). Two years after the sale, Bill works for Liberty and is making $5 million a year, while University is losing $5 million a year. Joe Kelly, University's new CEO, figures out that the contract that Bill Brown negotiated for University was highly favorable to Liberty and now University can't get out of it for another nine years.

Case Questions

1. Did Brown act unethically? If so, how? What should Brown have done? Why didn't he do it?
2. Did Edgar act competently? If not, what should he have done differently? Why didn't he do it?
3. What should the University CEO, Joe Kelly, do now?

Short Case M
The Great Mosaic: Multiculturalism at Seaview Nursing Home

James Castiglione and Anthony R. Kovner

Alice O'Connor is the new director of the Seaview Nursing Home (SNH), a large investor-owned facility in Far West City, which provides services to 98 ethnic groups speaking 68 different languages. Most of the top management jobs at SNH are held by white females. Although Far West City has a 23 percent Latino population, Latinos hold only a 6 percent representation in the higher levels of management at SNH. SNH has an affirmative action program and, as a result, staff members at lower levels come from a wide range of backgrounds. Twelve percent of SNH employees are classified as minorities.

According to Ms. O'Connor's predecessor, Una Light, SNH has had an exemplary affirmative action program, promoting diversity awareness, hiring more minority staff at lower-level positions, and being responsive to the health needs of the minority populations served by the nursing home.

SNH has a diversity awareness training program that has been offered 14 times over the last two years. The need for this program has been assessed through internal surveys and interviews of all staff. The purpose of these meetings is to increase the level of awareness and sensitivity of the staff of SNH as service providers; to promote awareness within the organization and increase the level of informed cross-cultural interactions among staff; and to expose potential problems and keep them from increasing in severity.

Only 8 percent of students who graduated last year from local accredited schools of nursing or healthcare administration were minorities. Latinos accounted for only 3 percent of graduates.

As part of becoming familiar with the organization, Ms. O'Connor has had conversations with each of SNH's middle managers. Anna Gonzales, who is Latino, feels that given the large minority population in the area, SNH is not doing enough to grant power to minority groups. She would like to be considered for the position of deputy director, currently occupied by a 60-year-old white female. Jim Leone, another of the middle managers, points out that white men have not occupied positions of power at SNH for the last 20 years, and that positions should be allocated strictly on the basis of merit.

Case Questions

1. Do you feel that SNH has been doing an adequate job in managing diversity?
2. What, if anything, do you think the new director should do differently?
3. How useful is the concept of "minorities" in managing diversity?

Short Case N
Case of the Crippled Children

Anthony R. Kovner

You are the new state health commissioner of a southern state. The legislature has recently passed a bill expanding eligibility and benefits for the state's crippled children's program without authorizing funds to pay for the services. The program is 25 percent underfunded now. There are 600 kids now on the waiting list, 150 more kids are being added each month. There are no priorities for care on the waiting list. The state is going through another budget crisis. A Program Advisory Committee, made up mostly of advocates for crippled children, has recommended saving money by cutting out the three physicians who direct and monitor the program and replacing them with a manager and an MD consultant. There are 5,000 children enrolled in the program, 2,000 get services by their own choice. The program has a $40 million budget. The Advisory Committee feels that they're not now "in the loop."

Case Question

1. What should the state health commissioner do now?

Reading List of Books
for Healthcare Managers

Bibliographic materials are scattered throughout the text. This short section is devoted to a selection of longer books for healthcare managers which we believe have a great deal to offer. It is a relatively short list, and the criteria for selection is as follows: (1) the book will be useful to the reflective manager, (2) the book is fun to read. The list is in alphabetical order.

* Bossidy, L., and R. Charan. 2002. *Execution: The Discipline of Getting Things Done.* New York: Crown.

  The authors focus on implementation. Fundamental building blocks include the leader's personal priorities, the social software of culture change and the leader's most important job, which is selecting and appraising people.

* Bridges, W. 1991. *Managing Transitions: Making the Most of the Change.* Reading MA: Perseus Books.

  This short book shows managers how to manage change with due emphasis on the emotional impact of change. The author directs his attention to leaving the organization stronger in the face of mergers, reorganizations, layoffs, shifts in strategy or service or culture.

* Christensen, C. M. 1997. *The Innovator's Dilemma: When New Technologies Cause Great Firms to Fail.* Boston: Harvard University Press.

  This book is about the failure of companies to stay atop their industries when they confront certain types of market and technological change. It is about well-managed companies that yet lose market dominance. The author suggests that there are times at which it is right not to listen to customers, right to invest in developing lower-performance products that promise lower margins, and right to pursue small rather than substantial markets.

- Greene, R. 1998. *The 48 Laws of Power*. New York: Viking.

  Primer on organizational politics. Some laws follow: never outshine the master, never put too much trust in friends, learn how to use enemies, conceal your intentions, always say less than necessary, court attention at all costs, think as you like but behave like others.

- Griffith, J. R. 1993. *The Moral Challenges of Health Care Management*. Chicago: Health Administration Press.

  Of course, everyone should read and own *The Well Managed Health Care Organization*, 5th edition, by John Griffith and Ken White, (Chicago: Health Administration Press 2002). Less widely known is Griffith's earlier book, which has three parts: theories of moral obligation, conflicting obligations, and improving virtue. The book is full of case studies and addresses the tough questions at both theoretical and operating levels. Read and reflect.

- Handy, C. 1998. *The Hungry Spirit*. New York: Broadway Books.

  This book is divided into three parts—a creaking capitalism, a life of our own, and toward a decent society—providing essential context for the healthcare manager. Handy forces you to examine the justification and limits of capitalism, how to conduct your life in modern large organizations, and how to improve your organization and your society. And he writes well. Also by the same author, read *Understanding Organizations* and *The Age of Unreason*.

- Herzlinger, R. E. 1997. *Market-Driven Health Care*. Reading, MA: Addison-Wesley.

  Herzlinger explains how the "true market . . . will provide the solution to the deep problems that plague the American health system." Her solution is creating "focused factories" that decentralize the modern hospital into centers for eye care, heart care, cancer care, and so forth. She leaves out what will and should happen to hospitals in the process.

- Kindig, D. A. 1997. *Purchasing Population Health: Paying for Results*. Ann Arbor, MI: The University of Michigan Press.

  Kindig suggests measuring health outcomes in terms of health adjusted life expectancy and paying providers relative to how they improve such outcomes. He argues that such a strategy will reallocate resources to health investments of greater value. What Kindig neglects to consider is that health expenditures equal health incomes. What is his proposal to mitigate the effects of what he suggests on provider incomes? Otherwise, where is he going to find the political wherewithal to enact his proposal?

- Maister, D. H. 1993. *Managing the Professional Service Firm.* New York: Free Press.

  Managers of healthcare organizations have a lot to learn from the management of other organizations in the business of providing services. Maister's insights are largely drawn from the management of law and consulting firms. For example, Maister suggests that managing client relations is immensely valuable and suggests that spending time with existing client executives (one thinks of doctors and payers) on top of what the organization's senior managers are already doing, "goes a long way in cementing relationships, assuring client satisfaction and uncovering new business issues with decision makers."

- Pointer, D. D., and J. E. Orlikoff. 2002. *Getting to Great: Principles of Health Care Organization Governance.* San Francisco: Jossey-Bass.

  Classic, practical "how to" book on improving the governance of healthcare organizations. It provides a model, principles and practices, recommendations on how to get started, checkups for assessing your board, and guidelines for implementing principle-based governance.

Index

About the Editors

Anthony R. Kovner, M.P.A., Ph.D., is currently professor of health policy and management at the Robert F. Wagner Graduate School of Public Service, New York University. He has served as senior program consultant to the Robert Wood Johnson Foundation and the W. K. Kellogg Foundation. Dr. Kovner is a member of the board of trustees of Lutheran Medical Center, The Augustana Nursing Home, and Health Plus in Brooklyn, New York. Before joining NYU, he was chief executive officer of the Newcomb Hospital of Vineland, New Jersey, and senior health consultant to the United Auto Workers Union in Detroit, Michigan. He is the author of *A Career Guide for the Health Services Manager*, 3rd Edition, published by Health Administration Press, and of *Healthcare Management in Mind: Eight Careers* (Springer, 2000).

Duncan Neuhauser, M.H.A., M.B.A., Ph.D., is the Charles Elton Blanchard, M.D., Professor of Health Management, Department of Epidemiology and Biostatistics, Medical School, Case Western Reserve University. He holds secondary professorships in internal medicine, family medicine, and organizational behavior and is the codirector of the Health Systems Management Center at his university. For 15 years he was the editor of *Medical Care*. His other books include *Coming of Age*, 2nd Edition (1994), a 60-year history of the American College of Healthcare Executives, and, with Edward McEachern, M.D., and Linda Headrick, M.D., *Clinical IQ: A Book of Readings* (JCAHO Press, 1996.) He is a member of the Institute of Medicine.